Secondary Metabolites for the Reduction of Oxidative Stress

Secondary Metabolites for the Reduction of Oxidative Stress

Editor

Andrea Ragusa

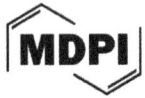

Basel • Beijing • Wuhan • Barcelona • Belgrade • Novi Sad • Cluj • Manchester

Editor
Andrea Ragusa
Department of Biological and
Environmental Sciences and
Technologies
University of Salento
Lecce
Italy

Editorial Office
MDPI
St. Alban-Anlage 66
4052 Basel, Switzerland

This is a reprint of articles from the Special Issue published online in the open access journal *Molecules* (ISSN 1420-3049) (available at: www.mdpi.com/journal/molecules/special_issues/ Secondary_Metabolites_Oxidative_Stress).

For citation purposes, cite each article independently as indicated on the article page online and as indicated below:

Lastname, A.A.; Lastname, B.B. Article Title. *Journal Name* **Year**, *Volume Number*, Page Range.

ISBN 978-3-7258-0344-6 (Hbk)
ISBN 978-3-7258-0343-9 (PDF)
doi.org/10.3390/books978-3-7258-0343-9

© 2024 by the authors. Articles in this book are Open Access and distributed under the Creative Commons Attribution (CC BY) license. The book as a whole is distributed by MDPI under the terms and conditions of the Creative Commons Attribution-NonCommercial-NoDerivs (CC BY-NC-ND) license.

Contents

About the Editor vii

Preface ix

Tianshuang Xia, Jiabao Zhang, Yunxiang Guo, Yiping Jiang, Fangliang Qiao, Kun Li, et al.
Humulus lupulus L. Extract Protects against Senior Osteoporosis through Inhibiting Amyloid β Deposition and Oxidative Stress in APP/PS1 Mutated Transgenic Mice and Osteoblasts
Reprinted from: Molecules 2023, 28, 583, doi:10.3390/molecules28020583 1

Gaurav Gajurel, Rokib Hasan and Fabricio Medina-Bolivar
Antioxidant Assessment of Prenylated Stilbenoid-Rich Extracts from Elicited Hairy Root Cultures of Three Cultivars of Peanut (Arachis hypogaea)
Reprinted from: Molecules 2021, 26, 6778, doi:10.3390/molecules26226778 15

Raghvendra A. Bohara, Nazish Tabassum, Mohan P. Singh, Giuseppe Gigli,
Andrea Ragusa and Stefano Leporatti
Recent Overview of Resveratrol's Beneficial Effects and Its Nano-Delivery Systems
Reprinted from: Molecules 2022, 27, 5154, doi:10.3390/molecules27165154 27

Danyang Zhang, Xia Li, Xiaoshi He, Yan Xing, Bo Jiang, Zhilong Xiu, et al.
Protective Effect of Flavonoids against Methylglyoxal-Induced Oxidative Stress in PC-12 Neuroblastoma Cells and Its Structure–Activity Relationships
Reprinted from: Molecules 2022, 27, 7804, doi:10.3390/molecules27227804 44

Mahban Rahimifard, Maryam Baeeri, Haji Bahadar, Shermineh Moini-Nodeh,
Madiha Khalid, Hamed Haghi-Aminjan, et al.
Therapeutic Effects of Gallic Acid in Regulating Senescence and Diabetes; an In Vitro Study
Reprinted from: Molecules 2020, 25, 5875, doi:10.3390/molecules25245875 55

Dong-Lin Yang, Yong Li, Shui-Qing Ma, Ya-Jun Zhang, Jiu-Hong Huang and Liu-Jun He
Compound 275# Induces Mitochondria-Mediated Apoptosis and Autophagy Initiation in Colorectal Cancer Cells through an Accumulation of Intracellular ROS
Reprinted from: Molecules 2023, 28, 3211, doi:10.3390/molecules28073211 70

Maria Salbini, Alessandra Quarta, Fabiana Russo, Anna Maria Giudetti, Cinzia Citti,
Giuseppe Cannazza, et al.
Oxidative Stress and Multi-Organel Damage Induced by Two Novel Phytocannabinoids, CBDB and CBDP, in Breast Cancer Cells
Reprinted from: Molecules 2021, 26, 5576, doi:10.3390/molecules26185576 86

Rosanna Mallamaci, Roberta Budriesi, Maria Lisa Clodoveo, Giulia Biotti, Matteo Micucci,
Andrea Ragusa, et al.
Olive Tree in Circular Economy as a Source of Secondary Metabolites Active for Human and Animal Health Beyond Oxidative Stress and Inflammation
Reprinted from: Molecules 2021, 26, 1072, doi:10.3390/molecules26041072 105

Biswajita Pradhan, Rabindra Nayak, Srimanta Patra, Bimal Prasad Jit, Andrea Ragusa
and Mrutyunjay Jena
Bioactive Metabolites from Marine Algae as Potent Pharmacophores against Oxidative Stress-Associated Human Diseases: A Comprehensive Review
Reprinted from: Molecules 2020, 26, 37, doi:10.3390/molecules26010037 128

Karyne Rangel, Fellipe O. Cabral, Guilherme C. Lechuga, João P. R. S. Carvalho, Maria H. S. Villas-Bôas, Victor Midlej and Salvatore G. De-Simone
Potent Activity of a High Concentration of Chemical Ozone against Antibiotic-Resistant Bacteria
Reprinted from: *Molecules* **2022**, 27, 3998, doi:10.3390/molecules27133998 153

Rakibul Islam, Rima Maria Corraya, Lara Pasovic, Ayyad Zartasht Khan, Hans Christian D. Aass, Jon Roger Eidet and Tor Paaske Utheim
The Effects of Prolonged Storage on ARPE-19 Cells Stored at Three Different Storage Temperatures
Reprinted from: *Molecules* **2020**, 25, 5809, doi:10.3390/molecules25245809 170

Evelina Moliteo, Monica Sciacca, Antonino Palmeri, Maria Papale, Sara Manti, Giuseppe Fabio Parisi and Salvatore Leonardi
Cystic Fibrosis and Oxidative Stress: The Role of CFTR
Reprinted from: *Molecules* **2022**, 27, 5324, doi:10.3390/molecules27165324 183

About the Editor

Andrea Ragusa

Andrea Ragusa graduated with a degree in Chemistry from the University of Parma (Italy) and obtained his PhD in Supramolecular Chemistry from the University of Southampton (UK) in 2005. After a 2-year postdoctoral Marie Curie stay at the Consejo Superior de Investigaciones Quimicas (CSIC, in Seville, Spain), he returned to Italy and worked at the National Nanotechnology Laboratory (NNL), at the Italian Institute of Technology (IIT), and then at the University of Salento (Lecce, Italy). Since 2018, he has been a Professor of Pharmaceutical Chemistry at the Department of Biological and Environmental Sciences and Technologies, and his research interests range from the study of the antioxidant properties of natural products to the exploitation of new targeted formulations for the selective release of bioactive and chemotherapeutic molecules.

Preface

Oxidative stress is a condition that occurs when there is an imbalance between the production of reactive oxygen species (ROS) and the body's ability to neutralize them. ROS are normally produced inside cells, and their amount is finely counterbalanced by antioxidant enzymes such as SOD, GPx, and catalase. However, when this homeostasis is interrupted and ROS levels are too high or antioxidant levels are too low, oxidative stress can occur.

Oxidative stress has been linked to a wide range of pathologies, including cardiovascular diseases, cancer, neurological disorders (e.g., Alzheimer's disease, Parkinson's disease, and multiple sclerosis), pulmonary diseases (e.g., asthma and chronic obstructive pulmonary disease), inflammatory diseases (e.g., arthritis and inflammatory bowel disease), and autoimmune diseases (e.g., lupus and rheumatoid arthritis). The exact mechanisms by which oxidative stress contributes to disease are complex and vary depending on the specific pathology. However, it is thought that oxidative stress can damage cells and tissues in a number of ways, including by damaging DNA and proteins, disrupting cellular signaling pathways, inducing inflammation, and causing cell death.

The growing body of evidence suggesting that oxidative stress may play a role in the initiation and progression of many chronic diseases has led to increased interest in developing strategies to reduce oxidative stress and protect against its harmful effects. One way to reduce oxidative stress is to follow a healthy diet rich in antioxidants, substances that can neutralize ROS and protect cells from damage. For example, fruit, vegetables, marine algae, and many traditional medicinal plants are rich in secondary metabolites with antioxidant properties, among others, as are many beverages obtained from natural products. Several molecules contained in these products, although at low concentrations, have already been shown to exert antioxidant activity, among others, both in vitro and in vivo.

In this collection, comprised of eight original research articles and four review articles, the latest research into oxidative stress and the exploitation of secondary metabolites for its reduction is reported.

Andrea Ragusa
Editor

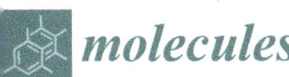

Article

Humulus lupulus L. Extract Protects against Senior Osteoporosis through Inhibiting Amyloid β Deposition and Oxidative Stress in APP/PS1 Mutated Transgenic Mice and Osteoblasts

Tianshuang Xia [1], Jiabao Zhang [1], Yunxiang Guo [1], Yiping Jiang [1], Fangliang Qiao [1], Kun Li [1], Nani Wang [2], Ting Han [1] and Hailiang Xin [1,*]

1 School of Pharmacy, Navy Medical University, Shanghai 200433, China
2 Department of Medicine, Zhejiang Academy of Traditional Chinese Medicine, Hangzhou 310007, China
* Correspondence: hailiangxin@163.com; Tel.: +86-021-81871309

Abstract: As aging progresses, β-amyloid (Aβ) deposition and the resulting oxidative damage are key causes of aging diseases such as senior osteoporosis (SOP). *Humulus lupulus* L. (hops) is an important medicinal plant widely used in the food, beverage and pharmaceutical industries due to its strong antioxidant ability. In this study, APP/PS1 mutated transgenic mice and Aβ-injured osteoblasts were used to evaluate the protective effects of hops extracts (HLE) on SOP. Mice learning and memory levels were assessed by the Morris water maze. Mice femurs were prepared for bone micro-structures and immunohistochemistry experiments. The deposition of Aβ in the hippocampus, cortex and femurs were determined by Congo red staining. Moreover, protein expressions related to antioxidant pathways were evaluated by Western blotting. It was found that HLE markedly improved learning abilities and ameliorated memory impairment of APP/PS1 mice, as well as regulated antioxidant enzymes and bone metabolism proteins in mice serum. Micro-CT tests indicated that HLE enhanced BMD and improved micro-architectural parameters of mice femur. More importantly, it was discovered that HLE significantly reduced Aβ deposition both in the brain and femur. Further in vitro results showed HLE increased the bone mineralization nodule and reduced the ROS level of Aβ-injured osteoblasts. Additionally, HLE increased the expression of antioxidant related proteins Nrf2, HO-1, NQO1, FoxO1 and SOD-2. These results indicated that *Humulus lupulus* L. extract could protect against senior osteoporosis through inhibiting Aβ deposition and oxidative stress, which provides a reference for the clinical application of hops in the prevention and treatment of SOP.

Keywords: amyloid β; *Humulus lupulus* L.; senior osteoporosis; APP/PS1 mice; oxidative stress

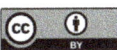

1. Introduction

Senior osteoporosis (SOP) is a type of metabolic disease characterized by osteopenia, bone micro-structure degeneration and fracture. Aging is a major pathogenic factor causing SOP. Along with aging, the body will induce oxidative stress through releasing excessive reactive oxygen species (ROS), further decreasing bone formation in osteoblasts and increasing bone resorption in osteoclasts, eventually leading to a bone homeostasis imbalance [1]. According to statistics, more than one-fifth of men and one-third of women in the world suffer from osteoporosis at the age of 50 or above [2]. Furthermore, it is estimated that the number of people suffering from osteoporosis in China will exceed 200 million by 2050 [3], which is a crucial public health problem to be solved. In recent years, there is increasing evidence suggesting that SOP patients are more likely to have memory impairment, even Alzheimer's disease (AD) [4], which is associated with oxidative stress and β-amyloid (Aβ) protein plaque deposition. However, these are all relatively unclear pathogeneses of SOP. Current clinical drug treatments for SOP mainly include estrogen therapy, bisphosphonates supplementation, as well as calcium and active vitamin D, which cause more side effects and lack a clear target. Therefore, there is a desperate need to elucidate the pathogenesis of SOP and to find appropriate alternative drugs for SOP with few adverse effects.

Humulus lupulus L. (hops) is an important medicinal plant widely used in the food, beverage and pharmaceutical industries due to its strong antioxidant capacity [5], and has long medicinal history in China for digestive diseases, tuberculosis, insomnia and forgetfulness. In Europe, hops is used for hot flushes during the menopause and postmenopausal osteoporosis [6]. In addition, hops has been proven to have a strong antioxidation effect and is a potential antioxidant [7,8]. It has been reported that phenolic acids (including hydroxybenzoic acids, hydroxycinnamic acids and hydroxyphenylpropanoic acids) and flavonoids (mainly anthocyanins, flavones, flavonols and isoflavonoids) are the main effective components of hops, which contribute to its antioxidant capacity. Our previous studies have also discovered that hops extract could prevent ovariectomy-induced osteoporosis in mice and regulate the activities of osteoblasts and osteoclasts through attenuating oxidative stress [9–11]. In addition, xanthohumol, a unique isoflavone in hops, has been found to have a potent effect on Aβ-induced oxidative damage and bone loss in APP/PS1 mice and osteoblasts [12,13]. These studies demonstrated that hops have potential as an antioxidant with anti-Aβ deposition and anti-SOP properties.

Aβ aggregation and deposition in the cerebrum is a significant pathological feature in AD patients. Aβ deposition can cause neurotoxicity and oxidative stress, which leads to wide neurodegeneration [14]. More researchers have found that Aβ not only exists in the cerebrum, but also in the bone [15], and Aβ_{42} is often abnormally elevated in osteoporosis patients [16]. In addition, progressively more clinical results have demonstrated that most senile dementia patients suffer from bone diseases and have a high risk of fractures [4]. SOP may be caused by Aβ deposition in femurs, which affect the activities of osteoblasts and osteoclasts [17]. More importantly, it has been discovered that in APP/PS1 mutated transgenic mice, both brain and bone tissues showed Aβ deposition accompanied with peroxidation injury, and antioxidants could improve the cognitive ability and bone loss caused by this Aβ deposition and oxidative damage [18]. It is therefore speculated that antioxidants may prevent bone loss caused by Aβ deposition and oxidative damage.

In view of the strong antioxidant effect of hops, the present study employed APP/PS1 mice to investigate the effect of hops on memory deficit and bone loss induced by Aβ deposition, and probed its potential mechanism using Aβ-injured osteoblasts, which can provide more references for the prevention and treatment of SOP.

2. Results

2.1. HLE Prevented Spatial Memory Deficit of APP/PS1 Mice

The Morris water maze (MWM) task was conducted to estimate whether hops extract could improve the long-term spatial memory of APP/PS1 mice. After 2 months administration, 11-month-old mice were prepared for the MWM task. The MWM task included two parts: task acquisition (days 1–5) and probe trial (day 6). During the experiment, the tank was videotaped from above, and all the relevant data were recorded. Detailed experimental steps are shown in "Section 4.3". As shown in Figure 1A, during 5-day training, the escape latency of mice to find and load upon the platform decreased progressively. From the third training day to the last training day, the latency of APP/PS1 mice was significantly longer than that of wild-type mice ($p < 0.001$), and the mice in treatment groups had a lower latency to load upon the platform compared with that of APP/PS1 mice during the last two training days ($p < 0.05$). On the probe test day, the swimming time spent in the target zone is shown in Figure 1B. We observed significant differences in swimming time between APP/PS1 mice and mice in treatment groups ($p < 0.05$). APP/PS1 mice swam for less time in the target zone than the wild-type mice, and the mice treated with HLE or N-acetyl-L-cysteine (NAC, a kind of antioxidant, used as positive control in this study) spent an increased amount of time in the target zone. Moreover, as shown in Figure 1C, it was observed that the number of platform crossings in APP/PS1 mice was significantly lower than that in the wild-type mice ($p < 0.001$), while treatment with HLE (2 g/kg) or

NAC significantly increased the number of platform crossings ($p < 0.05$). The swimming tracking showed that APP/PS1 mice mostly swam in the quadrant far from the target quadrant, while mice in wild-type group and other treatment groups mostly swam near the platform (Figure 1E). However, the treatment did not affect the swimming speed compared with APP/PS1 mice, as shown in Figure 1D ($p > 0.05$). These results suggested that HLE had a good effect on improving the learning and memory abilities and could prevent spatial memory deficit of APP/PS1 mice.

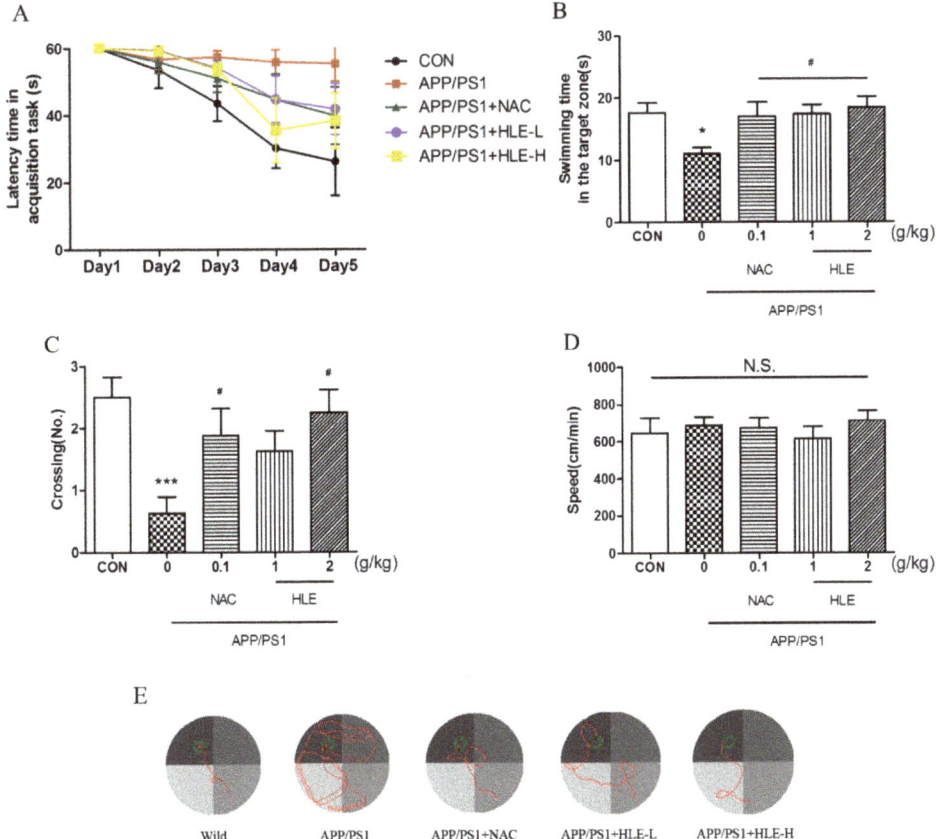

Figure 1. Effects of HLE on spatial memory impairment of APP/PS1 transgenic mice in the Morris water maze task. (**A**) Escape latency time of tested mice over 5 days of MWM task acquisition; (**B**) the swimming time; (**C**) the crossing numbers; (**D**) swimming speed in the target zone on the probe test day and (**E**) path taken by one random rat in each group during MWM probe trial ($n = 8$). (* $p < 0.05$, *** $p < 0.001$, compared with the control (CON) group; # $p < 0.05$, compared with the APP/PS1 group.)

2.2. HLE Reduced Aβ Deposition Both in the Brain and Bone of APP/PS1 Mice

To determine the effect of HLE on Aβ deposition, we applied Congo red strain to observe the pathological changes in Aβ plaque in the brain and femur. The brownish red or orange precipitates were positive for Aβ (Figure 2A). In the brain, Aβ plaque in mice hippocampi and cortexes was measured, and it was found that the amount of Aβ plaque in APP/PS1 group mice was significantly more than that of the wild-type group ($p < 0.001$). HLE or NAC markedly decreased the amount of Aβ plaque in hippocampi and cortexes of APP/PS1 mice ($p < 0.001$). Moreover, we observed more Aβ deposition in the femurs of APP/PS1 mice than in wild-type mice ($p < 0.01$), while HLE or NAC could ameliorate the accumulation of Aβ in femurs of APP/PS1 mice ($p < 0.01$) (Figure 2B–D). These results suggested that HLE could reduce Aβ deposition both in the brains and bones of APP/PS1 mice.

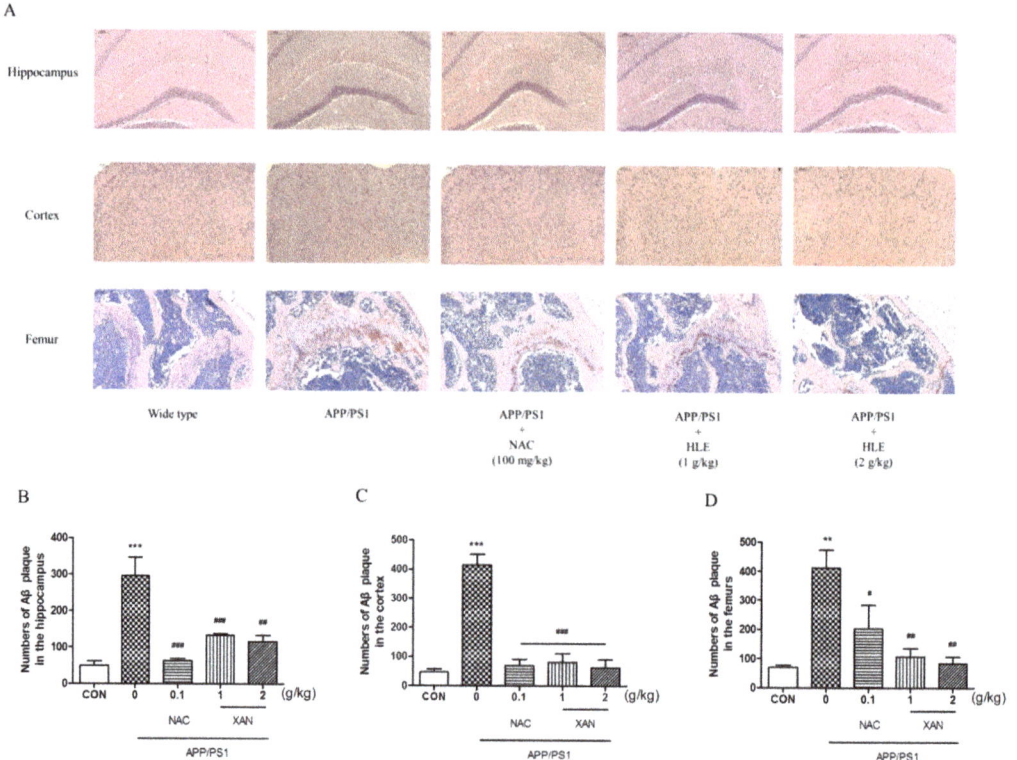

Figure 2. The effects of HLE on Aβ plaque in the hippocampus, cortex and femurs. (A) Congo red-positive plaque in the hippocampus, cortex or femurs of APP/PS1 mice; (B–D) quantitative analysis of amount of Aβ ($n = 3$). (** $p < 0.01$, *** $p < 0.001$, compared with the CON group; # $p < 0.05$, ## $p < 0.01$, ### $p < 0.001$ compared with the APP/PS1 group.)

2.3. HLE Improved Bone Mineral Density (BMD) and Bone Microarchitecture of APP/PS1 Mice

Micro-CT was conducted to observe the bone structural properties of trabecular bone and BMD in femurs. As shown in the micro-CT images (Figure 3A), there was larger gap space in the ROI region in APP/PS1 mice compared to mice in wild and treatment groups. As shown in Figure 3B, femur BMD in APP/PS1 mice was significantly decreased ($p < 0.01$), while HLE or NAC could reverse this decrease and enhance the BMD ($p < 0.05$). The bone volume fraction (BVF) indicates the ratio of bone volume to total volume. Figure 3C showed that the BVF of APP/PS1 mice was significantly decreased compared with that of wild-type mice ($p < 0.01$), while HLE or NAC could markedly increase the femur BVF in APP/PS1 mice ($p < 0.05$). In addition, as shown in Figure 3D–F, the morphologic parameters of trabecular number (Tb.N.) and trabecular thickness (Tb.Th.) decreased, while trabecular separation (Tb.Sp.) increased significantly in APP/PS1 mice when compared with those in wild group. On the contrary, HLE or NAC markedly reversed these changes in trabecular morphological parameters by increasing the Tb.N. and Tb.Th. and decreasing the Tb.Sp., indicating that HLE had an excellent bone protection effect.

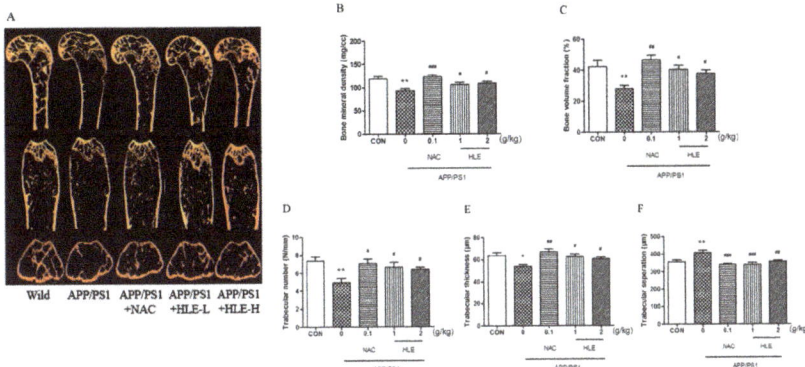

Figure 3. Effects of HLE on bone mineral density and the structures of trabecular bone in femurs of APP/PS1 mice. (**A**) Micro-CT images of the ROI region in the longitudinal section, transverse section and 3-D architecture; (**B–F**) trabecular bone parameter analysis of (**B**) BMD; (**C**) BVF; (**D**) Tb.N.; (**E**) Tb.Th.; and (**F**) Tb.Sp. in the distal femur region in APP/PS1 mice ($n = 8$). (* $p < 0.05$, ** $p < 0.01$, compared with the CON group; # $p < 0.05$, ## $p < 0.01$, ### $p < 0.001$ compared with the APP/PS1 group.)

2.4. HLE Relieved Oxidative Stress and Regulated Bone Metabolism in APP/PS1 Mice

As shown in Figure 4A, the superoxide dismutase (SOD) activity in the serum of APP/PS1 mice decreased to 4.341 ± 0.45 U/mL, significantly less than that of the wild-type mice (7.663 ± 0.34 U/mL) ($p < 0.001$). Moreover, osteocalcin (OCN), which plays an important role in regulating bone metabolism, was activated less in APP/PS1 mice (4.237 ± 0.41 ng/mL) than that in wild-type mice (11.250 ± 0.43 ng/mL) (Figure 4B, $p < 0.001$). HLE or NAC could increase the SOD and OCN levels of APP/PS1 mice, respectively ($p < 0.001$), and there were no significant differences between the two dose groups. Inflammatory cytokines interleukin-1β (IL-1β) and interleukin-6 (IL-6) levels in the serum of APP/PS1 mice significantly increased from 5.028 ± 0.46 ng/L and 35.51 ± 1.18 ng/L in wild-type mice to 19.42 ± 0.68 ng/L and 51.70 ± 2.27 ng/L ($p < 0.001$), respectively. After treatment, HLE or NAC reversed the high level of IL-1β and IL-6 in the serum of APP/PS1 mice to almost ordinary levels (Figure 4C,D, $p < 0.001$).

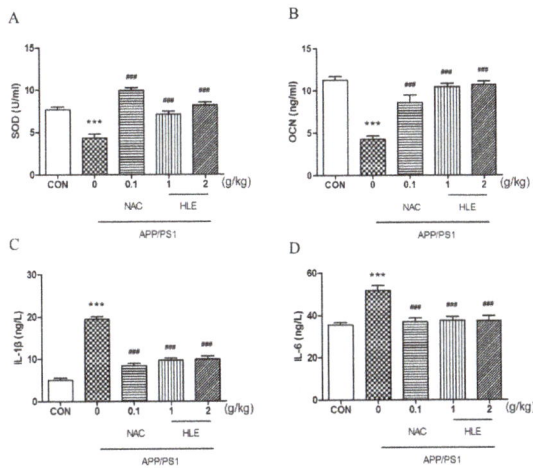

Figure 4. Effects of HLE on (**A**) SOD; (**B**) OCN; (**C**) IL-1β; and (**D**) IL-6 in serum of APP/PS1 mice by the Elisa test ($n = 8$). (*** $p < 0.001$, compared with the CON group; ### $p < 0.001$ compared with the APP/PS1 group).

The bone metabolism index osteoprotegerin (OPG) and oxidative stress indexes nuclear factor erythroid 2-related factor 2 (Nrf2), forkhead box O1 (FoxO1) and SOD-2 in mice femurs were measured by immunohistochemistry. As shown in Figure 5A, compared with wild-type mice, the expression of OPG in femurs of APP/PS1 mice was significantly reduced ($p < 0.01$). High doses of HLE significantly improved this inhibition ($p < 0.01$), indicating that endogenous Aβ reduced OPG content, and HLE might play a bone protective role by promoting the expression of OPG. As shown in Figure 5B–D, Nrf2, FoxO1 and SOD-2 expression in femurs of APP/PS1 mice was significantly reduced compared with that in wild-type mice ($p < 0.01$), while high doses of HLE could return it to a normal level ($p < 0.01$), suggesting that HLE might alleviate oxidative stress through regulating Nrf2 and FoxO1 pathways.

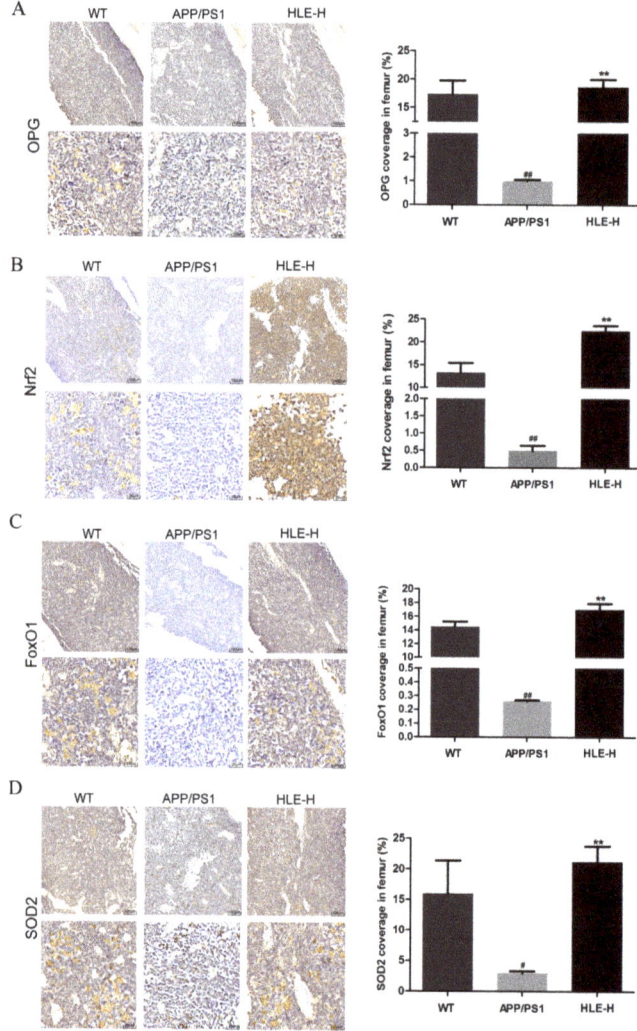

Figure 5. Effects of HLE on (**A**) OPG; (**B**) Nrf2; (**C**) FoxO1; and (**D**) SOD2 expression in femurs of APP/PS1 mice by immunohistochemistry ($n = 3$). (# $p < 0.05$, ## $p < 0.01$, compared with the WT group; ** $p < 0.01$ compared with the APP/PS1 group).

2.5. HLE Improved Cell Activities and Alleviated Oxidative Stress in Aβ-Injured Osteoblasts

To further verify the effect of hops on alleviating oxidative stress and promoting bone formation through inhibiting Aβ deposition, osteoblasts were injured by Aβ for in vitro study. Bone mineralization levels were measured by Alizarin red staining. As shown in Figure 6A, all doses of HLE significantly increased the bone mineralization nodule in Aβ-injured osteoblasts, proving that hops could promote bone mineralization and bone formation. As shown in Figure 6B, Aβ significantly improved the ROS release in osteoblasts, while HLE markedly reduced the ROS level in a dose-dependent manner ($p < 0.01$). In addition, oxidative stress related Nrf2 and FoxO1 pathways were measured by Western blotting. As shown in Figure 6C–E, Aβ markedly reduced the expression of Nrf2, heme oxygenase-1 (HO-1), NAD(P)H:quinone oxidoreductase 1 (NQO1), FoxO1 and SOD-2 compared to the control group. After treatment, HLE or NAC significantly reversed the decreased expression of Nrf2, HO-1, NQO1, FoxO1 and SOD-2 in Aβ-injured osteoblasts, indicating that HLE could alleviate oxidative stress caused by Aβ deposition through activating Nrf2 and FoxO1 pathways.

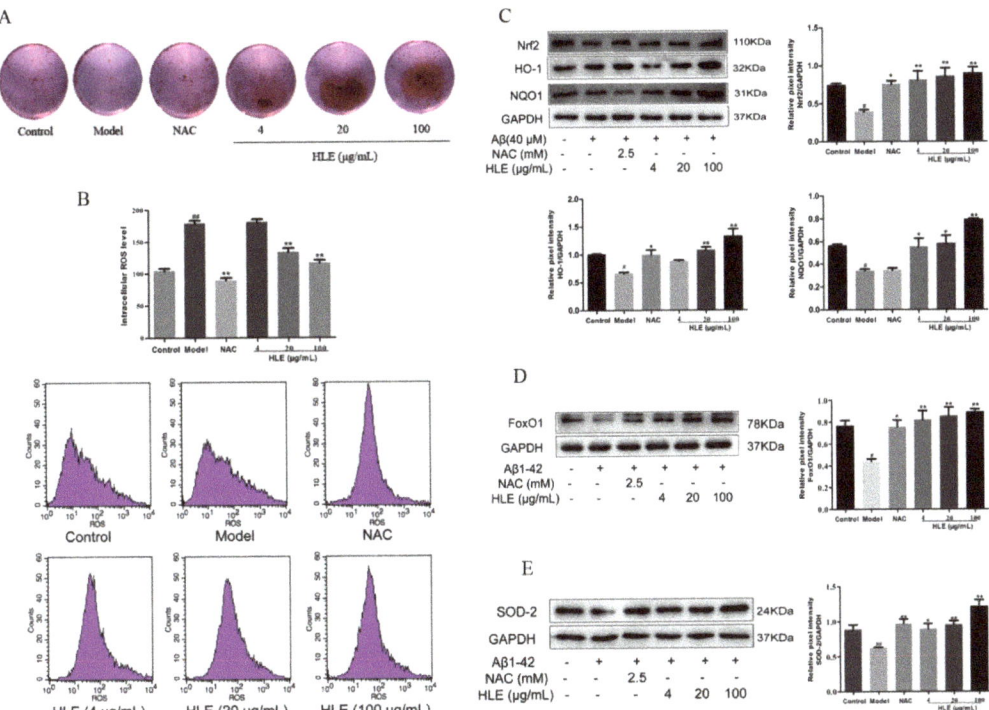

Figure 6. Effects of HLE on bone formation and oxidative stress in Aβ-injured osteoblastic MC3T3-E1 cells. (**A**) The bone mineralization nodule determined by Alizarin red staining; (**B**) intracellular ROS levels determined by flow cytometry; (**C–E**) relative expression of Nrf2, HO-1, NQO1, FxoO1 and SOD-2 determined by Western blotting ($n = 3$). (# $p < 0.05$, ## $p < 0.01$, compared with the CON group; * $p < 0.05$, ** $p < 0.01$ compared with the model group. Model group means osteoblasts only treated with Aβ).

3. Discussion

Osteoporosis is a degenerative chronic disease closely related to aging. It is crucial to fully recognize the potential risks and benefits of diagnosing and treating osteoporosis in elderly people. The high consumption of beer all over the world leads us to focus on hops plants that are essential in beer brewing, and our previous studies have detailed the potent effects of hops on relieving oxidative stress and alleviating bone loss. However, details of the mechanism of hops on preventing senior osteoporosis have not been clarified. In this study, it was determined for the first time that hops improved the learning ability and alleviated bone loss of APP/PS1 mice through inhibiting Aβ deposition in both the brain and bone. In vivo and in vitro experiments revealed hops could relieve Aβ-induced oxidative stress and protect against SOP.

In agreement with the clinical and epidemiological evidence, it has been found that Aβ deposition and the dysfunction of antioxidant system play an important role in the pathogenesis of SOP and AD [19]. Extracellular amyloid plaques and intracellular neurofibrillary tangles in the brain are primary indicators of AD. It has been demonstrated that the mutations in the APP gene, presenilin (PS) 1, potentially lead to early onset of AD [20]. In mice, the APP transgene combined with a PS1 transgene yielded Aβ plaques with earlier onset than the single transgenic sample [21]. Aβ directly or indirectly modulates mitochondrial function and induces oxidative stress, which in turn enhances Aβ synthesis and aggregation. In this study, APP/PS1 mutated transgenic mice were used to mimic the SOP condition, and we found that there was Aβ deposition not only in the brain but also in the femurs of APP/PS1 mice, which was an important trigger of memory impairment and osteoporosis. After treatment, it was discovered that hops could both alleviate memory impairment and attenuate bone loss. More importantly, the Aβ amount in mice hippocampi, cortexes and femurs were markedly decreased after treatment with HLE, proving that hops could alleviate senior osteoporosis and dementia in APP/PS1 mice through removing Aβ deposition.

The histomorphometric parameters of the trabecular bone obtained from micro-CT analysis can predict osteopenia and deterioration of bone quality, and BMD is known as the golden indicator for diagnosing osteoporosis [22]. The present study found that the femur BMD of APP/PS1 mice decreased significantly and the bone micro-structure was severely damaged, indicating that Aβ deposition led to bone loss. Hops could improve the micro-architecture, enhance the BMD, and increase the trabecular parameters in the femurs of APP/PS1 mice, suggesting that hops was effective in both preserving bone mass and rescuing the deterioration of bone micro-architecture when damaged by Aβ deposition. During bone remodeling, osteoblastic bone formation and osteoclastic bone resorption are a synergistic action. OCN and OPG are important enzymes characterized by the capacity of osteoblastic bone formation [23], while the concentrations of IL-1β and IL-6 in serum were associated with increased ROS and osteoclastic bone resorption [24]. IL-1β and IL-6 not only directly stimulate osteoclastogenesis and bone resorption but also stimulate RANKL production in osteoblastic cells in a synergistic fashion. In this study, hops can significantly increase the OCN and OPG expression and inhibit the serum IL-1β and IL-6 levels in APP/PS1 mice, indicating the potential of hops in maintaining bone homeostasis.

Aβ deposition could interfere with the mitochondria, which causes cells to stop breathing and subsequently oxidative stress [25,26]. Studies have increasingly shown that excessive oxidative stress can lead to memory impairment and induce osteoporosis. On one hand, excess ROS damages osteogenic activity and osteoblast dysfunction, eventually resulting in osteoporosis [27]. On the other hand, dementia is mainly caused by the accumulation of Aβ protein plaque and overexpression of hyperphosphorylated tau protein in neurons [28], all of which ultimately induce neurotoxic effects via the upregulation of ROS in the brain. Thus, oxidative stress is seen as a risk factor for both AD and SOP. In this process, SOD is the major enzymatic scavenger in the antioxidant-defense system. The transgenic mice with overexpression of APP mutant and deficiency of Mn-SOD had elevated oxidative stress and significantly increased levels of brain Aβ plaque. Conversely, Mn-SOD was overexpressed in APP/PS1 mice and they exhibited an increased antioxidant defense capability in the brain and a reduced level of Aβ plaque [29]. In our study, we observed significantly lower SOD activities in both the serum and femurs of APP/PS1 mice, and higher ROS levels in Aβ-injured osteoblasts. Fortunately, hops could increase the SOD level and reduce active oxygen release, thus relieving oxidative stress.

As a key redox-sensitive transcription factor, Nrf2 is conducive to maintaining cellular redox homeostasis and improving oxidative injury. Expressions of antioxidant enzymes SOD and CAT are intimately related with Nrf2 signaling activation [30]. The by-products catalyzed by HO-1 have potent ROS scavenging activity, while NQO1-induced by-products prevent DNA oxidative damage caused by environmental stress agents [31]. FoxO1, the major member in the Forkhead box O family, counteracts ROS generation by upregulating antioxidant enzymes. FoxO can also affect the proliferation and differentiation of osteoblasts through its regulation of the redox balance [32]. In this study, it was discovered that hops could increase the Nrf2, FoxO1 and SOD-2 expression in the femurs of APP/PS1 mice and promote the expression of Nrf2 and FoxO1 pathway-related proteins in Aβ-injured osteoblasts, suggesting that hops might alleviate oxidative stress and SOP through regulating Nrf2 and FoxO1 pathways.

Collectively, we have, for the first time, demonstrated that hops extract protects against Aβ-induced senior osteoporosis primarily by ameliorating memory impairment, enhancing BMD and trabecular bone structure and improving osteoblastic MC3T3-E1 cell activities in APP/PS1 mutated transgenic mice. As for its mechanism, removing Aβ deposition in the brain and bone and its inducing of oxidative stress plays a crucial role.

4. Materials and Methods

4.1. Reagents

Humulus lupulus L. was obtained from the Anguo Traditional Chinese medicine market (Hebei, China) and identified through microscope identification and HPLC to test its quality (Figure 7). An amount of 150 g *Humulus lupulus* L. was extracted by 2.25 L 75% ethanol at 80 °C for 2 h twice. The filtrate was concentrated at 40 °C under reduced pressure. The final extract was standardized by ICE-3 and xanthohumol, a special component in hops, to evaluate the quality by HPLC. The content of xanthohumol in the extract was 0.55%. The final extract was stored at -20 °C.

NAC and SOD assay kits were purchased from Shanghai Biyotime Biotechnology Co., Ltd. Enzyme-linked immunosorbent assay (ELISA) kits for determination of OCN, IL-1β and IL-6 were purchased from Nanjing Jiancheng Bioengineering Institute. Antibodies against Nrf2, HO-1, NQO1, FoxO1 and SOD-2 were purchased from Abcam. All materials were dissolved in 0.5% CMC-Na solution.

4.2. Animals and Treatment

Male APP/PS1 mutated transgenic mice (9 months old, 25–30 g) were obtained from the Nanjing Biomedical Research Institute of Nanjing University (Certificate No. SCXK 2015-0001, Nanjing, China), and housed four per cage, maintained under constant temperature (23 ± 1 °C) and humidity (60 ± 10%) under a 12 h light/dark cycle (light from 7:30 am to 7:30 pm). Mice were freely provided with water and food and divided equally into five groups of ten mice, namely CON, APP/PS1, APP/PS1 + NAC (100 mg/kg/d), APP/PS1 + HLE-L (1 g/kg/d) and APP/PS1 + HLE-H (2 g/kg/d). The selection of the drug doses in the experiment was based on our previous study [9]. The experimental dosage was adjusted according to the weight by 0.1 mL/g, and all drugs were given 6 days a week for 2 months. The wild mice were treated with the same volume of 0.5% CMC-Na solution by intragastric administration. In the end, mice were fasted for 12 h, followed by anesthetization by injection of 3 mL/kg 10% (w/v) chloral hydrate. Serums were centrifuged and stored at -80 °C for biochemical assay, and femurs were prepared for micro-CT and immunohistochemistry experiments. All studies were conducted in accordance with the NIH publication and approved by the Committee on Ethics of Medical Research Second Military Medical University.

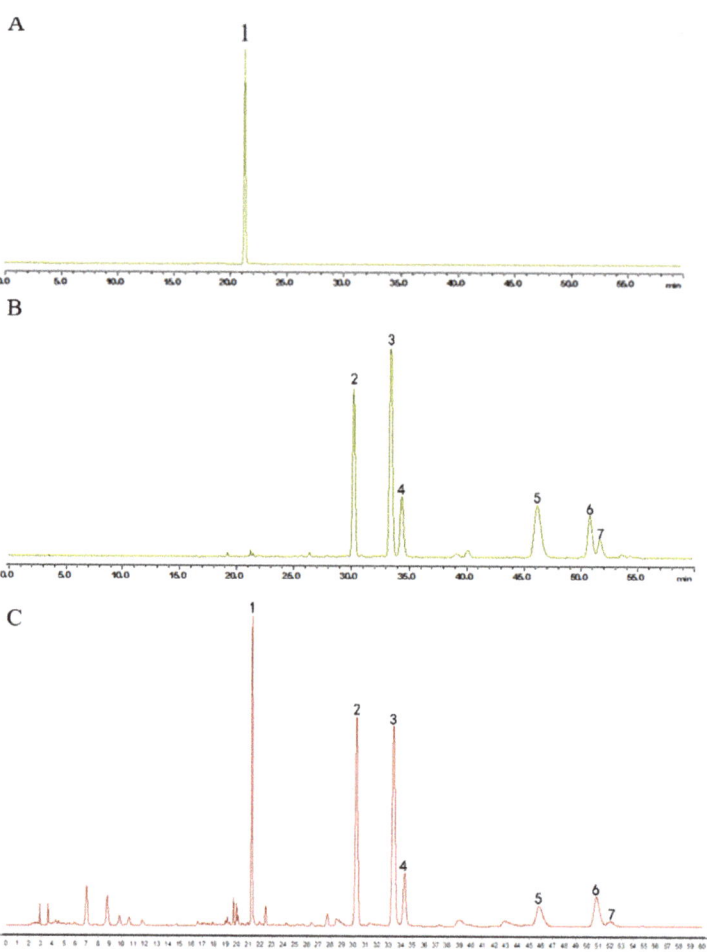

Figure 7. HPLC chromatogram of (**A**) xantholhumol; (**B**) the mixed standard control and (**C**) the hops extract. The content of xanthohumol in the extract was 0.55%. (1. xanthohumol; 2. cohumulone; 3. humulone; 4. adhumulone; 5. colupulone; 6. lupulone; 7. adlupulone).

4.3. Morris Water Maze Task

The Morris water maze task was employed to test spatial learning and memory ability of mice in this study [33]. The task consisted of a circular pool (180 cm in diameter and 45 cm in height) and a transparent escape platform (9 cm in diameter and 29 cm in height). The platform was submerged 1 cm below the surface of the water and placed in one quadrant named the target quadrant. Four visual cues were placed around the tank (one triangle, one square, one circle and one hexagon) and the water in the pool was maintained at $24 \pm 1\ ^\circ C$, and contained titanium white powder. On the first day, all test mice were habituated to swimming for 60 s freely in the tank without the escape platform. During the next five days, the mice were trained to swim to the platform placed in the center of the target quadrant within 60 s, with three trials per day in a section, and the interval between the two trails was 30 min. The time (latency) spent searching for platform was recorded. On the probe test day, the animals were admitted to freely swim in the tank without the platform for 60 s, and the time spent in the target quadrant, the number of crossings of the platform and the swimming velocity were recorded.

4.4. Congo Red Staining

After mice were sacrificed, the whole brain and right femurs were picked and fixed in 4% paraformaldehyde, then placed in 30% sucrose solution until they sunk to the bottom. The tissue was continuously cut, and every slice (10 µm, three sections for one mouse) was stained with Congo red to determine the total amount of Aβ plaque, as described previously [13]. In the end, the hippocampus, cortex and femur slices were mounted on slides for detection using an Olympus microscope with DP-70 software.

4.5. Micro-CT and Biochemical Marker Measurement

Mice femur micro-architecture was measured with a micro-CT scanner (GE eXplore Locus SP). BMD and trabecular bone parameters of BVF, Tb.N., Tb.Th. and Tb.Sp. were auto calculated by the computer.

Mice serum was centrifuged at 3000 r/min for 10 min, and the supernatant was collected for the biochemical markers assay. The SOD, OCN, IL-1β and IL-6 levels were measured by commercially available assay kits in accordance with the manufacturer's instructions.

4.6. Immunohistochemistry

The femur section was separated for immunohistochemistry by xylene and hydrated in ethanol of graded concentrations. The cross-section was bathed in sodium citrate buffer (pH = 6.0) and heated. Then, the section was incubated in 3% hydrogen peroxide for 25 min and 3% BSA solution for 30 min, successively. After that, the sections were incubated with primary and secondary antibodies at 4 °C, successively. Finally, slides were incubated by a DAB staining kit and stained with hematoxylin-eosin, and the positive section was stained brown-yellow. The coverage of positive staining was calculated with Image-pro plus software.

4.7. Cell Cultures and Treatment

Osteoblastic MC3T3-E1 cells were purchased from the typical Culture Committee Cell Library of the Chinese Academy of Sciences, Shanghai, China, and cultured in DMEM containing 10% FBS in a humidified atmosphere of 5% CO_2 at 37 °C. When reaching 80% confluence, osteoblasts could be used for follow-up studies. According to the experiment design, osteoblasts were incubated overnight and then pretreated with different concentration of HLE (4, 20 and 100 µg/mL) or NAC (2.5 mM) for 4 h. After that, the plate was removed from the incubator and 1 µL of 1 mM $Aβ_{1-42}$ oligomer mother liquor was added to each well, resulting in a final concentration of 10 µM Aβ. Osteoblasts were incubated for another 44 h, and cell growth in the orifice without the treatment was used as the control group.

4.8. Osteoblastic Mineralization and ROS Analysis

The cultured osteoblasts were added to 24-well plates overnight (5×10^4 cells/well) and then cultured with osteogenic differentiation medium (10 nM dexamethasone, 50 µg/mL ascorbic acid and 10 mM β-glycerophosphate) for 18 days. Then, cells were cultured in HLE or NAC, which contained 10 µM Aβ, for another 2 days. Osteoblasts were fixed in ice-cold 4% paraformaldehyde for 10 min, and then dyed with 0.1% Alizarin red solution at 37 °C for 30 min. After washing, osteoblasts were completely dissolved in 10% cetylpyridinium chloride for 15 min, and then measured at 570 nm.

For intracellular ROS measurements, osteoblasts were treated with reagents for 48 h and then incubated with 5 µM DCFHDA for 30 min at room temperature. Finally, the intracellular ROS level was analyzed with a flow cytometer according to the instructions of the ROS Assay Kit.

4.9. Western Blotting

Osteoblasts were seeded in 6-well plates with a density of 1×10^5 cells/mL. After 48 h treatment, the osteoblasts were lysed and centrifuged at 12,000 r/min for 10 min. The cell lysis solution was separated onto 10% sodium dodecyl sulfate-polyacrylamide gels and electrically blotted onto a polyvinylidene fluoride membrane. Membranes were blocked with 5% BSA for 1 h and then incubated with primary antibodies overnight at 4 °C. These targets were immunoblotted in the same membrane from which GAPDH was immunoblotted. After that, TBST was used to wash membranes three times, and the membranes were incubated with horseradish peroxidase-conjugated goat anti-rabbit secondary antibodies at 37 °C for 1 h. Membranes were visualized by enhanced chemiluminescent (ECL) reagents and imaged using the Gel imaging system. For protein bands with similar KD values, we used the removal solution to remove the previous protein imprint, and then carried out another incubation for other antibodies.

4.10. Statistical Analysis

All data were expressed as mean ± standard error of mean (SEM). Statistical significance was set at $p < 0.05$ and determined by one-way analysis of variance and the Student–Newman–Keuls test for multiple comparisons. GraphPad Prism (version 5.0) was used for statistical analysis.

Author Contributions: H.X., T.X. and T.H. conceived and designed the research; T.X., J.Z., Y.G. and Y.J. performed the in vivo experiments; F.Q. and K.L. performed the in vitro experiments; T.X. and N.W. analyzed the data; T.X. and J.Z. wrote the manuscript. All authors have read and agreed to the published version of the manuscript.

Funding: This research was funded by the National Natural Science Foundation of China (82174079, 82004015) and Project of Science and Technology Commission of Shanghai Municipality (21S21902600).

Institutional Review Board Statement: The animal study protocol was approved by Committee on Ethics of Medical Research Second Military Medical University on 2019/09/25 (No. 201930921).

Informed Consent Statement: Not applicable.

Data Availability Statement: The data presented in this study are available on request from the corresponding author.

Acknowledgments: We thank the support of the National Natural Science Foundation of China (82174079, 82004015) and Project of Science and Technology Commission of Shanghai Municipality (21S21902600).

Conflicts of Interest: The authors declare no conflict of interest.

References

1. Shi, Y.; Liu, X.Y.; Jiang, Y.P.; Zhang, J.B.; Zhang, Q.Y.; Wang, N.N.; Xin, H.L. Monotropein attenuates oxidative stress via Akt/mTOR-mediated autophagy in osteoblast cells. *Biomed. Pharmacother.* **2020**, *121*, 109566. [CrossRef]
2. Ishikawa, K.; Nagai, T.; Sakamoto, K.; Ohara, K.; Eguro, T.; Ito, H.; Toyoshima, Y.; Kokaze, A.; Toyone, T.; Inagaki, K. High bone turnover elevates the risk of denosumab-induced hypocalcemia in women with postmenopausal osteoporosis. *Ther. Clin. Risk Manag.* **2016**, *12*, 1831–1840. [CrossRef] [PubMed]
3. Si, L.; Winzenberg, T.M.; Jiang, Q.; Chen, M.; Palmer, A.J. Projection of osteoporosis-related fractures and costs in China: 2010-2050. *Osteoporos Int.* **2015**, *26*, 1929–1937. [CrossRef] [PubMed]
4. Amouzougan, A.; Lafaie, L.; Marotte, H.; Dénariè, D.; Collet, P.; Pallot-Prades, B.; Thomas, T. High prevalence of dementia in women with osteoporosis. *Jt. Bone Spine* **2017**, *84*, 611–614. [CrossRef]
5. Di Sotto, A.; Checconi, P.; Celestino, I.; Locatelli, M.; Carissimi, S.; De Angelis, M.; Rossi, V.; Limongi, D.; Toniolo, C.; Martinoli, L.; et al. Antiviral and Antioxidant Activity of a Hydroalcoholic Extract from *Humulus lupulus* L. *Oxid. Med. Cell Longev.* **2018**, *2018*, 5919237. [CrossRef] [PubMed]
6. Sasaoka, N.; Sakamoto, M.; Kanemori, S.; Kan, M.; Tsukano, C.; Takemoto, Y.; Kakizuka, A. Long-term oral administration of hop flower extracts mitigates Alzheimer phenotypes in mice. *PLoS ONE* **2014**, *9*, e87185. [CrossRef] [PubMed]
7. Lela, L.; Ponticelli, M.; Caddeo, C.; Vassallo, A.; Ostuni, A.; Sinisgalli, C.; Faraone, I.; Santoro, V.; De Tommasi, N.; Milella, L. Nanotechnological exploitation of the antioxidant potential of *Humulus lupulus* L. extract. *Food Chem.* **2022**, *393*, 133401. [CrossRef]

8. Önder, F.C.; Ay, M.; Sarker, S.D. Comparative study of antioxidant properties and total phenolic content of the extracts of Humulus lupulus L. and quantification of bioactive components by LC-MS/MS and GC-MS. *J. Agric. Food Chem.* **2013**, *61*, 10498–10506. [CrossRef]
9. Xia, T.S.; Lin, L.Y.; Zhang, Q.Y.; Jiang, Y.P.; Li, C.H.; Liu, X.Y.; Qin, L.P.; Xin, H.L. Humulus lupulus L. Extract Prevents Ovariectomy-Induced Osteoporosis in Mice and Regulates Activities of Osteoblasts and Osteoclasts. *Chin. J. Integr. Med.* **2021**, *27*, 31–38. [CrossRef]
10. Sun, X.L.; Xia, T.S.; Zhang, S.Y.; Zhang, J.B.; Xu, L.C.; Han, T.; Xin, H.L. Hops extract and xanthohumol ameliorate bone loss induced by iron overload via activating Akt/GSK3β/Nrf2 pathway. *J. Bone Miner. Metab.* **2022**, *40*, 375–388. [CrossRef]
11. Sun, X.L.; Xia, T.S.; Jiang, Y.P.; Wang, N.N.; Xu, L.C.; Han, T.; Xin, H.L. Humulus lupulus L. extract and its active constituent xanthohumol attenuate oxidative stress and nerve injury induced by iron overload via activating AKT/GSK3β and Nrf2/NQO1 pathways. *J. Nat. Med.* **2022**. Online ahead of print. [CrossRef]
12. Xia, T.S.; Liu, X.Y.; Wang, N.N.; Jiang, Y.P.; Bai, H.H.; Xu, W.M.; Feng, K.M.; Han, T.; Xin, H.L. PI3K/AKT/Nrf2 signalling pathway is involved in the ameliorative effects of xanthohumol on amyloid β-induced oxidative damage and bone loss. *J. Pharm. Pharmacol.* **2022**, *74*, 1017–1026. [CrossRef] [PubMed]
13. Sun, X.L.; Zhang, J.B.; Guo, Y.X.; Xia, T.S.; Xu, L.C.; Rahmand, K.; Wang, G.P.; Li, X.J.; Han, T.; Wang, N.N.; et al. Xanthohumol ameliorates memory impairment and reduces the deposition of β-amyloid in APP/PS1 mice via regulating the mTOR/LC3II and Bax/Bcl-2 signalling pathways. *J. Pharm. Pharmacol.* **2021**, *73*, 1230–1239. [CrossRef] [PubMed]
14. Brier, M.R.; Gordon, B.; Friedrichsen, K.; McCarthy, J.; Stern, A.; Christensen, J.; Owen, C.; Aldea, P.; Su, Y.; Hassenstab, J.; et al. Tau and Aβ imaging, CSF measures, and cognition in Alzheimer's disease. *Sci. Transl. Med.* **2016**, *8*, 338ra66. [CrossRef]
15. Kulas, J.A.; Franklin, W.F.; Smith, N.A.; Manocha, G.D.; Puig, K.L.; Nagamoto-Combs, K.; Hendrix, R.D.; Taglialatela, G.; Barger, S.W.; Combs, C.K. Ablation of amyloid precursor protein increases insulin-degrading enzyme levels and activity in brain and peripheral tissues. *Am. J. Physiol. Endocrinol. Metab.* **2019**, *316*, E106–E120. [CrossRef]
16. Gatineau, E.; Polakof, S.; Dardevet, D.; Mosoni, L. Similarities and interactions between the ageing process and high chronic intake of added sugars. *Nutr. Res. Rev.* **2017**, *30*, 191–207. [CrossRef] [PubMed]
17. Cui, S.; Xiong, F.; Hong, Y.; Jung, J.U.; Li, X.S.; Liu, J.Z.; Yan, R.; Mei, L.; Feng, X.; Xiong, W.C. APPswe/Aβ regulation of osteoclast activation and RAGE expression in an age-dependent manner. *J. Bone Miner. Res.* **2011**, *26*, 1084–1098. [CrossRef]
18. Zhao, L.; Liu, S.; Wang, Y.; Zhang, Q.Y.; Zhao, W.J.; Wang, Z.J.; Yin, M. Effects of Curculigoside on Memory Impairment and Bone Loss via Anti-Oxidative Character in APP/PS1 Mutated Transgenic Mice. *PLoS ONE* **2015**, *10*, e0133289. [CrossRef] [PubMed]
19. Park, L.; Uekawa, K.; Garcia-Bonilla, L.; Koizumi, K.; Murphy, M.; Pistik, R.; Younkin, L.; Younkin, S.; Zhou, P.; Carlson, G.; et al. Brain Perivascular Macrophages Initiate the Neurovascular Dysfunction of Alzheimer Aβ Peptides. *Circ. Res.* **2017**, *121*, 258–269. [CrossRef] [PubMed]
20. Selkoe, D.J.; Hardy, J. The amyloid hypothesis of Alzheimer's disease at 25 years. *EMBO Mol. Med.* **2016**, *8*, 595–608. [CrossRef]
21. Webster, S.J.; Bachstetter, A.D.; Nelson, P.T.; Schmitt, F.A.; Van Eldik, L.J. Using mice to model Alzheimer's dementia: An overview of the clinical disease and the preclinical behavioral changes in 10 mouse models. *Front Genet.* **2014**, *5*, 88. [CrossRef] [PubMed]
22. Xia, T.S.; Dong, X.; Jiang, Y.P.; Lin, L.Y.; Dong, Z.M.; Shen, Y.; Xin, H.L.; Zhang, Q.Y.; Qin, L.P. Metabolomics Profiling Reveals Rehmanniae Radix Preparata Extract Protects against Glucocorticoid-Induced Osteoporosis Mainly via Intervening Steroid Hormone Biosynthesis. *Molecules* **2019**, *24*, 253. [CrossRef] [PubMed]
23. Chatziravdeli, V.; Katsaras, G.N.; Lambrou, G.I. Gene Expression in Osteoblasts and Osteoclasts Under Microgravity Conditions: A Systematic Review. *Curr. Genom.* **2019**, *20*, 184–198. [CrossRef] [PubMed]
24. Guan, Y.J.; Li, J.; Yang, X.; Du, S.; Ding, J.; Gao, Y.; Zhang, Y.; Yang, K.; Chen, Q. Evidence that miR-146a attenuates aging- and trauma-induced osteoarthritis by inhibiting Notch1, IL-6, and IL-1 mediated catabolism. *Aging Cell.* **2018**, *17*, e12752. [CrossRef]
25. Ng, J.; Kaur, H.; Collier, T.; Chang, K.; Brooks, A.E.S.; Allison, J.R.; Brimble, M.A.; Hickey, A.; Birch, N.P. Site-specific glycation of Aβ1-42 affects fibril formation and is neurotoxic. *J. Biol. Chem.* **2019**, *294*, 8806–8818. [CrossRef] [PubMed]
26. Moskovitz, J.; Du, F.; Bowman, C.F.; Yan, S.S. Methionine sulfoxide reductase A affects β-amyloid solubility and mitochondrial function in a mouse model of Alzheimer's disease. *Am. J. Physiol. Endocrinol. Metab.* **2016**, *310*, E388–E393. [CrossRef] [PubMed]
27. Manolagas, S.C. From estrogen-centric to aging and oxidative stress: A revised perspective of the pathogenesis of osteoporosis. *Endocr. Rev.* **2010**, *31*, 266–300. [CrossRef] [PubMed]
28. Hardas, S.S.; Sultana, R.; Clark, A.M.; Beckett, T.L.; Szweda, L.I.; Murphy, M.P.; Butterfield, D.A. Oxidative modification of lipoic acid by HNE in Alzheimer disease brain. *Redox Biol.* **2013**, *1*, 80–85. [CrossRef] [PubMed]
29. Ferrer, I.; Boada Rovira, M.; Sánchez Guerra, M.L.; Rey, M.J.; Costa-Jussá, F. Neuropathology and pathogenesis of encephalitis following amyloid-beta immunization in Alzheimer's disease. *Brain Pathol.* **2004**, *14*, 11–20. [CrossRef] [PubMed]
30. Feng, H.; Wang, L.; Zhang, G.X.; Zhang, Z.W.; Guo, W. Oxidative stress activated by Keap-1/Nrf2 signaling pathway in pathogenesis of preeclampsia. *Int. J. Clin. Exp. Pathol.* **2020**, *13*, 382–392.
31. González-Burgos, E.; Carretero, M.E.; Gómez-Serranillos, M.P. Diterpenoids isolated from Sideritis species protect astrocytes against oxidative stress via Nrf2. *J. Nat. Prod.* **2012**, *75*, 1750–1758. [CrossRef] [PubMed]

32. Xu, W.M.; Liu, X.Y.; He, X.H.; Jiang, Y.P.; Zhang, J.B.; Zhang, Q.Y.; Wang, N.N.; Qin, L.P.; Xin, H.L. Bajitianwan attenuates D-galactose-induced memory impairment and bone loss through suppression of oxidative stress in aging rat model. *J. Ethnopharmacol.* **2020**, *261*, 112992. [CrossRef] [PubMed]
33. Liao, Y.; Bae, H.J.; Park, J.H.; Zhang, J.; Koo, B.; Lim, M.K.; Han, E.H.; Lee, S.H.; Jung, S.Y.; Lew, J.H.; et al. Aster glehni Extract Ameliorates Scopolamine-Induced Cognitive Impairment in Mice. *J. Med. Food* **2019**, *22*, 685–695. [CrossRef] [PubMed]

Disclaimer/Publisher's Note: The statements, opinions and data contained in all publications are solely those of the individual author(s) and contributor(s) and not of MDPI and/or the editor(s). MDPI and/or the editor(s) disclaim responsibility for any injury to people or property resulting from any ideas, methods, instructions or products referred to in the content.

Article

Antioxidant Assessment of Prenylated Stilbenoid-Rich Extracts from Elicited Hairy Root Cultures of Three Cultivars of Peanut (*Arachis hypogaea*)

Gaurav Gajurel [1,2], Rokib Hasan [1,2] and Fabricio Medina-Bolivar [1,3,*]

[1] Arkansas Biosciences Institute, Arkansas State University, Jonesboro, AR 72467, USA; gaurav.gajurel@smail.astate.edu (G.G.); mdrokib.hasan@smail.astate.edu (R.H.)
[2] Molecular Biosciences Graduate Program, Arkansas State University, Jonesboro, AR 72467, USA
[3] Department of Biological Sciences, Arkansas State University, Jonesboro, AR 72467, USA
* Correspondence: fmedinabolivar@astate.edu; Tel.: +1-8706804319

Abstract: Peanut produces prenylated stilbenoids upon biotic stress. However, the role of these compounds against oxidative stress have not been thoroughly elucidated. To this end, the antioxidant capacity of extracts enriched in prenylated stilbenoids and derivatives was studied. To produce these extracts, hairy root cultures of peanut cultivars Hull, Tifrunner, and Georgia Green were co-treated with methyl jasmonate, cyclodextrin, hydrogen peroxide, and magnesium chloride and then the stilbenoids were extracted from the culture medium. Among the three cultivars, higher levels of the stilbenoid derivatives arachidin-1 and arachidin-6 were detected in cultivar Tifrunner. Upon reaction with 2,2-diphenyl-1picrylhydrazyl, extracts from cultivar Tifrunner showed the highest antioxidant capacity with an IC_{50} of 6.004 µg/mL. Furthermore, these extracts had significantly higher antioxidant capacity at 6.25 µg/mL and 3.125 µg/mL when compared to extracts from cultivars Hull and Georgia Green. The stilbenoid-rich extracts from peanut hairy roots show high antioxidant capacity and merit further study as potential nutraceuticals to promote human health.

Keywords: stilbenoid-rich extract; prenylated stilbenoids; arachidin; peanut; antioxidant; elicitation; hairy root

1. Introduction

Reactive oxygen species (ROS) are continually produced by living organisms during cellular metabolism. At physiological concentration, ROS may be required for the normal function of the cell. However, excess accumulation of ROS can cause oxidative stress, damaging the cellular macromolecules like DNA, lipids, and proteins, and eventually lead to disease conditions. In humans, the harmful effect of ROS has been associated with the occurrence of more than 100 diseases, including neurodegenerative disease, heart-related disease, diabetes, and cancer [1–3]. Antioxidants protect the living system from the harmful effect of ROS by scavenging them directly or indirectly [4]. In the past few years, plant-derived stilbenoids and their derivatives have gained considerable interest as a source of antioxidants due to their diverse chemical structure and biological activities with potential application as pharmacological agents [5].

Stilbenoids are a group of polyphenolic compounds that can be found in a limited number of plant families, including those of grapevine (Vitaceae), peanut (Fabaceae), and blueberry (Ericaceae). These compounds are phytoalexins that are produced upon infection by fungus and other pathogens to protect the host plant against them. Thus, the peanut plant produces stilbenoids as a defense response to biotic stress and more than 45 stilbenoids and their derivatives have been reported in peanut tissues subjected to biotic stresses [6–10]. The first described peanut stilbenoids include resveratrol and the prenylated stilbenoids arachidin-1, arachidin-3, and isopentadienyl trihydroxystilbene [11].

Among these stilbenoids, the most studied is resveratrol due to its biological properties beneficial to human health including antioxidant, cardioprotective, anticancer, antiaging, and others. Despite the wide range of bioactivities of resveratrol, this stilbenoid has shown limited bioavailability in vivo due to its rapid metabolism into glucuronide and sulfate metabolites [12]. Interestingly, natural resveratrol analogs such as the prenylated stilbenoids may have increased bioavailability due to favorable metabolic profiles as demonstrated by in vitro assays [13]. Additionally, prenylated stilbenoids have shown to exhibit enhanced or equivalent antioxidant, anti-inflammatory, and anti-adipogenic activities when compared to resveratrol [14–16].

Hairy root cultures of peanut cv. Hull was established previously using *Agrobacterium rhizogenes* to enhance the production of non-prenylated and prenylated stilbenoids [17]. The hairy roots when treated with a combination of methyl jasmonate (MeJA), cyclodextrin (CD), hydrogen peroxide, and magnesium chloride secrete several stilbenoids and their derivatives into the culture medium and thus these compounds can be extracted from the culture medium [18]. This stilbenoid-rich extract from peanut hairy root culture medium is rich in the non-prenylated stilbenoid resveratrol and prenylated stilbenoids arachidin-5, arachidin-1, arachidin-2, arachidin-3, and others with diverse biological activity (Figure 1). Similarly, treatment of hairy roots from peanut cv. Kalasin 2 with chitosan, MeJA, and CD induced a large amount of arachidin-1 and arachidin-3 [19]. However, a study comparing the biological properties of stilbenoid-rich extracts from hairy roots of different peanut cultivars have not been done thoroughly.

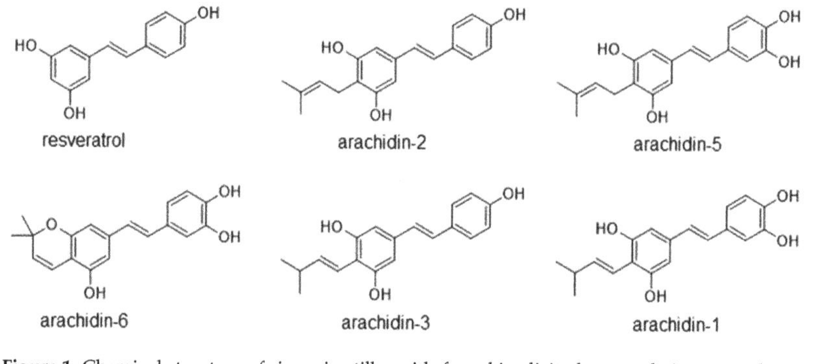

Figure 1. Chemical structure of six main stilbenoids found in elicited peanut hairy root culture. All compounds are shown in their *trans*-isomer.

In this study, we compared the antioxidant property as determined by DPPH (2,2-diphenyl-1-picrylhydrazyl) assay of stilbenoid-rich extracts obtained from elicited peanut hairy root cultures of three cultivars, i.e., Tifrunner, Hull, and Georgia Green. In addition, a comparative study of the yield of stilbenoids and their derivatives in these three cultivars of peanut was performed. We established a hairy root line from the whole-genome sequenced peanut cv. Tifrunner, and reported the production of prenylated stilbenoids and the ring-prenylated piceatannol derivative arachidin-6 in this cultivar for the first time.

2. Results and Discussion

2.1. Development and Characterization of Peanut cv. Tifrunner Hairy Roots

The peanut hairy root platform provides a potential platform for the bioproduction of prenylated stilbenoids and elucidation of new genes involved in the biosynthetic pathway of these compounds [11]. Recently, the whole genome of peanut cv. Tifrunner has been sequenced providing the potential to discover candidate genes of interest in this economically important crop [20]. Thus, the hairy root system of the whole genome sequence cultivar would provide valuable information to further elucidate the biosynthetic pathway for prenylated stilbenoids. In present work, hairy root culture of peanut cv. Tifrunner was established and treated with the combination of elicitors for stilbenoid profiling. Additionally, the antioxidant properties of the stilbenoid-rich extract from elicited hairy roots from three cultivars were compared for their potential application as nutraceuticals to promote human health.

Several hairy root lines of peanut cv. Tifrunner were produced by infecting leaves from 4-week-old seedlings with *A. rhizogenes* ATCC 15834. The wounded leaves were cultured and subcultured on MSV medium with antibiotics for 3 to 5 weeks until the development of hairy roots to avoid overgrowth of *Agrobacterium*. Tifrunner hairy root line 1 (Figure 2) was selected based on its sustained growth in liquid culture. PCR analysis of line 1 was performed for confirming the presence of *aux1* and *rolC* genes, indicating the integration of the two T-DNA, T_L-DNA, and T_R-DNA, from Ri plasmid of *A. rhizogenes* ATCC 15834 into the plant genome. Furthermore, PCR amplification of the *virD2* gene was negative suggesting the absence of any *Agrobacterium* in the root tissue (Supplementary Materials Figure S1).

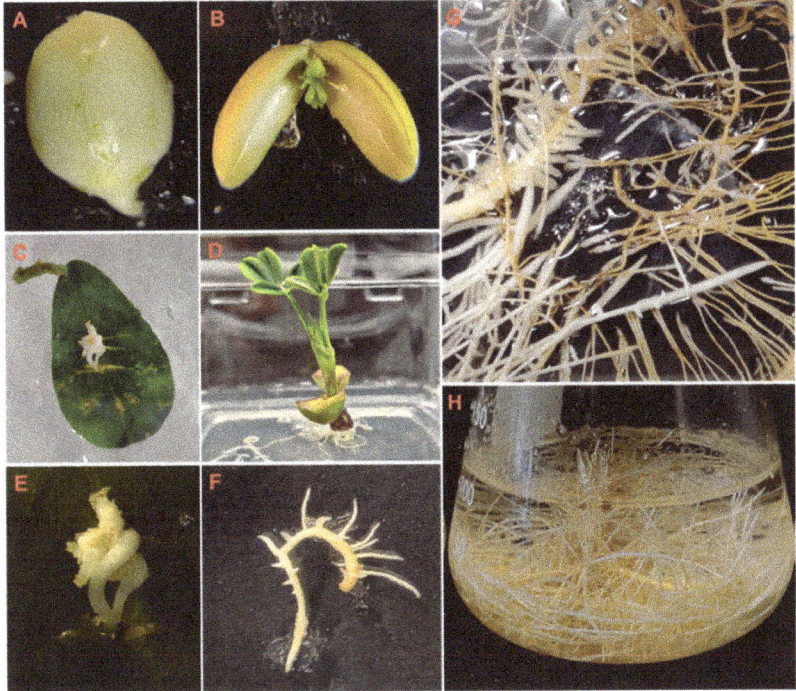

Figure 2. Germination and establishment of hairy root cultures of peanut cv. Tifrunner. (**A**): Seed germination; (**B**): One-week-old seedling; (**D**): Three-week-old seedling; (**C,E**): Hairy root development from leaf infected with *Agrobacterium rhizogenes*; (**F**): Branching of hairy roots after excision from the leaf; (**G**): Phenotype of hairy root line 1 on semi-solid medium; (**H**): Phenotype hairy root line 1 in liquid medium after 15 days in culture.

2.2. Production of Prenylated Stilbenoids in Hairy Roots of Peanut cvs. Tifrunner, Hull, and Georgia Green

The hairy root cultures of peanut cvs. Tifrunner, Hull, and Georgia Green were elicited as described before for comparison of their stilbenoid profile and yields. Notably, the color of the medium changed from clear to yellow in the hairy root cultures of all three cultivars suggesting the secretion of stilbenoids in the culture medium after elicitation treatment

(Figure 3) [17]. The stilbenoid content in the culture medium after 168 h elicitation treatment was analyzed using HPLC (Figure 4). Accordingly, all three hairy roots were able to secrete resveratrol and different prenylated stilbenoids like arachidin-5, arachidin-1, arachidin-2, and arachidin-3 into the medium upon elicitation. The production of these stilbenoids suggests that the stilbenoid-specific prenyltransferase responsible for their biosynthesis might be expressed in these three cultivars of peanuts [11].

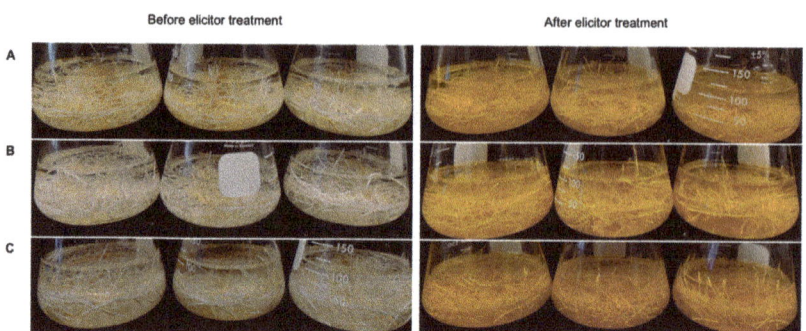

Figure 3. Elicitation of hairy root cultures. Changes in the phenotype of (**A**): Peanut cv. Tifrunner hairy root line 1; (**B**): Peanut cv. Hull line 3; (**C**): Peanut cv. Georgia Green after 168 h of treatment with different elicitors: 125 µM methyl jasmonate (MeJA), 18 g/L cyclodextrin (CD), 3 mM hydrogen peroxide (H_2O_2) and 1 mM magnesium chloride ($MgCl_2$) in a 100 mL elicitation medium.

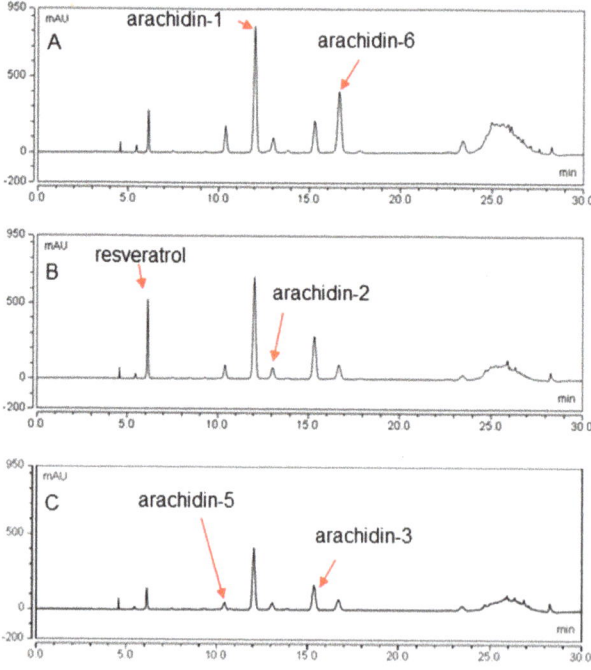

Figure 4. Comparison of secreted stilbenoid profiles among three different cultivars of peanut hairy root cultures. HPLC chromatograms of culture medium extract of hairy root cultures of (**A**): Peanut cv. Tifrunner; (**B**): Peanut cv. Hull line 3; (**C**): Peanut cv. Georgia Green after 168 h elicitor treatment. All chromatograms were monitored at 340 nm.

The yield of arachidin-5, arachidin-1, and arachidin-2 was higher in the medium of the Tifrunner hairy root culture when compared to the other two cultivars. Interestingly, the yield of resveratrol and arachidin-3 was higher in cultivar Hull (Figure 5). The yield of arachidin-5 in cv. Tifrunner was 24.07 ± 4.33 mg/L which was approximately 2.2- and 4.7-fold higher than in Hull and Georgia Green hairy roots, respectively. Similarly, the yield of arachidin-1 in cv. Tifrunner was 169.73 ± 25.17 mg/L which was significantly higher than in Hull and Georgia Green, respectively. The yield of arachidin-2 in cv. Tifrunner was 31.75 ± 5.59 mg/L which was approximately 1.4- and 2.3-fold higher than in Hull and Georgia Green, respectively. The yield of resveratrol in cv. Hull was 44.1 ± 3.3 mg/L which was significantly higher than Tifrunner and Georgia Green hairy roots, respectively. Whereas the yield of arachidin-3 in cv. Hull was 52.24 ± 3.66 mg/L which was approximately 1.2- and 1.7-fold higher than in Tifrunner and Georgia Green hairy root respectively (Figure 5).

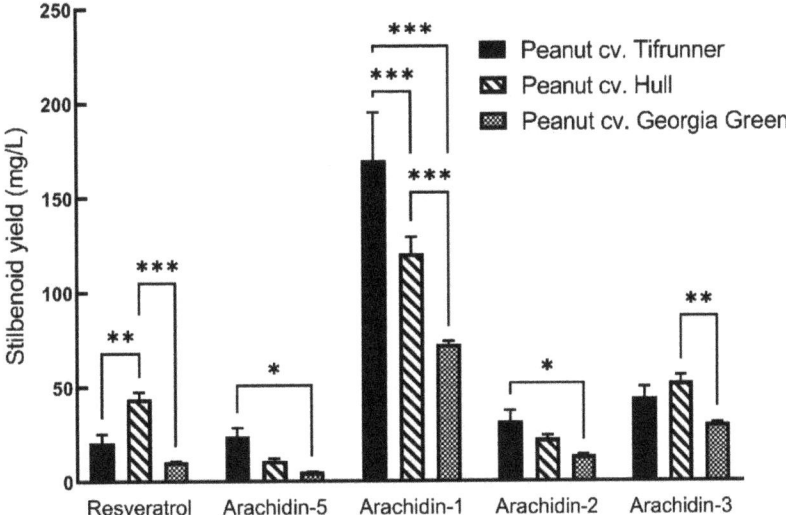

Figure 5. Comparison of stilbenoid yield in hairy root cultures of peanut cultivars Tifrunner, Hull (line 3), and Georgia Green. Yield is expressed in mg/L and each bar represents the average of three technical replicates of stilbenoids extracted from 0.9 L elicited medium. Error bars represent standard deviation. Statistical analysis was performed with two-way ANOVA with Tukey's multiple-comparisons test. The asterisks above the connecting line represent a significant difference when compared to the stilbenoid yield among the three cultivars (*, $p < 0.033$; **, $p < 0.002$; ***, $p < 0.001$).

Particularly in the Tifrunner cultivar, arachidin-1 and arachidin-6 were the predominant stilbenoids when compared to the Georgia Green and Hull cultivars. We identified arachidin-6 in the ethyl acetate extract of the culture medium by comparing characteristic UV spectrum (λ_{max}), and mass spectrometric analysis of arachidin-6 from *Rhizopus*-elicited peanut seedlings [21] (Supplementary Materials Figures S3–S5). A total of 5.3 mg of arachidin-6 (λ_{max} = 344 nm), was purified from the peanut cv. Tifrunner hairy root culture medium using semi-preparative HPLC method (Supplementary Materials Figure S2). As shown in Table 1, the precursor ion of the isolated compound ([M − H]$^-$, m/z 309) provided the main fragment with a [M − H]$^-$ of m/z 265 in MS^2 which suggested that the purified compound was arachidin-6 as described in fungal-challenged peanut. Interestingly, arachidin-6 has been reported to show moderate antimicrobial activity against methicillin-resistant *Staphylococcus aureus* with a minimum inhibitory concentration ranging from 50 to 75 µg/mL [21]. The difference in yield of stilbenoids suggests that the enzymes responsible for the production of these compounds are expressed at different levels among the hairy roots from different cultivars. To our knowledge, this is the first study to show the production of stilbenoids in peanut cv. Tifrunner.

Table 1. Tandem mass spectrometry analysis of arachidin-6 detected in ethyl acetate extract from the medium of elicited peanut cv. Tifrunner hairy root culture. Analysis was done by HPLC-PDA-electronspray ionization-MS^3.

t_R (Min)	UV Max (nm)	[M − H]$^-$	MS^2 Ions [a]	MS^3 Ions	[M + H]$^+$	MS^2 Ions [a]	MS^3 Ions
16.57	344	309	291, **265**, 294	159, 249	311	**201**, 283, 296	159, 173, 183

[a] MS^2 ions in boldface were the most abundant ions and were subjected to MS^3 fragmentation. t_R: HPLC retention time.

The first stilbenoidspecific prenyltransferases, AhR4DT-1 and AhR3′DT-1, involved in the prenylation of stilbenoids have been identified from peanut. Specifically, AhR4DT-1 catalyzes the transfer of a 3,3-dimethylallyl group to the C-4 carbon of the A-ring of resveratrol and piceatannol, producing arachidin-2 and arachidin-5, respectively. AhR3′DT-1 can use resveratrol as substrate to add a 3,3-dimethylallyl group to the C-3′ of the B ring. However, the biosynthetic steps for the production of arachidin-1 and arachidin-3 have not been elucidated yet [11]. The Tifrunner hairy root line might provide a platform to further elucidate the biosynthetic pathway for prenylated stilbenoids and their derivatives in peanut.

2.3. Comparison of Antioxidant Activity of Stilbenoid-Rich Extract from Hairy Roots of Three Peanut Cultivars

The antioxidant activities of the extract obtained from the culture medium of elicited hairy roots of peanut cvs. Tifrunner, Hull, and Georgia Green were compared using the scavenging effect of DPPH. DPPH scavenging assay is economic, reliable, efficient, and sensitive method for measuring the antioxidant activity of non-enzymatic antioxidants such as stilbenoids [2,22]. After incubation of DPPH solution with a stilbenoid-rich extract from different cultivars for 30 min, the violet color of DPPH changed to yellow confirming reduction of DPPH for all extract concentrations above 1.5625 µg/mL.

Interestingly, the stilbenoid-rich extract of peanut cv. Tifrunner had a higher scavenging effect on DPPH radical when compared to the stilbenoid-rich extract of peanut cvs. Hull and Georgia Green at all concentrations. The DPPH scavenging rate for the stilbenoid-rich extract from all three extracts was highest at the extract concentration of 100 µg/mL and the scavenging rate decreased gradually as the concentration of the extract decreased. At 100 µg/mL, the DPPH scavenging rate of stilbenoid-rich extract from the Tifrunner cultivar was 90.67 ± 0.64%. Whereas the rate was 82.94 ± 0.75% and 76.80 ± 1.51% for Hull and Georgia Green, respectively. Interestingly, the extract from Tifrunner hairy roots had significantly higher ($p < 0.05$) antioxidant capacity at a lower concentration of 6.25 µg/mL and 3.125 µg/mL when compared to stilbenoid-rich extract of the other two cultivars (Figure 6). The DPPH scavenging ability at concentrations of 6.25 µg/mL and 3.125 µg/mL for the extract of Tifrunner were 61.70 ± 10.74% and 41.24 ± 9.12%, for Hull were 42.26 ± 5.96% and 26.70 ± 6.45%, and for Georgia Green were 37.20 ± 13.41% and 23.15 ± 7.98% respectively. The DPPH scavenging rate of stilbenoid-rich extracts from all three cultivars was lowest at 0.78125 µg/mL.

The Tifrunner extract had the highest amount of prenylated stilbenoids such as arachidin-1 (207.5 ± 7.35 µg/mg), arachidin-2 (39.15 ± 0.98 µg/mg), arachidin-3 (75.28 ± 7.39 µg/mg), and arachidin-5 (30.92 ± 1.52 µg/mg) in terms of dry weight of the extract whereas Hull extract had highest amount of resveratrol (60.56 ± 1.19 µg/mg) (Table 2). The higher DPPH scavenging rate for Tifrunner stilbenoid-rich extract might correlate to a higher amount of prenylated stilbenoids present in the extract as compared to the other two cultivars. Overall, Tifrunner stilbenoid-rich extract had the highest DPPH scavenging rate followed by Hull and then Georgia Green extract.

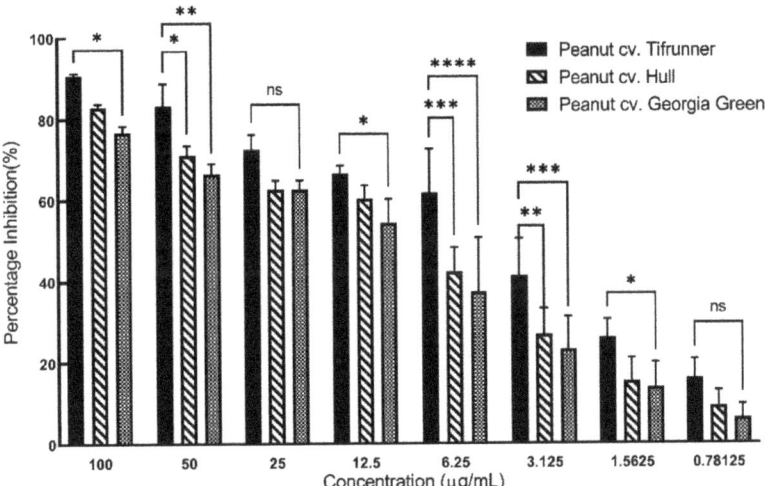

Figure 6. Comparison of total antioxidant capacity of medium extracts from hairy root cultures of peanut cultivars Tifrunner, Hull (line 3), and Georgia Green at different concentrations. Antioxidant capacity was evaluated by the DPPH assay method. Values are the average of three independent experiments, each performed in technical triplicate. Error bar represents standard deviation. Statistical analysis was performed with two-way ANOVA with Tukey's multiple-comparisons test. The asterisks above the connecting line represent a significant difference when compared to the total antioxidant activity among three cultivars (*, $p < 0.033$; **, $p < 0.002$; ***, $p < 0.001$; ****, $p < 0.0001$; ns, not significant).

Table 2. Amount of stilbenoid per dry weight of the extract (μg/mg) in three different cultivars of peanuts.

Stilbenoids	μg/mg DW [a]		
	Tifrunner	Hull	Georgia Green
Resveratrol	29.47 ± 1.40	60.56 ± 1.19	12.52 ± 0.29
Arachidin-5	30.92 ± 1.52	13.5 ± 0.29	6.9 ± 0.13
Arachidin-1	207.5 ± 7.35	162.37 ± 1.33	108.76 ± 1.53
Arachidin-2	39.15 ± 0.98	28.21 ± 1.97	19.74 ± 2.21
Arachidin-3	75.28 ± 7.39	72.24 ± 2.05	46.78 ± 0.52

[a] Data are the means ± SD of the experiments performed in technical triplicate.

Based on the DPPH antioxidant assay, the IC_{50} value for the stilbenoid-rich extract from all three extracts was calculated (Figure 7). The IC_{50} value for the stilbenoid-rich extract from the Tifrunner cultivar was 6.004 μg/mL, from the Hull cultivar was 8.147 μg/mL and from Georgia Green was 7.768 μg/mL respectively. The IC_{50} value represents the amount of stilbenoid-rich extract required to decrease the initial concentration of DPPH by 50%. The lowest IC_{50} value was found for the stilbenoid-rich extract from Tifrunner hairy roots suggesting that the extract had higher radical scavenging activity as compared to extract from the other two cultivars. Thus, stilbenoid-rich extract from Tifrunner hairy root had higher antioxidant activity followed by Georgia Green and Hull in terms of IC_{50} value.

Previously, the ethanolic extract of peanut sprouts rich in stilbenoids, such as resveratrol, arachidin-1, and arachidin-3, showed antioxidant and anti-inflammatory activities [23]. The antioxidant activity of stilbenoid-rich extract have been previously reported from peanut hairy roots treated with paraquat, MeJA, and CD and peanut hairy roots treated with cadmium, MeJA, and CD [24,25]. In this study, the IC_{50} value of the stilbenoid-rich extract of peanut hairy roots was lower in comparison to the phenolic extract of grape pomace from five different red grape cultivars with IC$_{50}$ values ranging from 14.45 µg/mL to 38.93 µg/mL suggesting higher antioxidant properties of peanut hairy root extracts [26].

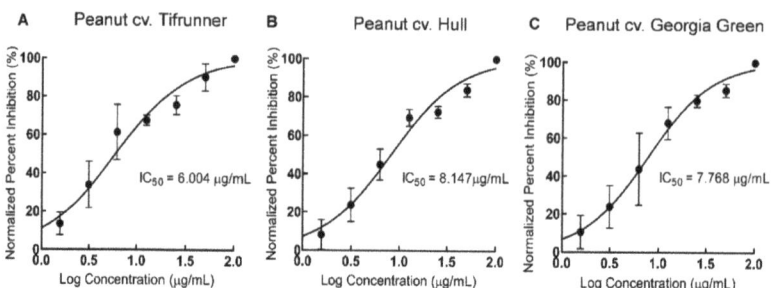

Figure 7. Concentration-dependent inhibitory effect of culture medium extracts from hairy root cultures of peanut cultivars. Tifrunner (**A**), Hull (**B**) (line 3), and Georgia Green (**C**) on DPPH based antioxidant assay. Data are represented as mean ± SD of three independent experiments, each performed in technical triplicate.

The in vivo study of bio-elicited peanut sprout powder rich in stilbene compounds such as resveratrol, arachidin-1, arachidin-3, and isopentadienylresveratrol suggested that the extract inhibits testosterone-mediated benign prostatic enlargement [27]. Similarly, in vivo study of peanut sprout extracts rich in resveratrol and its glycosides have been reported to have anti-obesity properties [28]. The stilbenoid-rich extracts from elicited peanut hairy root cultures could be further studied to explore their role as functional antioxidant ingredients using in vivo models.

3. Materials and Methods

3.1. Seed Sterilization and Germination of Peanut cv. Tifrunner

Seeds of peanut cv. Tifrunner (accession No. PI 644011, USDA) were obtained from USDA-ARS Plant Genetic Resources Conservation Unit (Griffin, GA, USA). The shells of the seeds were removed, and then the seeds were surface sterilized by soaking in 0.1% Palmolive detergent for 2 min followed by vigorous shaking in 50% Clorox solution for 15 min and rinsed using sterilized distilled water 4–5 times. The seeds were placed on plates containing modified Murashige and Skoog medium (MSV) medium with 3% sucrose and 0.4% phytagel and cultured under dark conditions until germination. After germination, the plates were transferred to the photoperiod incubator (16 h light/8 h dark) until the emergence of true leaves [17]. Next, the peanut seedlings were transferred to Phytatray^{TM} boxes (Millipore Sigma, Saint Louis, MO, USA) and kept in the photoperiod incubator for further growth. All cultures were done at 24 °C.

3.2. Establishment of Hairy Root Cultures of Peanut cv. Tifrunner

Leaves from the in vitro seedlings were excised and wounded with a scalpel containing *Agrobacterium rhizogenes* strain ATCC 15834. The wounded leaves were cultured on MSV medium and incubated for a week (till *Agrobacterium* growth was observed on the leaves). The leaves were then transferred to MSV medium with 250 mg/L cefotaxime and maintained in this medium until hairy roots were developed. Among several hairy root lines established, line 1 was selected for its sustained and vigorous growth. Molecular analyses were done to confirm hairy root establishment. Genomic DNA was extracted from these roots and PCR analyses were performed for *rolC*, *aux1*, and *virD2* genes as described before [29]. To establish hairy root cultures, ten 2–3 cm long tips were excised and cultured in 250 mL flasks containing 50 mL of MSV medium with 3% sucrose. The flasks were incubated in an orbital shaker incubator (Innova 44R, New Brunswick Scientific, Hauppauge, NY, USA) at 90 rpm and 28 °C under continuous darkness.

3.3. Growth Conditions and Elicitation of Peanut Hairy Root Cultures of cvs. Tifrunner, Hull, and Georgia Green

Hairy roots of peanut cvs. Hull and Georgia Green were established previously and maintained in 250 mL media flasks with 50 mL of MSV medium [17,30]. The hairy root cultures were grown till the mid-log stage prior to elicitation [17,30]. The spent medium was discarded and replaced with 100 mL of MSV medium containing 3% sucrose with 125 µM methyl jasmonate (MeJA), 18 g/L cyclodextrin (CD), 3 mM hydrogen peroxide (H_2O_2), and 1 mM magnesium chloride ($MgCl_2$) as described before [18]. All elicitation was carried out under continuous darkness at 28 °C for 168 h.

3.4. Extraction and Analysis of Stilbenoids

For each of the 3 cultivars, i.e., Tifrunner, Hull, and Georgia Green, the 168 h-elicited medium of nine flasks were combined before extraction. The extraction was performed by partitioning the elicited medium with ethyl acetate twice at a ratio of 1:1 first time and 2:1 second time in a separatory funnel by mixing them by vigorous shaking. The obtained organic upper phase was transferred to a round bottom flask and dried using a rotary evaporator (Büchi, rotavapor R-2000, Flawil, Switzerland). The extract was dissolved in 10 mL methanol. An aliquot of the extract was diluted and analyzed by HPLC. The recovery of each stilbenoid from the elicited medium of the combined nine flasks using ethyl acetate ranged from 79% to 83%.

Quantitative analysis of stilbenoids was performed using HPLC as described before [31]. Briefly, the chromatography was done in a Sunfire^{TM} C18, 5 µm, 4.6 × 250 mm column (Waters, Milford, MA, USA) at 40 °C and a flow rate at 1.0 mL/min. The HPLC system was controlled by Chromeleon software (Thermo Scientific, Waltham, MA, USA). The mobile phase consisted of methanol (A) and 0.5% formic acid (B). The column was initially calibrated with B for 1 min. Then a linear gradient was performed from 60% A to 65% A for 1–20 min, 65% A and 35% B to 100% B for 20–25 min, and 100% B for 25–30 min. Calibration curves for reference compounds were established at A_{320} for resveratrol (Biophysica, La Jolla, CA, USA) ($y = 1.2596x + 4.9349$, $R^2 = 0.999$, limit of quantitatation (LOQ): 16.74 mg/L, and limit of detection (LOD): 5.524 mg/L), arachidin-2 ($y = 0.7009x + 1.7334$, $R^2 = 0.994$, LOQ: 14.44 mg/L, LOD: 4.76 mg/L), and arachidin-5 ($y = 1.041x + 2.1378$, $R^2 = 0.996$, LOQ: 7.15 mg/L, LOD: 2.36 mg/L) and at A_{340} for arachidin-1 ($y = 0.748x + 1.589$, $R^2 = 0.997$, LOQ: 5.44 mg/L, LOD: 1.80 mg/L) and arachidin-3 ($0.8464x + 1.3747$, $R^2 = 0.998$, LOQ: 6.52 mg/L, LOD: 2.15 mg/L). Limit of quantitation (LOQ) and limit of detection (LOD) were determined as described before [32]. Production of arachidin reference standards was described previously [33].

Liquid chromatography-mass spectrometry qualitative analysis of stilbenoids was done using an UltiMate 3000 rapid separation LC system (Thermo Scientific, Waltham, MA, USA). The separation method was similar to the HPLC conditions described above. The LTQ XL linear ion trap mass spectrophotometer (Thermo Scientific, Waltham, MA, USA) with an electrospray ionization source was used for obtaining structural information of stilbenoids following the method described previously [34]. Briefly, all mass spectra were performed in positive and negative modes with ion spray voltage at 4 kV, sheath gas at 45 arbitrary units and capillary temperature at 300 °C. Full scans were recorded in the mass range m/z 50 to 2000. The collision energy of 35% was applied in collision-induced dissociation. The data was recorded and analyzed by Xcalibur software (Thermo Scientific, Waltham, MA, USA).

3.5. DPPH Antioxidant Assay

A microplate DPPH (2,2-diphenyl-1-picrylhydrazyl) assay was carried out using 200 µg/mL culture medium extract of peanut hairy roots cvs. Tifrunner, Hull, and Georgia Green using a protocol established by Patrick Roberto in the Medina-Bolivar laboratory [35]. First, 200 µL of 200 µg/mL of extract was added to three separate wells on row A of the 96 well plates followed by the addition of 100 µL of methanol to the first three wells of rows B-H of the 96 well plates. The 100 µL sample in row A was transferred from row A to row B, row B to row C and the process was repeated until the very last row. Finally, 100 µL of 100 µM DPPH was added to all the wells with samples on the 96 well plate. The control was a mixture of 100 µL of methanol and 100 µL of 100 µM DPPH and the blank contained 100 µL methanol. The reaction mixture was incubated in dark at room temperature for 30 min. Finally, the absorbance was measured after exactly 30 min at 515 nm on a BioTek absorbance microplate well reader using the Gen5 data analysis software [36]. The percentage inhibition was calculated using the formula below:

$$\text{Percent scavenging} = 1 - \left(\frac{\text{Abs (sample)} - \text{Abs (blank)}}{\text{Abs (control)} - \text{Abs (blank)}} \right) \quad (1)$$

The data were fit into sigmoidal dose-response inhibition curves with non-linear regression and IC_{50} values were calculated in GraphPad Prism version 9.10 software (San Diego, CA, USA).

3.6. Purification and Identification of Arachidin-6 in Peanut Hairy Root Culture

For purification of arachidin-6, 900 mL of elicited medium was obtained from a pool of about 9 flasks of 168 h elicited peanut cv. Tifrunner hairy root culture. The medium was partitioned with an equal volume of ethyl acetate twice in a 2-L separatory funnel. The organic phase was recovered and dried in rotavapor (Buchi, Flawil, Switzerland), and the crude extract (approximately 1.14 g) was further used for semi-preparative HPLC.

For semi-preparative HPLC, a Sunfire® C18 OBD™ Prep, 10 × 250 mm column (Waters, Milford, MA, USA) at 40 °C and a flow rate at 4.0 mL/min were used. The HPLC system was controlled by Chromeleon software (Thermofisher). The mobile phase consisted of methanol (A) and 0.5% formic acid (B). The mobile phase consisted of methanol (A) and 0.5% formic acid (B). A linear gradient started from 40% A to 50% A for 2 min, then from 50% A to 70% A for 2–50 min, and 100% A for 50–55 min. Based on retention time and UV, arachidin-6 peak was collected and dried under nitrogen gas for subsequent MS analysis as described above.

3.7. Statistical Analysis

Two-way ANOVA with Tukey's multiple-comparison tests was performed for data in Figures 5 and 6 with GraphPad Prism 9 software, version 9.10.

4. Conclusions

In conclusion, the antioxidant activity of stilbenoid-rich extracts obtained from elicited hairy roots of three cultivars of peanut was compared. The extract from cv. Tifrunner had significantly higher radical scavenging activity even at lower concentrations when compared to extracts of the other two cultivars. The higher antioxidant activity in Tifrunner stilbenoid-rich extract suggested that there might be a correlation between the level of stilbenoids and antioxidant properties in the hairy root extract. The hairy root of whole-genome sequenced peanut cv. Tifrunner was established and characterized for the first time and may provide a potential platform for further elucidation of the biosynthetic pathway of these prenylated stilbenoids. The antioxidant stilbenoid-rich extract from peanut could be further studied for its potential implication as nutraceuticals for promoting human health.

Supplementary Materials: The following are available online, Figure S1: PCR analysis of Tifrunner hairy root line 1 with primers targeting the rolC, aux1, and virD2 genes. Plasmid pRi15834 was used as positive control and ddH2O was used as negative control. Figure S2: Purification of arachidin-6. (A) semi-preparative HPLC profile of ethyl acetate extract of peanut cv. Tifrunner (B) HPLC profile of purified arachidin-6. Figure S3: UV spectrum of arachidin-6. Figure S4: MS ion chromatogram of arachidin-6 under negative mode. Figure S5: MS ion chromatogram of arachidin-6 under positive mode.

Author Contributions: Conceptualization, G.G. and F.M.-B.; methodology, G.G., R.H. and F.M.-B.; formal analysis, G.G. and F.M.-B.; investigation, G.G., R.H. and F.M.-B.; resources, F.M.-B.; writing—original draft preparation, G.G.; writing—review and editing, F.M.-B.; visualization, G.G. and F.M.-B.; supervision, F.M.-B.; project administration, F.M.-B.; funding acquisition, F.M.-B. All authors have read and agreed to the published version of the manuscript.

Funding: This research was funded by the Arkansas Biosciences Institute (Fund No. 200156).

Institutional Review Board Statement: Not applicable.

Informed Consent Statement: Not applicable.

Data Availability Statement: The data of this study are available upon request.

Conflicts of Interest: The authors declare no competing financial interest.

Sample Availability: Not available.

References

1. Apel, K.; Hirt, H. Reactive oxygen species: Metabolism, oxidative stress, and signal transduction. *Annu. Rev. Plant Biol.* **2004**, *55*, 373–379. [CrossRef]
2. Gulcin, İ. Antioxidants and antioxidant methods: An updated overview. *Arch. Toxicol.* **2020**, *94*, 651–715. [CrossRef]
3. Tang, S.Y.; Whiteman, M.; Peng, Z.F.; Jenner, A.; Yong, E.L.; Halliwell, B. Characterization of antioxidant and antiglycation properties and isolation of active ingredients from traditional chinese medicines. *Free Radic. Biol. Med.* **2004**, *36*, 1575–1587. [CrossRef]
4. Halliwell, B.; Murcia, M.A.; Chirico, S.; Aruoma, O.I. Free radicals and antioxidants in food and in vivo: What they do and how they work. *Crit. Rev. Food Sci. Nutr.* **1995**, *35*, 7–20. [CrossRef]
5. Dávid, C.Z.; Hohmann, J.; Vasas, A. Chemistry and pharmacology of Cyperaceae stilbenoids: A Review. *Molecules* **2021**, *26*, 2794. [CrossRef]
6. Sobolev, V.S. Localized production of phytoalexins by peanut (*Arachis hypogaea*) kernels in response to invasion by *Aspergillus* species. *J. Agric. Food Chem.* **2008**, *56*, 1949–1954. [CrossRef]
7. Sobolev, V.S. Production of phytoalexins in peanut (*Arachis hypogaea*) seed elicited by selected microorganisms. *J. Agric. Food Chem.* **2013**, *61*, 1850–1858. [CrossRef]
8. Sobolev, V.S.; Khan, S.I.; Tabanca, N.; Wedge, D.E.; Manly, S.P.; Cutler, S.J.; Coy, M.R.; Becnel, J.J.; Neff, S.A.; Gloer, J.B. Biological activity of peanut (*Arachis hypogaea*) phytoalexins and selected natural and synthetic stilbenoids. *J. Agric. Food Chem.* **2011**, *59*, 1673–1682. [CrossRef]
9. Sobolev, V.S.; Potter, T.L.; Horn, B.W. Prenylated stilbenes from peanut root mucilage. *Phytochem. Anal.* **2006**, *17*, 312–322. [CrossRef] [PubMed]
10. Wu, Z.; Song, L.; Huang, D. Food grade fungal stress on germinating peanut seeds induced phytoalexins and enhanced polyphenolic antioxidants. *J. Agric. Food Chem.* **2011**, *59*, 5993–6003. [CrossRef]
11. Yang, T.; Fang, L.; Sanders, S.; Jayanthi, S.; Rajan, G.; Podicheti, R.; Thallapuranam, S.K.; Mockaitis, K.; Medina-Bolivar, F. Stilbenoid prenyltransferases define key steps in the diversification of peanut phytoalexins. *J. Biol. Chem.* **2018**, *293*, 28–46. [CrossRef]
12. Yang, T.; Fang, L.; Medina-Bolivar, F. Production and biosynthesis of bioactive stilbenoids in hairy root cultures. In *Production of Plant Derived Natural Compounds through Hairy Root Culture*; Malik, S., Ed.; Springer International Publishing: Cham, Switzerland, 2017; pp. 45–64.
13. Brents, L.; Medina-Bolivar, F.; Seely, K.; Nair, V.; Bratton, S.; Ñopo-Olazabal, L.; Patel, R.; Liu, H.; Doerksen, R.; Prather, P.; et al. Natural prenylated resveratrol analogs arachidin-1 and -3 demonstrate improved glucuronidation profiles and have affinity for cannabinoid receptors. *Xenobiotica* **2011**, *42*, 139–156. [CrossRef]
14. Chang, J.-C.; Lai, Y.-H.; Djoko, B.; Wu, P.-L.; Liu, C.-D.; Liu, Y.-W.; Chiou, R.Y.-Y. Biosynthesis enhancement and antioxidant and anti-inflammatory activities of peanut (*Arachis hypogaea* L.) arachidin-1, arachidin-3, and isopentadienylresveratrol. *J. Agric. Food Chem.* **2006**, *54*, 10281–10287. [CrossRef] [PubMed]
15. Huang, C.-P.; Au, L.-C.; Chiou, R.Y.-Y.; Chung, P.-C.; Chen, S.-Y.; Tang, W.-C.; Chang, C.-L.; Fang, W.-H.; Lin, S.-B. Arachidin-1, a peanut stilbenoid, induces programmed cell death in human leukemia HL-60 cells. *J. Agric. Food Chem.* **2010**, *58*, 12123–12129. [CrossRef]
16. Zhang, L.; Ravipati, A.S.; Koyyalamudi, S.R.; Jeong, S.C.; Reddy, N.; Smith, P.T.; Bartlett, J.; Shanmugam, K.; Münch, G.; Wu, M.J. Antioxidant and anti-inflammatory activities of selected medicinal plants containing phenolic and flavonoid Compounds. *J. Agric. Food Chem.* **2011**, *59*, 12361–12367. [CrossRef]
17. Condori, J.; Sivakumar, G.; Hubstenberger, J.; Dolan, M.C.; Sobolev, V.S.; Medina-Bolivar, F. Induced biosynthesis of resveratrol and the prenylated stilbenoids arachidin-1 and arachidin-3 in hairy root cultures of peanut: Effects of culture medium and growth stage. *Plant Physiol. Biochem.* **2010**, *48*, 310–318. [CrossRef]

18. Fang, L.; Yang, T.; Medina-Bolivar, F. Production of prenylated stilbenoids in hairy root cultures of peanut (*Arachis hypogaea*) and its wild relatives *A. ipaensis* and *A. duranensis* via an optimized elicitation procedure. *Molecules* **2020**, *25*, 509. [CrossRef]
19. Chayjarung, P.; Poonsap, W.; Pankaew, C.; Inmano, O.; Kongbangkerd, A.; Limmongkon, A. Using a combination of chitosan, methyl jasmonate, and cyclodextrin as an effective elicitation strategy for prenylated stilbene compound production in *Arachis hypogaea* L. hairy root culture and their impact on genomic DNA. *Plant Cell Tissue Organ Cult.* **2021**, *147*, 117–129. [CrossRef]
20. Agarwal, G.; Clevenger, J.; Pandey, M.K.; Wang, H.; Shasidhar, Y.; Chu, Y.; Fountain, J.C.; Choudhary, D.; Culbreath, A.K.; Liu, X.; et al. High-density genetic map using whole-genome resequencing for fine mapping and candidate gene discovery for disease resistance in peanut. *Plant Biotechnol. J.* **2018**, *16*, 1954–1967. [CrossRef] [PubMed]
21. de Bruijn, W.J.C.; Araya-Cloutier, C.; Bijlsma, J.; de Swart, A.; Sanders, M.G.; de Waard, P.; Gruppen, H.; Vincken, J.-P. Antibacterial prenylated stilbenoids from peanut (*Arachis hypogaea*). *Phytochem. Lett.* **2018**, *28*, 13–18. [CrossRef]
22. Moon, J.-K.; Shibamoto, T. Antioxidant assays for plant and food components. *J. Agric. Food Chem.* **2009**, *57*, 1655–1666. [CrossRef] [PubMed]
23. Limmongkon, A.; Nopprang, P.; Chaikeandee, P.; Somboon, T.; Wongshaya, P.; Pilaisangsuree, V. LC-MS/MS profiles and interrelationships between the anti-inflammatory activity, total phenolic content and antioxidant potential of Kalasin 2 cultivar peanut sprout crude extract. *Food Chem.* **2018**, *239*, 569–578. [CrossRef] [PubMed]
24. Pilaisangsuree, V.; Anuwan, P.; Supdensong, K.; Lumpa, P.; Kongbangkerd, A.; Limmongkon, A. Enhancement of adaptive response in peanut hairy root by exogenous signalling molecules under cadmium stress. *J. Plant Physiol.* **2020**, *254*, 153278. [CrossRef] [PubMed]
25. Wongshaya, P.; Chayjarung, P.; Tothong, C.; Pilaisangsuree, V.; Somboon, T.; Kongbangkerd, A.; Limmongkon, A. Effect of light and mechanical stress in combination with chemical elicitors on the production of stilbene compounds and defensive responses in peanut hairy root culture. *Plant Physiol. Biochem.* **2020**, *157*, 93–104. [CrossRef] [PubMed]
26. Ruberto, G.; Renda, A.; Daquino, C.; Amico, V.; Spatafora, C.; Tringali, C.; Tommasi, N.D. Polyphenol constituents and antioxidant activity of grape pomace extracts from five Sicilian red grape cultivars. *Food Chem.* **2007**, *100*, 203–210. [CrossRef]
27. Cheng, P.; Chiu, P.; Chang, J.; Lin, S.; Li, Y.; Lo, D.; Lai, L.; Wu, S.; Chiou, R. Inhibition of testosterone-mediated benign prostatic enlargement of orchiectomized Sprague-Dawley rats by diets supplemented with bio-elicited peanut sprout powder (BPSP) and three new BPSP-extracted natural compounds identified. *J. Funct. Foods* **2021**, *79*, 104383. [CrossRef]
28. Kim, S.; Seo, J.; Kim, B.; Kim, H.; Lee, H.; Kim, J. Anti-obesity activity of peanut sprout extract. *Food Sci. Biotechnol.* **2014**, *23*, 601–607. [CrossRef]
29. Medina-Bolivar, F.; Condori, J.; Rimando, A.M.; Hubstenberger, J.; Shelton, K.; O'Keefe, S.F.; Bennett, S.; Dolan, M.C. Production and secretion of resveratrol in hairy root cultures of peanut. *Phytochemistry* **2007**, *68*, 1992–2003. [CrossRef]
30. Balmaceda, C. Efecto de la Cicodextrina y el Metil Jamonato en la Producción de Resveratrol y sus Análogos Prenilados Araquidina-1 y Araquidina-3 Empleando Raices en Cabellera de Mani. Licentiate Thesis, Universidad Peruana Cayetano Heredia, Lima, Peru, 2011.
31. Yang, T.; Fang, L.; Nopo-Olazabal, C.; Condori, J.; Nopo-Olazabal, L.; Balmaceda, C.; Medina-Bolivar, F. Enhanced production of resveratrol, piceatannol, arachidin-1, and arachidin-3 in hairy root cultures of peanut co-treated with methyl jasmonate and cyclodextrin. *J. Agric. Food Chem.* **2015**, *63*, 3942–3950. [CrossRef]
32. Shrivastava, A. Methods for the determination of limit of detection and limit of quantitation of the analytical methods. *Chron. Young Sci.* **2011**, *2*, 21–25. [CrossRef]
33. Ball, J.M.; Medina-Bolivar, F.; Defrates, K.; Hambleton, E.; Hurlburt, M.E.; Fang, L.; Yang, T.; Nopo-Olazabal, L.; Atwill, R.L.; Ghai, P.; et al. Investigation of stilbenoids as potential therapeutic agents for rotavirus gastroenteritis. *Adv. Virol.* **2015**, *2015*, 293524. [CrossRef] [PubMed]
34. Marsh, Z.; Yang, T.; Nopo-Olazabal, L.; Wu, S.; Ingle, T.; Joshee, N.; Medina-Bolivar, F. Effect of light, methyl jasmonate and cyclodextrin on production of phenolic compounds in hairy root cultures of *Scutellaria lateriflora*. *Phytochemistry* **2014**, *107*, 50–60. [CrossRef] [PubMed]
35. Roberto, P. Antioxidant Characterization of Peanut Hairy Roots Extracts Enriched with Prenylated Stilbenoids. Master's Thesis, Arkansas State University, Jonesboro, AR, USA, 2020.
36. Sharma, O.P.; Bhat, T.K. DPPH antioxidant assay revisited. *Food Chem.* **2009**, *113*, 1202–1205. [CrossRef]

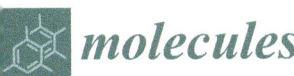

Review

Recent Overview of Resveratrol's Beneficial Effects and Its Nano-Delivery Systems

Raghvendra A. Bohara [1,2,*], Nazish Tabassum [3], Mohan P. Singh [3], Giuseppe Gigli [4,5], Andrea Ragusa [4,6] and Stefano Leporatti [4,*]

1. CÚRAM, SFI Research Centre For Medical Devices, National University of Ireland Galway, H91 W2TY Galway, Ireland
2. Centre for Interdisciplinary Research, D.Y. Patil Education Society, Deemed to be University, Kolhapur 416006, India
3. Centre of Biotechnology, University of Allahabad, Prayagraj 211002, India
4. CNR NANOTEC—Istituto di Nanotecnologia, 73100 Lecce, Italy
5. Department of Mathematics and Physics, University of Salento, 73100 Lecce, Italy
6. Department of Biological and Environmental Sciences and Technologies, University of Salento, 73100 Lecce, Italy
* Correspondence: raghvendrabohara@gmail.com (R.A.B.); stefano.leporatti@nanotec.cnr.it (S.L.)

Highlights:

1. Resveratrol is an antioxidant and exhibits numerous potential therapeutic applications. However, it suffers from low water-solubility, degradation, and poor bioavailability. The conventional dosage form of resveratrol shows various limitations, such as prolonged therapy, erratic bioavailability, and absence of effective drug concentrations in tissues.
2. Nanocarrier-based delivery systems are being studied extensively to target tissues and cells to improve the therapeutic potential of poorly soluble molecules by enhancing their bioavaila-bility, solubility, and retention time.
3. Resveratrol can act as a potential anti-cancer agent and lowers the progression of cancer disease.

Abstract: Natural polyphenols have a wide variety of biological activities and are taken into account as healthcare materials. Resveratrol is one such natural polyphenol, belonging to a group known as stilbenoids (STBs). Resveratrol (3,5,4′-trihydroxy-*trans*-stilbene) is mainly found in grapes, wine, nuts, and berries. A wide range of biological activities has been demonstrated by resveratrol, including antimicrobial, antioxidant, antiviral, antifungal, and antiaging effects, and many more are still under research. However, as with many other plant-based polyphenol products, resveratrol suffers from low bioavailability once administered in vivo due to its susceptibility to rapid enzyme degradation by the body's innate immune system before it can exercise its therapeutic influence. Therefore, it is of the utmost importance to ensure the best use of resveratrol by creating a proper resveratrol delivery system. Nanomedicine and nanodelivery systems utilize nanoscale materials as diagnostic tools or to deliver therapeutic agents in a controlled manner to specifically targeted locations. After a brief introduction about polyphenols, this review overviews the physicochemical characteristics of resveratrol, its beneficial effects, and recent advances on novel nanotechnological approaches for its delivery according to the type of nanocarrier utilized. Furthermore, the article summarizes the different potential applications of resveratrol as, for example, a therapeutic and disease-preventing anticancer and antiviral agent.

Keywords: resveratrol; polyphenols; drug delivery; nanocarriers; nanomedicine

Citation: Bohara, R.A.; Tabassum, N.; Singh, M.P.; Gigli, G.; Ragusa, A.; Leporatti, S. Recent Overview of Resveratrol's Beneficial Effects and Its Nano-Delivery Systems. *Molecules* **2022**, *27*, 5154. https://doi.org/10.3390/molecules27165154

Academic Editor: Luciano Saso

Received: 1 August 2022
Accepted: 10 August 2022
Published: 12 August 2022

Publisher's Note: MDPI stays neutral with regard to jurisdictional claims in published maps and institutional affiliations.

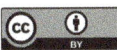

Copyright: © 2022 by the authors. Licensee MDPI, Basel, Switzerland. This article is an open access article distributed under the terms and conditions of the Creative Commons Attribution (CC BY) license (https://creativecommons.org/licenses/by/4.0/).

1. Introduction

Plant-based natural products are commonly used as an alternative to modern medicines. Since the beginning of human life, herbal medicines have developed and continued to exist until today. Awareness of this herbal medicine is considered to be the foundation of modern medicine [1]. The use of state-of-the-art technologies, such as purification techniques and computer bioinformatics tools, has helped to classify the plant's active ingredients and the molecular pathways that are potentially affected [2]. Natural materials display impressive qualities, such as excellent chemical diversity, biological and chemical activities with a macromolecular precision, and absent or low toxicity. These properties make them ideal candidates for developing novel drugs [3]. Additionally, theoretical studies have helped to envisage drug–target interactions and to build new drug generations, such as in the targeted drug discovery and drug delivery [4]. Despite the enormous potential of phytocomponents, the pharmaceutical companies are not so active in investing and researching with this approach. One possible reason is the lack of an in-depth molecular mechanism understanding and of viable carriers that ensure onsite delivery. These concerns have been extensively addressed in the recent years. Detailed molecular work has been carried out to study the in-depth action of plant-based natural materials [3,4]. However, concerns associated with the toxicity of some metabolites and their interaction with the desired target are still a problem, thus requiring additional studies to find viable alternatives. Hence, many natural compounds are not clearing the preclinical and Phase I clinical trials [5–7]. The possible solution to this problem can be the development of a nanocarrier system which can carry natural compounds and ensure their onsite delivery without causing toxicity [8]. Recently, nanotechnology has demonstrated these capabilities and it is considered to be the future of drug delivery systems. One successful example is the development of liposomal doxorubicin (Doxil^R), which has shown massive success in treating metastatic breast cancer [9].

Different carriers, micelles, liposomes, and nanoparticles (NPs) have been developed as natural product delivery systems, and they have shown promising results [10]. However, concerns related to polyphenols' nanoencapsulation have been reported due to the varying structures, solubility, and fast oxidation under physiological conditions [11]. Therefore, it is crucial to consider these impairing alterations on the polyphenol molecules when designing the nanocarrier.

Among the different natural polyphenols, resveratrol (RES) has shown immense potential due to excellent antioxidant, anticancer, antihypertensive, anti-inflammatory, and antiplatelet aggregation cardioprotective activities [12–15]. Because of these interesting properties, there is a sudden interest in exploring the full potential of this molecule (Figure 1).

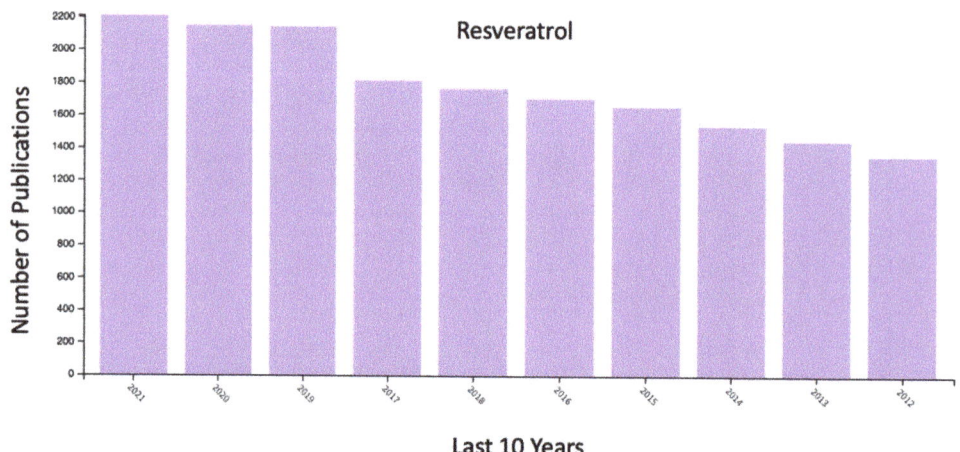

Figure 1. Cumulative research articles related to resveratrol grouped by year (2012–2020), as determined by the Web of Science® database (last accessed on 30 June 2022).

This review article, after a brief introduction about natural polyphenols, focuses on the chemistry of RES and nanotechnology's role in the development of RES delivery systems. The use of RES as anticancer drug is also discussed to understand how the carrier system can play a vital role in exploring the potential of natural phytochemicals, such as RES (see Figure 2).

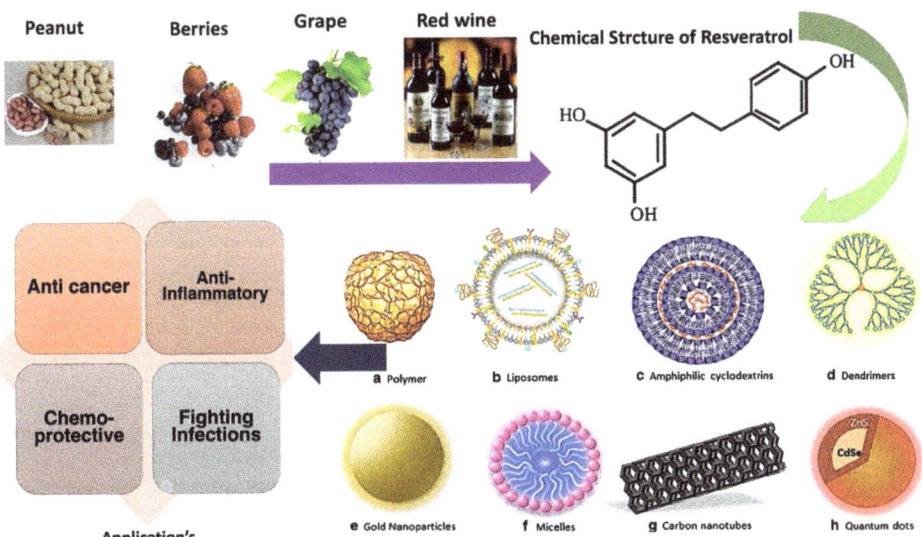

Figure 2. Scheme showing the main sources of *trans*-resveratrol, its chemical structure, the types of nanoformulations used to deliver it, and its beneficial health effects and applications.

2. Natural Polyphenols

Polyphenols are a phytochemical group with chemical properties and different structures ranging from simple molecules to polymers with high molecular weight [16]. Polyphenols are secondary plant metabolites, and their primary role is to attract pollinators and protect plants from insects, ultraviolet radiation, and microbial infection [17]. Polyphenols comprise a phenolic system with at least one phenyl ring and one or more hydroxyl substituents. Polyphenols are present in vegetables, fruits, herbs, spices, beverages such as tea and wine, chocolates, and whole grains [18].

Classification of Polyphenols

Generally, polyphenols are mainly categorized into flavonoids and nonflavonoids, but according to the aglycone chemical structures, they can be also classified as phenolic acids, lignans, and stilbenes [16].

Flavonoids. It is the largest group of phenolic compounds and mostly present in fruits. The structures consist of two aromatic rings bound with a three-carbon bridge to form an oxygenated heterocycle. The biological activities, such as anticancer, anti-inflammatory, and antioxidant ones, depend on the flavonoids' structural difference and glycosylation pattern [19]. Based on the number, position of the –OH groups and degree of oxidation of the central ring, flavonoids can be further divided into subclasses of flavones, flavonols, flavanones, flavanols, isoflavones, and anthocyanidin. Flavones, such as apigenin and luteolin, are found in celery, parsley, and some herbs. The polymethoxylated flavones (e.g., tangeretin and nobiletin) are found only in the tissues and peels of citrus fruit, such as oranges, grapefruit, and tangerines. The flavones' characteristic feature is to have methylated –OH groups, which increases their metabolic stability and enhances their oral bioavailability [20]. Flavonols are one of the most ubiquitous flavonoids found in capers, saffron, dried Mexican oregano, yellow and red onions, and spinach.

Two representatives of this subclass are quercetin and kaempferol. Naringenin and hesperetin are valuable flavanones found in food. The maximum concentrations of flavanones are present in citrus fruits and dried herbs, and they are responsible for the bitter taste of fruits [21]. Isoflavones are present in legumes, and the chief source is soybeans, having substantial amounts of daidzein and genistein. Isoflavones show pseudo-hormonal characteristics because of their structural similarity to oestrogen, and their supplements can bind to the oestrogenic receptors and, as such, be used as potential substitutes for conventional hormone therapy [22]. Among all flavonoids, flavanols are the most complex subclass, being able to form monomers, oligomers, polymers, and other derivative compounds. They are responsible for the bitterness of chocolate and the acid-based character of some fruits and beverages. Anthocyanidins are a subgroup of flavonoids responsible for the colour of flowers, leaves, fruits, and roots. Pelargonidin, delphinidin, peonidin, petunidin, malvidin, and cyanidin are common anthocyanidins distributed in fruits and vegetables [23].

Phenolic acids. They can be divided into two groups, led by benzoic and cinnamic acid. Gallic and ellagic acid are the essential derivatives of benzoic acid, and they are found in cranberries, raspberries, pomegranates, and nuts. On the other hand, cinnamic acids' essential derivatives are ferulic, coumaric, caffeic, and sinapic acid [24].

Lignans. The highest amount of lignans is found in flaxseeds, grains, and certain vegetables. In plants, they are typically found as glycosides and are converted by intestinal bacteria to give metabolites having oestrogenic activity [25].

Stilbenes. They are phytoalexins produced by plants in response to injury and infections. In the human diet, they are present in low quantities, and only resveratrol is essential for the human health. Grapes and red wine are an important dietary source of resveratrol. Resveratrol is directly connected to the French paradox. It was observed that French people consume high amounts of saturated fatty acids but they hardly suffer from cardiovascular diseases, having a lower death rate than other European countries. It is thus supposed that the daily consumption of red wine plays a significant role in preventing heart diseases [26].

3. Chemistry of Resveratrol

Resveratrol is a stilbenoid polyphenol with two phenol rings linked to each other by an ethylene bridge. The IUPAC name of resveratrol is E-5-(4-hydroxystyryl)benzene-1,3-diol, but both geometric isomers of resveratrol, the cis and the trans, can be found (Figure 3).

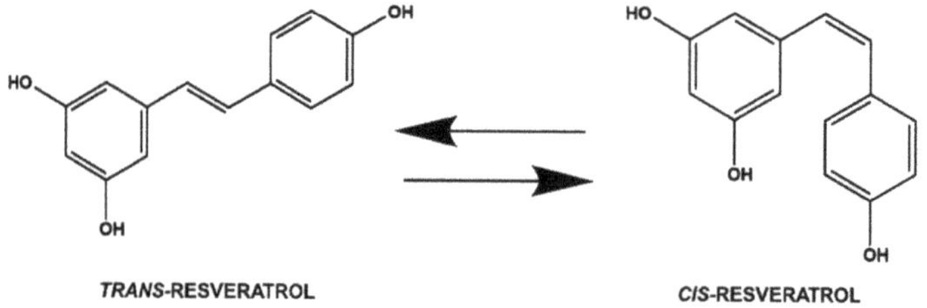

Figure 3. Chemical structures of *trans*- and *cis*-resveratrol.

After exposure to the UV radiation, the *trans* isomer can transform into the *cis* one. However, the *trans* form is dominant because of its occurrence, and it is also more interesting because of its many biological activities. The *trans* form induces cell differentiation, cell cycle arrest, apoptosis, and increased antiproliferation in cancerous cells [27]. The stability of *trans*-resveratrol powder depends on humidity (75%) and temperature (40 °C) in the presence of air. The isomerization of *trans*-resveratrol is influenced by irradiation time, wavelength, temperature, pH, and physical status of the molecule. Waterhouse and coworkers investigated the reaction kinetics [28]. *trans*-Resveratrol's stability is 42 h in neutral aqueous buffer and 28 days in acidic media when protected from light. At pH 10.0 the initial half-life for *trans*-resveratrol is nearly 1.6 h. The bioavailability of resveratrol is very low. Therefore, modification of its structure has received great attention from the scientific community and various resveratrol derivatives have been synthesized. Nanoformulations containing resveratrol have been considered as a promising approach for retaining its biological functions until delivery [28]. To enhance the oral bioavailability, two delivery systems of resveratrol, i.e., stable lipid nanoparticles and nanostructured lipid carriers, have been developed [29]. Moreover, as compared with the free form, resveratrol nanoparticles improve its solubility and increase its antioxidant potential [30].

In 1940, resveratrol was first isolated from white hellebore (*Veratrum grandiflorum* O. Loes) roots. After that, in 1963, it was isolated from *Polygonum cuspidatum* roots, which are used as antiplatelet and anti-inflammatory agents in traditional Chinese and Japanese medicine [31]. Resveratrol acts as a phytoalexin in plants synthesized in response to UV irradiation, mechanical injury, and fungal attacks. In industry, resveratrol is generally prepared by chemical or biotechnological synthesis from yeasts of *Saccharomyces cerevisiae* [32]. Ninety-two new resveratrol derivatives have been reported from the *Leguminosae, Paeoniaceae, Dipterocarpaceae, Vitaceae, Gnetaceae, Cyperaceae, Polygonaceae Gramineae*, and *Poaceae* families. Among these families, *Dipterocarpaceae* alone contains more than 50 resveratrol derivatives, and it is from seven genera [33]. Because of the broad range of pharmacological effects, resveratrol is sold on the market as a nutritional supplement [34].

4. Designing of Nanocarriers for Resveratrol Delivery

Nanocarriers are drug carrier systems usually having <500 nm particle size [35]. They have high surface-area-to-volume ratios, the ability to alter bioactivity of drugs, enhanced pharmacokinetics and biodistribution, and potential site-specific delivery, due to which they have already shown promising results as therapeutic agents in the drug delivery area [36]. In anticancer therapy, several problems arise when chemotherapeutics are delivered through conventional administration routes, such as low specificity, high toxicity, and induction of drug resistance, thus reducing the therapeutic value of most anticancer drugs [37]. To overcome this obstacle, nanocarrier-based platforms have been used to deliver anticancer drugs into the tumours and disturb the tumour microenvironment's pathophysiology, thus improving the therapeutic efficiency [38].

Types of nanocarriers. Nanocarriers can be categorized into three different categories: organic, inorganic, and hybrid nanocarriers. Organic nanocarriers comprise solid-lipid nanocarriers (SLNs), liposomes, dendrimers, polymeric nanoparticles (PNPs), virus-based nanoparticles (VNPs), and polymeric micelles (PMs), whereas inorganic polymers include mesoporous silica nanoparticles (MSNs) and carbon nanotubes (CNTs) (Figure 2).

Organic nanocarriers. SLNs increase controlled drug delivery, lack biotoxicity, present high drug-carrying efficiency and good stability, improve the bioavailability of poorly water-soluble drugs, and can be easily produced large scale [39]. SLN nanocarriers have been exploited to deliver anticancer drugs, such as methotrexate, docetaxel, paclitaxel, 5-fluorouracil (5-FU), and doxorubicin [40,41]. Liposome nanocarriers have shown several advantages over conventional therapy. They can increase delivery of the drug, prevent early degradation of the encapsulated drug, improve the performance of the drugs, are cost-effective formulations, and represent an effective treatment with reduced toxicity. They are generally used as carriers for drugs, vaccines, cosmetics, and nutraceuticals [42]. Dendrimers are spherically-shaped, monodispersed macromolecules with an average diameter of 1.5–14.5 nm and unique characteristics [43]. Lai et al. used dendrimers to enhance the efficacy of doxorubicin [44]. They used photochemical internalization technology to enhance the cytotoxicity to cancerous tissue. Polymeric nanoparticles (PNPs) are solid biodegradable polymers, nanosized colloidal particles ranging from 10 to 1000 nm [45]. Based on the structure, PNPs are categorized as nanospheres and nanocapsules. Nanospheres are a type of PNPs entrap the drug in the polymer matrix whereas, in nanocapsules, the drug is dispersed in the liquid core of oil or water encapsulated by a solid polymeric membrane [46]. PNPs are highly versatile. Examples of PNPs as a carrier for anticancer molecules are PLGA, PCL, chitosan, PLA, and alginate NPs [47,48]. Polymeric micelles (PMs) are 10–100 nm nanosized colloidal particles formed by the self-assembly of synthetic amphiphilic copolymers in an aqueous solution [49]. They have a core–shell structure with a hydrophobic core and hydrophilic shell [50]. The hydrophobic core of PMs captures the hydrophobic drugs and controls the drug release, thus increasing their water-solubility, whereas the hydrophilic shell of the PMs stabilizes the core and controls the in vivo pharmacokinetics [51]. Various chemotherapeutic agents, such as methotrexate, paclitaxel, docetaxel, cisplatin, and doxorubicin, have successfully been formulated in PMs for cancer treatment. Poloxamer-based micelles, PEGylated polyglutamic acid micelles, PEG-PLA micelles, and PEG-PAA micelles have been used as delivery systems [52]. VNPs are self-assembled protein cages with a diameter <100 nm, having uniform nanostructures. Recently, VNPs have been widely explored for various applications, such as drug delivery, vaccination, imaging, gene therapy, and targeting [53].

Inorganic nanocarriers. From the last few years, silica materials hold great promises in nanomedicine due to their straightforward and cost-effective synthesis and functionalization, and their multiple uses. Among silica materials, mesoporous silicas are catching the attention of researchers in drug delivery because of their honeycomb-like structure with hundreds of pores ranging from 2 to 50 nm, with narrow pore size and versatility of loading large amounts of drugs [54]. MSNs possess promise as nanoscale drug carriers because of good biocompatibility, controllable pore diameters, high specific surface area and pore volume, high loading capacity, and good chemical stability, which enhances therapeutic efficacy and decreases the toxicity of drugs [47]. Paclitaxel, camptothecin, doxorubicin, and methotrexate anticancer drugs have been effectively delivered via MSNs [55]. CNTs have a nanoneedle shape, hollow monolithic structure, high mechanical strength, electrical and thermal conductivities, and the ability of easy surface modification [56]. The needle-like shape of CNTs crosses the cell membrane and enters into the cell. One of the drawbacks of CNTs is insufficient water solubility, as well as their toxicity. However, after surface-functionalization, CNTs become water-soluble, biocompatible, less toxic, serum-stable, and ideal nanocarriers for cancer therapy [57]. Examples of the application of CNTs in anticancer drug delivery are methotrexate, paclitaxel, cisplatin, carboplatin, doxorubicin, and mitomycin C [58].

Hybrid nanocarriers. Hybrid nanocarriers have been developed to combine the properties of organic and inorganic materials. Surface coating with polyethyleneimine (PEI) increased the cellular uptake of MSNs for efficient nucleic acid delivery [59]. These hybrid nanocarriers prevented premature release of the loaded drug, multidrug resistance, extended the retention of hydrophilic drug cargo, and yielded stimuli-responsive drug release. Desai and co-workers reported the intracellular delivery of zoledronic acid in breast cancer cells [60]. Han et al. developed doxorubicin-loaded, hybrid, lipid-capped MSNs with pH and redox-responsive release of the drug cargo. These hybrid nanocarriers increased the uptake of doxorubicin, thus improving its accumulation, efficiency, and cytotoxicity [61].

The solubility of resveratrol has been shown to be very low, leading to low bioavailability [15] Hence, while designing delivery system for resveratrol, efforts should be made to enhance its bioavailability. This aim has been attempted by using cyclodextrin complexes, dendrimers, liposomes, self-nano-emulsifying drug delivery systems, solid lipid nanoparticles, nanosuspensions, nanocapsules, microparticles and both nano- and micro-encapsulation (Table 1).

Table 1. Brief overview of most important type of nanocarriers used for delivering resveratrol.

Nano System	Effect	Key Properties	Reference
Liposomes	Antioxidant activity	Enhanced solubility and stability of curcumin and resveratrol. Minimum particle size, lower polydispersity index and high encapsulation efficiency	[62]
	Anticancer activity	HepG2 cells exhibited a higher uptake of encapsulated-RES than the free form	[63]
Dendrimers	Enhanced RES solubility and stability in aqueous solution. Dendrimers can be engineered to control pharmacokinetics and target for oral, mucosal, transdermal, or parenteral administration	(PAMAM) dendrimer assembly overcame the problems of low bioavailability and poor water solubility	[64]
Solid lipid nanoparticles	In vitro cytotoxicity against C6 glioma cell lines	The resveratrol-TPGS-SLNs showed 11.12 and 9.37-times higher area under the curve (AUC) and plasma half-life, respectively, than the unprocessed resveratrol. Additionally, the concentration of resveratrol-TPGS-SLNs in the brain was found to be 9.23-times higher compared to free resveratrol	[65]
Polymeric nanoparticles	Fatty liver disorder	The prepared poly(lactic-*co*-glycolic acid) (PLGA) nanoparticles containing resveratrol increased its stability and solubility, yielding better in vitro results as compared to free drug	[66]

5. Prophylactic and Therapeutic Applications of Resveratrol

Cancer remains one of the main reasons for mortality in the world. Despite cutting-edge research, the mortality rate has not improved in the last 5 years. More than 1.6 million new cancer diagnoses and approximately 600,000 cancer-related deaths are expected in the United States of America in 2016 alone [67]. Despite the use of novel approaches, such as monoclonal antibodies (MABs) and personalized chemotherapy, the clinical outcomes are not satisfying [68,69]. The complexity of the diseases may justify the failure of cancer treatments. Carcinogenesis is a complicated and multistep process which involves molecular and cellular alterations, which are distinct but closely connected phases of initiation, promotion, and progression [70–72] (see Figure 4).

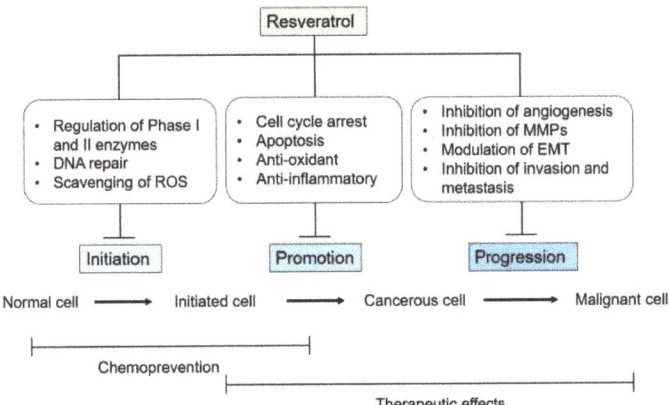

Figure 4. Schematic diagram summarizing the potential mechanisms underlying resveratrol's anti-cancer effects (adapted from [15]).

A possible reason for the failure of current cancer therapies, including chemotherapy, radiation, surgery, and immunosuppression, is emergency resistance [73]. Natural molecules are devoid of developing resistance, and delivering therapeutic effects without side effects remains a primary objective in the fight against cancer.

5.1. Resveratrol in Cancer Prevention and Treatment

Recent research has suggested that resveratrol can prevent the events linked to the initiation of tumours, which plays a vital role in developing resistance towards the current line of therapeutics. This characteristic of resveratrol has attracted great attention toward this molecule compared to other natural polyphenols. Another important mode of action is the prevention of free radical formation induced by 12-O-tetradecanoylphorbol-13-acetate (TPA). It has been seen over the course that TPA is one of the primary carcinogens mostly seen in the liquid tumours (e.g., in human leukaemia HL-60 cells) [74]. The various antioxidant properties of resveratrol have already been described previously [75,76]. Resveratrol is an excellent scavenger of hydroxyls and superoxides as well as the radicals induced by metals/enzymes and generated by cells [77]. It also protects against lipid peroxidation within cell membranes and damages DNA resulting from reactive oxygen species (ROS) [78]. Furthermore, resveratrol can function as an antimutagen, as shown by the inhibition of the mutagenicity of N-methyl-N'-nitro-N-nitrosoguanidine in the *Salmonella typhimurium* strain TA100 [79]. It has been proposed that resveratrol can be a possible chemo preventive agent, and its antimutagenic and anticarcinogenic properties have been demonstrated in several models [80]. Moreover, resveratrol showed a protective role in preclinical models of osteoarthritis and rheumatoid arthritis by reducing the production of pro-inflammatory and pro-degradative soluble factors, and through modulation of cellular and humoural responses [81].

Furthermore, resveratrol could enhance oxidative stress in adjuvant-arthritis (AA) rats and increase mtROS production by reducing the autophagy protein Beclin1, LC3A/B, and oxidative stress protein MnSOD, favouring the apoptosis of FLSs [82] (see Figure 5 for details).

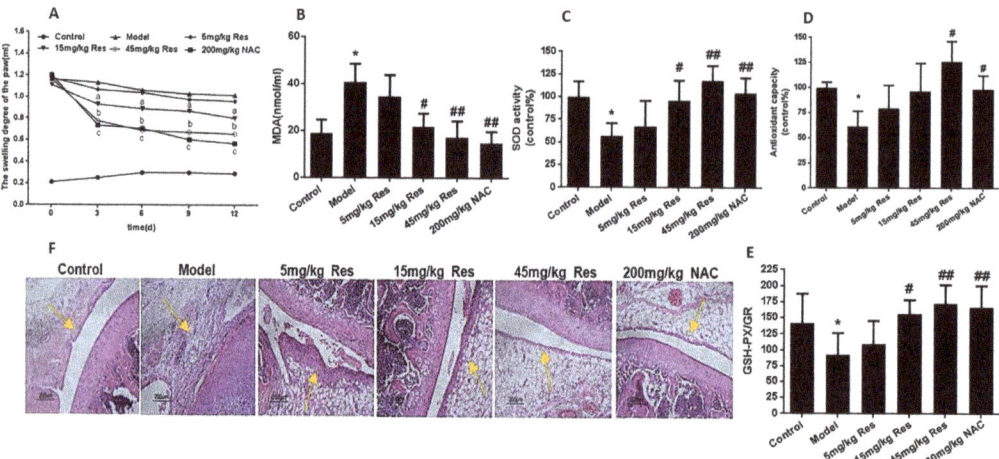

Figure 5. Resveratrol reduced oxidative injury in AA rats after injecting FCA 20 days, treated with 5 mg/kg, 15 mg/kg, 45 mg/kg resveratrol and 200 mg/kg N-acetyl-L-cysteine (NAC) for 12 days by continuous intragastric administration. (**A**) Swelling degree of the paw in SD rats after intragastric administration. (**B**) Lipoperoxide levels in the serum from six groups rats. (**C**) SOD activity in serum from six groups of rats. (**D**) Antioxidant capacity in serum from six groups of rats. (**E**) The ratio of glutathione peroxidase and glutathione reductase in serum from six groups of rats. (**F**) HE staining of knee joint in AA rats after administration resveratrol. Values are the means ± SD of at least three independent experiments. * $p < 0.05$ versus control; # $p < 0.05$, ## $p < 0.01$ versus model. (Reproduced with permission from [82]).

Resveratrol reduced the expression of heme oxygenase-1 (HO-1) and nuclear factor-E2-related factor 2 (Nrf2), and increased the expression of matrix metalloproteinase (MMP)-2, MMP-9, cyclooxygenase-2, and Toll-like receptor-4 in rats and further inhibited the formation of osteoclasts, the production of inflammation-related proteins, and of circulating ROS in periodontitis rats [83]. Treatment of monosodium iodoacetate (MIA)-injected rats with resveratrol (5 or 10 mg per kg BW) considerably reduced hyperalgesia and reduced the vertical and horizontal movements, additionally reducing any increase in the COX-2 and iNOS mRNA signalling pathways [84]. Very recently, it was also reported that in human bone mesenchymal stem cells, resveratrol suppressed interleukin-1β and thus downregulated metalloproteinase-13 mRNA expression and that it upregulated the chondrocyte markers (aggrecan, Col2, and Sox9 mRNA expression) [85].

5.2. Resveratrol in Wound Healing

Inflammation, proliferation, maturation, and remodelling are the four phases related to tissue integrity process after injury. The proliferation phase, starting within few days after injury, presents healing processes such as angiogenesis, granulation tissue formation, collagen deposition, and epithelialization [86]. Resveratrol seems to be a promising treatment approach, interacting with the healing cascade at different levels [87–89]. Several studies suggest that resveratrol could increase wound healing [87,90,91]. Figure 6 shows RES-induced angiogenesis blocked by PI3K and MEK inhibitors in HUVEC cells, as investigated by Wang et al. [88].

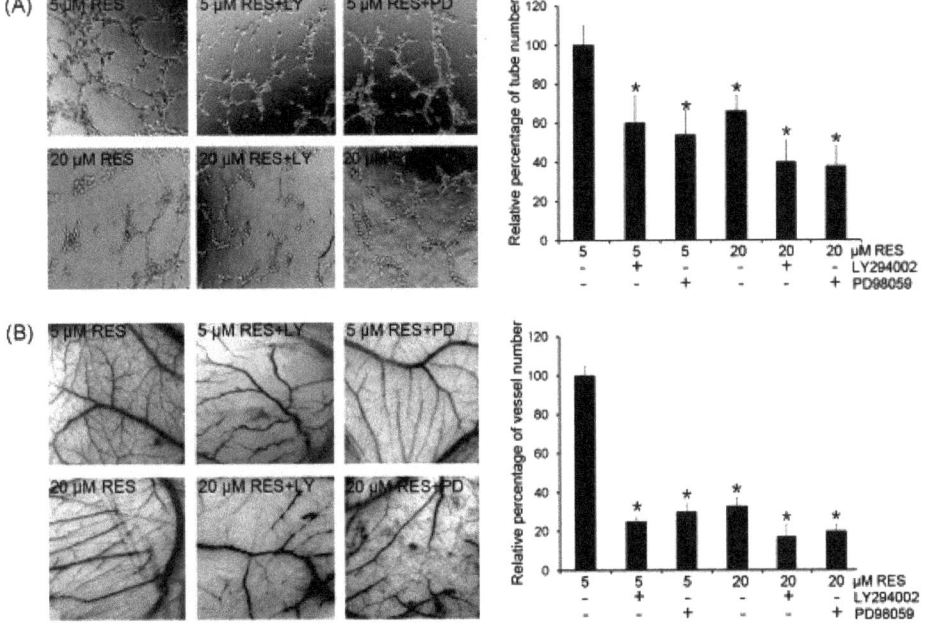

Figure 6. RES-induced angiogenesis was blocked by a PI3K inhibitor and an MEK inhibitor. (**A**) HUVECs were seeded on growth factor-reduced Matrigel-coated plate. Cells were treated with RES (5 μM or 20 μM) in the absence or presence of LY294002 (LY) or PD98059 (PD). The number of tube-like structures was scored. * $p < 0.05$ when compared to 5 μM RES treatment. (**B**) RES-induced angiogenesis was blocked by the PI3K inhibitor and MEK inhibitor in vivo by CAM assay. Cells were treated with RES (5 μM or 20 μM) in the absence or presence of LY294002 (LY) or PD98059 (PD). The number of branching vessels was scored. Each experiment was repeated three times. * $p < 0.05$ when compared to 5 μM RES treatment. (Reproduced with permission from [88]).

Resveratrol-induced vascular endothelial growth factor (VEGF) expression can regulate tissue regeneration and revascularization in wounds. Furthermore, it inhibits the expression of tumor necrosis factor-α (TNF-α), a pro-inflammatory factor [92–94]. In fact, VEGF has a broad spectrum of wound healing activities, such as increased cell migration, collagen deposition, capillary growth, and epithelialization [93]. An increase of pro-inflammatory markers such as interleukin (IL)-1β, IL-6, and TNF-α leads to an upregulation of matrix metalloproteinases (MMP), particularly increased in chronic wounds [95]. MMPs degrade local extracellular matrix (ECM), impairing cell migration in wounds [96]. In resveratrol-treated patients TNF-α, IL-1β, IL-6, MMP-2, -3, -9, and C-reactive protein (CRP) were reduced [97–100].

Moreover, resveratrol has also a significant impact on the regulation of inflammation and consequently in processes related to skin repair [101]. In vitro investigations showed that due to its antioxidant properties resveratrol can influence cell proliferation, ultrastructural preservation, and migration quality [102,103], whereas in vivo studies reported a significant improvement in wound healing properties [104].

5.3. Resveratrol as Cardioprotective Agent

Resveratrol is a natural compound with anti-inflammatory effects. Xiuyue Huo et al. evaluated the cardio protective effects of RES in a diabetic rat model with coronary heart disease [105]. RES maintained pancreatic tissue, reducing levels of glucose and triglyceride glycerides in serum. Inflammatory factors were also suppressed by RES. TLR4/MyD88/NF-kB signalling pathway was downregulated after RES treatment [105]. To confirm the cardioprotective effects of RES, the authors harvested heat tissues from rats and examined pathological changes using H&E staining. They demonstrated that RES can offer protective effects on cardiovascular tissues in diabetic rats. By downregulating a wide range of inflammatory factors, RES strongly improved coronary injuries from inflammation. Based on this effect, RES might show a beneficial outcome or has a promising effect in diabetic cases with coronary heart disease according to its protective effects on cardiovascular tissues [105].

Resveratrol and its analogues have been shown in preclinical studies to protect against cancer treatment-induced cardiovascular toxicity. They have also been reported to possess significant anticancer properties on their own and to enhance the anticancer effect of other cancer treatments. Thus, they hold significant promise to protect the cardiovascular system and fight the cancer at the same time [106]. Thus, they hold significant promise to protect the cardiovascular system and fight the cancer at the same time. Despite the very promising preclinical findings of resveratrol as a cardioprotective agent, there are still several questions that need to be answered before advancing resveratrol into clinical trials. Considering the possible hormetic dose–response properties of resveratrol [107], it is important to show that the same dose of resveratrol can protect the heart and fight cancer. On the other hand, to determine the effect of resveratrol on the pharmacokinetics and tissue distribution of chemotherapeutic agents, considering the potential of resveratrol to alter several drug metabolizing enzymes is also rather important [108].

5.4. Resveratrol in Fighting Infections

Resveratrol has been reported to show anti-inflammatory, cardioprotective, and antiproliferative properties and also to affect many viruses like retroviruses, influenza A virus, and polyomavirus by altering cellular pathways influencing viral replication itself. Epstein–Barr Virus (EBV), the agent causing mononucleosis, relates to different proliferative diseases and establishes a latent and/or a lytic infection. De Leo and co-workers [109] examined the antiviral activity of RES against the EBV replicative cycle and studied the molecular targets involved. In a cellular context that allows in vitro EBV activation and lytic cycle progression, they found that RES inhibited EBV lytic genes expression and the production of viral particles in a dose-dependent manner. They demonstrated that RES decreased reactive oxygen species (ROS) levels, inhibited protein synthesis, and suppressed the EBV-induced activation of the redox-sensitive transcription factors NF–kB and AP-1 [109]. RES action causes downregulation of EBV-lytic genes at the post-transcriptional level by influencing multiple cellular targets. The molecular mechanisms involved could be divided in three parts: (1) inhibition of protein synthesis, (2) decrement of ROS levels, and (3) fast suppression of NF–kB and AP-1 activities, augmented by EBV-lytic cycle reactivation [109]. With this work, De Leo and co-authors constructed the basis for evaluating the antiviral activity of RES against EBV infection, envisaging the possibility to extend it to other types of infections.

In a recent article, Palomera-Ávalos et al. [110] demonstrated that RES induced higher expression in cytokines with regard to LPS. Oxidative stress (OS) markers indicated non-significant changes after LPS or RES, although for the RES-treated groups a slight increment in several study parameters was observed, reaching significance for NF–kB protein levels and iNOS expression. The authors focused on the role of long-term resveratrol treatment as a tool to increase brain defenses in ageing animals against acute LPS proinflammatory stimuli. Their results showed an improvement in cellular response against LPS injury cellular modulation response in the ageing brain. Finally, they concluded that resveratrol treatment induced a different cellular response in ageing animals when they encountered acute inflammatory stimuli [110].

Shevelev and co-workers have compared the antimicrobial activity of resveratrol (a stilbene), dihydroquercetin, and dihydromyricetin (two flavonols) extracted from the bark and wood of conifers against the dermatophytes *Staphylococcus aureus*, *Pseudomonas aeruginosa*, and *Candida albicans*. This study suggests a significantly higher bactericidal activity of polyphenols in comparison with those traditionally used against *S. aureus* at 24.2 mM [111].

It has been shown that RES can block the critical pathways involved in SARS-CoV-2 pathogenesis, including control of both RAS and ACE2, and body immune activation, and downregulate pro-inflammatory cytokine release. It was also discovered to activate SIRT1 and p53 signalling pathways and increase cytotoxic T lymphocytes (CTLs) and natural killer (NK) immune cells. RES has also been a fetal hemoglobin stimulator and a potent antioxidant capable of blocking ROS [112,113].

RES also blocked MERS-CoV replication in vitro by inhibiting RNA synthesis and had other pleiotropic consequences, and it inhibited viral replication and reduced the death risk in piglets infected with the duck enteritis virus [114]. Similarly, Lin et al. (2017) showed that resveratrol can prevent MERS-CoV infections in a Vero E6 cell model. Two resveratrol concentrations of 250 and 125 µM were investigated, demonstrating that resveratrol can reduce the cell death induced by infection at this concentration range [115] (see Figure 7). Currently there is no evidence that RES has been used to treat SARS-CoV-2; however, available studies may envisage that it could be a strategic adjunctive antiviral agent to use in synergy with others.

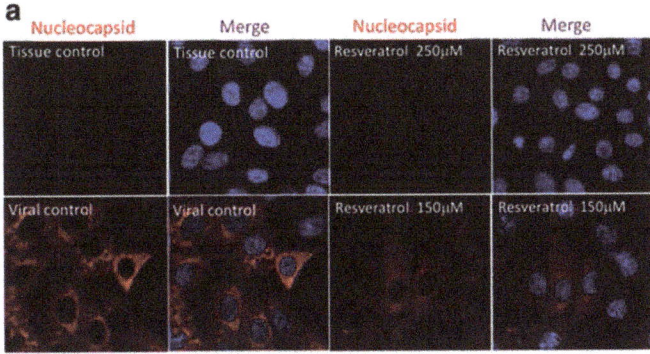

Figure 7. *Cont.*

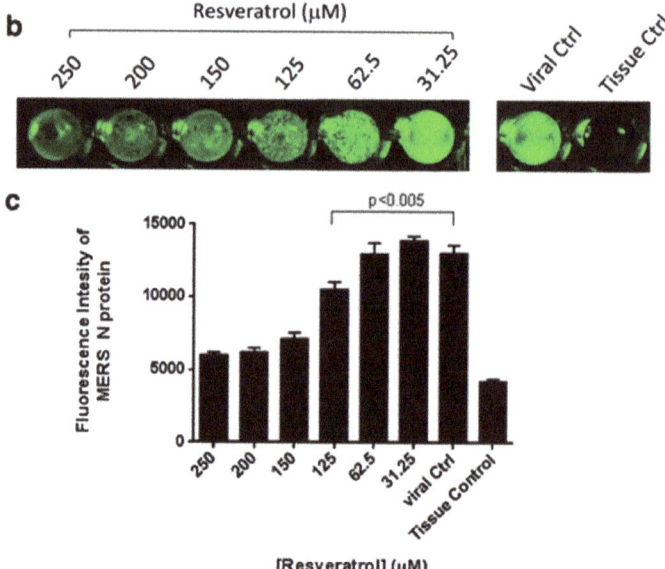

Figure 7. Resveratrol reduced nucleocapsid expression of MERS-CoV. Vero E6 cells were infected by MERS-CoV (M.O.I. 0.1) and treated with resveratrol for 24 h followed by 4% paraformaldehyde fixation for immunofluorescent assays. (**a**) Nucleocapsid expressions were examined with confocal microscope at 680× magnification. DAPI was used for nucleus staining. (**b**) Intracellular staining of MERS nucleocapsid expressions were visualized by Odyssey® CLx Imaging system. (**c**) Quantification results of fluorescent intensities of MERS nucleocapsid proteins were determined by Odyssey® CLx Imaging software. (Reproduced with permission from Ref. [115]).

6. Conclusions

Resveratrol is a very promising natural molecule because of its enormous therapeutic potential. However, the potential of resveratrol has not been fully explored due to its poor bioavailability. In the past two decades, nano-based delivery systems have created new hopes for delivering numerous drug molecules. Regardless of the encouraging results in preclinical trials, the suitability of resveratrol for humans has encountered only inadequate accomplishment, mostly due to its incompetent systemic delivery and, subsequently, its low bioavailability enterohepatic recirculation. Whether or not enterohepatic recirculation of resveratrol contributes expressively to the complete pharmacological action needs to be determined. To overcome these issues, it has been shown that encapsulating resveratrol into nanocarriers drastically improves the obstacles to its physicochemical characteristics. Furthermore, nanocarriers can enhance the bioavailability and permeability of resveratrol molecules, which are otherwise challenging to deliver orally.

7. Current Limitations and Future Perspectives

Several resveratrol-based nanoformulations are being explored for clinical applications. Despite these achievements, the 'ideal' resveratrol delivery system still needs to be disclosed. Significant progress has been made over last few years for developing the next generations of resveratrol-based nanocarriers that will play an essential role in curing human diseases and improving healthcare. The main limitations of these nanocarriers rely on difficulties in increasing bioavailability and targeting. By developing and designing novel nanovectors, one may also take into account the obstacles related to overcoming biological barriers in delivering cargos as well as the impendence to maintain intact or still-active, large quantities of RES during the transport to the target. For these reasons, additional studies (in vitro and more in vivo) are needed, and they will allow the development of novel strategies to overcome such challenges still limiting the use of resveratrol for therapy and/or prevention in deadly diseases such as cancer.

Author Contributions: Conception, drafting, writing, revision and final approval, R.A.B.; writing, editing and final approval, N.T. and M.P.S.; revision and final approval, G.G. and A.R.; funding, G.G.; revision and final approval, S.L. All authors have read and agreed to the published version of the manuscript.

Funding: G.G., A.R., and S.L. are grateful to the Tecnopolo per la medicina di precisione (TecnoMed Puglia)—Regione Puglia: DGR no. 2117 del 21/11/2018, CUP: B84I18000540002 and Tecnopolo di Nanotecnologia e Fotonica per la medicina di precisione (TECNOMED)—FISR/MIUR-CNR: delibera CIPE no. 3449 del 7-08-2017, CUP: B83B17000010001. R.B. acknowledge the financial support of Science Foundation Ireland (SFI) and is co-funded under the European Regional Development Fund under grant no 13/RC/2073_P2.

Institutional Review Board Statement: Not applicable.

Informed Consent Statement: Not applicable.

Data Availability Statement: Not applicable.

Conflicts of Interest: The authors declare that the research was conducted in the absence of any commercial or financial relationships that could be construed as a potential conflict of interest.

References

1. Siegel, R.L.; Miller, K.D.; Jemal, A. Cancer Statistics. *CA Cancer J. Clin.* **2017**, *67*, 7–30. [CrossRef] [PubMed]
2. Okimoto, R.A.; Bivona, T.G. Recent advances in personalized lung cancer medicine. *Pers. Med.* **2014**, *11*, 309–321. [CrossRef] [PubMed]
3. Krepler, C.; Xiao, M.; Sproesser, K.; Brafford, P.A.; Shannan, B.; Beqiri, M.; Liu, Q.; Xu, W.; Garman, B.; Nathanson, K.L.; et al. Personalized Preclinical Trials in BRAF Inhibitor-Resistant Patient-Derived Xenograft Models Identify Second-Line Combination Therapies. *Clin. Cancer Res.* **2016**, *22*, 1592–1602. [CrossRef] [PubMed]
4. Hong, W.K.; Sporn, M.B. Recent advances in chemoprevention of Cancer. *Science* **1997**, *278*, 1073–1077. [CrossRef] [PubMed]
5. Sethi, G.; Shanmugam, M.K.; Ramachandran, L.; Kumar, A.P.; Tergaonkar, V. Multifaceted link between Cancer and inflammation. *Biosci. Rep.* **2012**, *32*, 1–15. [CrossRef] [PubMed]
6. Chai, E.Z.; Siveen, K.S.; Shanmugam, M.K.; Arfuso, F.; Sethi, G. Analysis of the intricate relationship between chronic inflammation and Cancer. *Biochem. J.* **2015**, *468*, 1–15. [CrossRef] [PubMed]
7. Sethi, G.; Tergaonkar, V. Potential pharmacological control of the NF-κB pathway. *Trends Pharmacol. Sci.* **2009**, *30*, 313–321. [CrossRef] [PubMed]
8. Janakiram, N.B.; Mohammed, A.; Madka, V.; Kumar, G.; Rao, C.V. Prevention and treatment of cancers by immune modulating nutrients. *Mol. Nutr. Food Res.* **2016**, *60*, 1275–1294. [CrossRef] [PubMed]
9. Sharma, S.; Stutzman, J.D.; Kelloff, G.J.; Steele, V.E. Screening of potential chemopreventive agents using biochemical markers of carcinogenesis. *Cancer Res.* **1994**, *54*, 5848–5855. [PubMed]
10. Martinez, J.; Moreno, J.J. Effect of resveratrol, a natural polyphenolic compound, on reactive oxygen species and prostaglandin production. *Biochem. Pharmacol.* **2000**, *59*, 865–870. [CrossRef]
11. Leonard, S.S.; Xia, C.; Jiang, B.H.; Stinefelt, B.; Klandorf, H.; Harris, G.K.; Shi, X. Resveratrol scavenges reactive oxygen species and effects radical-induced cellular responses. *Biochem. Biophys. Res. Commun.* **2003**, *309*, 1017–1026. [CrossRef] [PubMed]
12. Kim, H.J.; Chang, E.J.; Bae, S.J.; Shim, S.M.; Park, H.D.; Rhee, C.H.; Park, J.H.; Choi, S.W. Cytotoxic and antimutagenic stilbenes from seeds of *Paeonia lactiflora*. *Arch. Pharm. Res.* **2002**, *25*, 293–299. [CrossRef] [PubMed]
13. Sgambato, A.; Ardito, R.; Faraglia, B.; Boninsegna, A.; Wolf, F.I.; Cittadini, A. Resveratrol, a natural phenolic compound, inhibits cell proliferation and prevents oxidative DNA damage. *Mutat. Res.* **2001**, *496*, 171–180. [CrossRef]
14. Attia, S.M. Influence of resveratrol on oxidative damage in genomic DNA and apoptosis induced by cisplatin. *Mutat. Res.* **2012**, *741*, 22–31. [CrossRef] [PubMed]
15. Ko, J.H.; Sethi, G.; Um, J.Y.; Shanmugam, M.K.; Arfuso, F.; Kumar, A.P.; Bishayee, A.; Ahn, K.S. The role of resveratrol in cancer therapy. *Int. J. Mol. Sci.* **2017**, *18*, 2589. [CrossRef] [PubMed]
16. Singla, R.K.; Dubey, A.K.; Garg, A.; Sharma, R.K.; Fiorino, M.; Ameen, S.M.; Haddad, M.A.; Al-Hiary, M. Natural polyphenols: Chemical classification, definition of classes, subcategories, and structures. *J. AOAC Int.* **2019**, *102*, 1397–1400. [CrossRef]
17. Wink, M. Plant secondary metabolites modulate insect behavior-steps toward addiction? *Front. Physiol.* **2018**, *9*, 364. [CrossRef]
18. Laganà, P.; Anastasi, G.; Marano, F.; Piccione, S.; Singla, R.K.; Dubey, A.K.; Delia, S.; Coniglio, M.A.; Facciolà, A.; Di Pietro, A.; et al. Phenolic Substances in Foods: Health Effects as Anti-Inflammatory and Antimicrobial Agents. *J. AOAC Int.* **2019**, *102*, 1378–1387. [CrossRef]

19. Wang, T.Y.; Li, Q.; Bi, K.S. Bioactive flavonoids in medicinal plants: Structure, activity and biological fate. *Asian J. Pharma. Sci.* **2018**, *13*, 12–23. [CrossRef]
20. Evans, M.; Sharma, P.; Guthrie, N. Bioavailability of citrus polymethoxylated flavones and their biological role in metabolic syndrome and hyperlipidemia. In *Readings in Advanced Pharmacokinetics-Theory, Methods and Applications*; Intech Open: London, UK, 2012. [CrossRef]
21. Testai, L.; Calderone, V. Nutraceutical value of citrus flavanones and their implications in cardiovascular disease. *Nutrients* **2017**, *9*, 502. [CrossRef]
22. Yu, J.; Bi, X.; Yu, B.; Chen, D. Isoflavones: Anti-inflammatory benefit and possible caveats. *Nutrients* **2016**, *8*, 361. [CrossRef] [PubMed]
23. Khoo, H.E.; Azlan, A.; Tang, S.T.; Lim, S.M. Anthocyanidins and anthocyanins: Colored pigments as food, pharmaceutical ingredients, and the potential health benefits. *Food Nutr. Res.* **2017**, *61*, 1361779. [CrossRef] [PubMed]
24. Saibabu, V.; Fatima, Z.; Khan, L.A.; Hameed, S. Therapeutic potential of dietary phenolic acids. *Adv. Pharmacol. Sci.* **2015**, *2015*, 823539. [CrossRef]
25. Rodríguez-García, C.; Sánchez-Quesada, C.; Toledo, E.; Delgado-Rodríguez, M.; Gaforio, J.J. Naturally lignan-rich foods: A dietary tool for health promotion? *Molecules* **2019**, *24*, 917. [CrossRef] [PubMed]
26. El Khawand, T.; Courtois, A.; Valls, J.; Richard, T.; Krisa, S. A review of dietary stilbenes: Sources and bioavailability. *Phytochem. Rev.* **2018**, *17*, 1007–1029. [CrossRef]
27. Salehi, B.; Mishra, A.P.; Nigam, M.; Sener, B.; Kilic, M.; Sharifi-Rad, M.; Fokou, P.V.T.; Martins, N.; Sharifi-Rad, J. Resveratrol: A double-edged sword in health benefits. *Biomedicines* **2018**, *6*, 91. [CrossRef]
28. Trela, B.C.; Waterhouse, A.L. Resveratrol: Isomeric molar absorptivities and stability. *J. Agric. Food Chem.* **1996**, *44*, 1253–1257. [CrossRef]
29. Gokce, E.H.; Korkmaz, E.; Dellera, E.; Sandri, G.; Bonferoni, M.C.; Ozer, O. Resveratrol-loaded solid lipid nanoparticles versus nanostructured lipid carriers: Evaluation of antioxidant potential for dermal applications. *Int. J. Nanomed.* **2012**, *7*, 1841. [CrossRef]
30. Chen, J.; Wei, N.; Lopez-Garcia, M.; Ambrose, D.; Lee, J.; Annelin, C.; Peterson, T. Development and evaluation of resveratrol, Vitamin E, and epigallocatechin gallate loaded lipid nanoparticles for skin care applications. *Eur. J. Pharm. Biopharm.* **2017**, *117*, 286–291. [CrossRef]
31. Nawaz, W.; Zhou, Z.; Deng, S.; Ma, X.; Ma, X.; Li, C.; Shu, X. Therapeutic versatility of resveratrol derivatives. *Nutrients* **2017**, *9*, 1188. [CrossRef]
32. Li, M.; Kildegaard, K.R.; Chen, Y.; Rodriguez, A.; Borodina, I.; Nielsen, J. De novo production of resveratrol from glucose or ethanol by engineered Saccharomyces cerevisiae. *Metab. Eng.* **2015**, *32*, 1–11. [CrossRef] [PubMed]
33. Burns, J.; Yokota, T.; Ashihara, H.; Lean, M.E.; Crozier, A. Plant foods and herbal sources of resveratrol. *J. Agric. Food Chem.* **2002**, *50*, 3337–3340. [CrossRef] [PubMed]
34. Risuleo, G. Resveratrol: Multiple activities on the biological functionality of the cell. In *Nutraceuticals*; Academic Press: Cambridge, MA, USA, 2016; pp. 453–464. [CrossRef]
35. Neubert, R.H.H. Potentials of new nanocarriers for dermal and transdermal drug delivery. *Eur. J. Pharm. Biopharm.* **2011**, *77*, 1–2. [CrossRef]
36. How, C.W.; Rasedee, A.; Manickam, S.; Rosli, R. Tamoxifen-loaded nanostructured lipid carrier as a drug delivery system: Characterization, stability assessment and cytotoxicity. *Colloids Surf. B. Biointerfaces* **2013**, *112*, 393–399. [CrossRef] [PubMed]
37. Wong, H.L.; Bendayan, R.; Rauth, A.M.; Li, Y.; Wu, X.Y. Chemotherapy with anticancer drugs encapsulated in solid lipid nanoparticles. *Adv. Drug Deliv. Rev.* **2007**, *59*, 491–504. [CrossRef] [PubMed]
38. Wang, A.Z.; Langer, R.; Farokhzad, O.C. Nanoparticle delivery of cancer drugs. *Annu. Rev. Med.* **2012**, *63*, 185–198. [CrossRef] [PubMed]
39. Zeb, A.; Qureshi, O.S.; Kim, H.S.; Kim, M.S.; Kang, J.H.; Park, J.S.; Kim, J.K. High payload itraconazole-incorporated lipid nanoparticles with modulated release property for oral and parenteral administration. *J. Pharm. Pharmacol.* **2017**, *69*, 955–966. [CrossRef] [PubMed]
40. Kakkar, D.; Dumoga, S.; Kumar, R.; Chuttani, K.; Mishra, A.K. PEGylated solid lipid nanoparticles: Design, methotrexate loading and biological evaluation in animal models. *Med. Chem. Comm.* **2015**, *6*, 1452–1463. [CrossRef]
41. Qureshi, O.S.; Kim, H.S.; Zeb, A.; Choi, J.S.; Kim, H.S.; Kwon, J.E.; Kim, M.S.; Kang, J.H.; Ryou, C.; Park, J.S.; et al. Sustained release docetaxel-incorporated lipid nanoparticles with improved pharmacokinetics for oral and parenteral administration. *J. Microencapsul.* **2017**, *34*, 250–261. [CrossRef] [PubMed]
42. Deshpande, P.P.; Biswas, S.; Torchilin, V.P. Current trends in the use of liposomes for tumor targeting. *Nanomedicine* **2013**, *8*, 1509–1528. [CrossRef]
43. Basu, S.; Sandanaraj, B.S.; Thayumanavan, S. Molecular recognition in dendrimers. In *Encyclopedia of Polymer Science and Technology*; John Wiley & Sons, Inc.: Hoboken, NJ, USA, 2002. [CrossRef]
44. Lai, P.S.; Lou, P.J.; Peng, C.L.; Pai, C.L.; Yen, W.N.; Huang, M.Y.; Young, T.H.; Shieh, M.J. Doxorubicin delivery by polyamidoamine dendrimer conjugation and photochemical internalization for cancer therapy. *J. Control. Release.* **2007**, *122*, 39–46. [CrossRef] [PubMed]

45. Zielińska, A.; Carreiró, F.; Oliveira, A.M.; Neves, A.; Pires, B.; Venkatesh, D.N.; Durazzo, A.; Lucarini, M.; Eder, P.; Silva, A.M.; et al. Polymeric nanoparticles: Production, characterization, toxicology and ecotoxicology. *Molecules* **2020**, *25*, 3731. [CrossRef]
46. ud Din, F.; Aman, W.; Ullah, I.; Qureshi, O.S.; Mustapha, O.; Shafique, S.; Zeb, A. Effective use of nanocarriers as drug delivery systems for the treatment of selected tumors. *Int. J. Nanomed.* **2017**, *12*, 7291. [CrossRef] [PubMed]
47. Wang, W.; Chen, S.; Zhang, L.; Wu, X.; Wang, J.; Chen, J.F.; Le, Y. Poly (lactic acid)/chitosan hybrid nanoparticles for controlled release of anticancer drug. *Mater Sci. Eng. C* **2015**, *46*, 514–520. [CrossRef] [PubMed]
48. Anitha, A.; Deepa, N.; Chennazhi, K.P.; Lakshmanan, V.K.; Jayakumar, R. Combinatorial anticancer effects of curcumin and 5-fluorouracil loaded thiolated chitosan nanoparticles towards colon cancer treatment. *Biochim. Biophys. Acta* **2014**, *1840*, 2730–2743. [CrossRef] [PubMed]
49. Zhu, Y.; Liao, L. Applications of nanoparticles for anticancer drug delivery: A review. *J. Nanosci. Nanotechnol.* **2015**, *15*, 4753–4773. [CrossRef] [PubMed]
50. Biswas, S.; Kumari, P.; Lakhani, P.M.; Ghosh, B. Recent advances in polymeric micelles for anticancer drug delivery. *Eur. J. Pharm. Sci.* **2016**, *83*, 184–202. [CrossRef] [PubMed]
51. Gothwal, A.; Khan, I.; Gupta, U. Polymeric micelles: Recent advancements in the delivery of anticancer drugs. *Pharm. Res.* **2016**, *33*, 18–39. [CrossRef] [PubMed]
52. Ren, J.; Fang, Z.; Yao, L.; Dahmani, F.Z.; Yin, L.; Zhou, J.; Yao, J. A micelle-like structure of poloxamer–methotrexate conjugates as nanocarrier for methotrexate delivery. *Int. J. Pharma.* **2015**, *487*, 177–186. [CrossRef]
53. Zhang, W.; Li, M.; Zhou, W.; Zhang, X.; Li, F. Self-assembly, biosynthesis, functionalization and applications of virus-based nanomaterials. *Synth. Biol. J.* **2020**, *1*, 298. [CrossRef]
54. Slowing, I.I.; Vivero-Escoto, J.L.; Wu, C.W.; Lin, V.S.Y. Mesoporous silica nanoparticles as controlled release drug delivery and gene transfection carriers. *Adv. Drug Del. Rev.* **2008**, *60*, 1278–1288. [CrossRef] [PubMed]
55. Rosenholm, J.M.; Peuhu, E.; Bate-Eya, L.T.; Eriksson, J.E.; Sahlgren, C.; Lindén, M. Cancer-cell-specific induction of apoptosis using mesoporous silica nanoparticles as drug-delivery vectors. *Small* **2010**, *6*, 1234–1241. [CrossRef] [PubMed]
56. Ng, C.M.; Loh, H.S.; Muthoosamy, K.; Sridewi, N.; Manickam, S. Conjugation of insulin onto the sidewalls of single-walled carbon nanotubes through functionalization and diimide-activated amidation. *Int. J. Nanomed.* **2016**, *11*, 1607. [CrossRef]
57. Vardharajula, S.; Ali, S.Z.; Tiwari, P.M.; Eroğlu, E.; Vig, K.; Dennis, V.A.; Singh, S.R. Functionalized carbon nanotubes: Biomedical applications. *Int. J. Nanomed.* **2012**, *7*, 5361. [CrossRef]
58. Rout, G.K.; Shin, H.S.; Gouda, S.; Sahoo, S.; Das, G.; Fraceto, L.F.; Patra, J.K. Current advances in nanocarriers for biomedical research and their applications. *Artif. Cells Nanomed. Biotechnol.* **2018**, *46*, 1053–1062. [CrossRef]
59. Prabhakar, N.; Zhang, J.; Desai, D.; Casals, E.; Gulin-Sarfraz, T.; Näreoja, T.; Westermarck, J.; Rosenholm, J.M. Stimuli-responsive hybrid nanocarriers developed by controllable integration of hyperbranched PEI with mesoporous silica nanoparticles for sustained intracellular siRNA delivery. *Int. J. Nanomed.* **2016**, *11*, 6591. [CrossRef] [PubMed]
60. Desai, D.; Zhang, J.; Sandholm, J.; Lehtimäki, J.; Grönroos, T.; Tuomela, J.; Rosenholm, J.M. Lipid bilayer-gated mesoporous silica nanocarriers for tumor-targeted delivery of zoledronic acid in vivo. *Mol. Pharm.* **2017**, *14*, 3218–3227. [CrossRef] [PubMed]
61. Han, N.; Zhao, Q.; Wan, L.; Wang, Y.; Gao, Y.; Wang, P.; Wang, Z.; Zhang, J.; Jiang, T.; Wang, S. Hybrid lipid-capped mesoporous silica for stimuli-responsive drug release and overcoming multidrug resistance. *ACS Appl. Mater. Interfaces* **2015**, *7*, 3342–3351. [CrossRef]
62. Huang, M.; Liang, C.; Tan, C.; Huang, S.; Ying, R.; Wang, Y.; Wang, Z.; Zhang, Y. Liposome co-encapsulation as a strategy for the delivery of curcumin and resveratrol. *Food Funct.* **2019**, *10*, 6447–6458. [CrossRef] [PubMed]
63. Jagwani, S.; Jalalpure, S.; Dhamecha, D.; Jadhav, K.; Bohara, R. Pharmacokinetic and pharmacodynamic evaluation of resveratrol loaded cationic liposomes for targeting hepatocellular carcinoma. *ACS Biomater. Sci. Eng.* **2020**, *6*, 4969–4984. [CrossRef]
64. Chauhan, A.S. Dendrimer nanotechnology for enhanced formulation and controlled delivery of resveratrol. *Ann. N. Y. Acad. Sci.* **2015**, *1384*, 134–140. [CrossRef] [PubMed]
65. Vijayakumar, M.R.; Kumari, L.; Patel, K.K.; Vuddanda, P.R.; Vajanthri, K.Y.; Mahto, S.K.; Singh, S. Intravenous administration of trans-resveratrol-loaded TPGS-coated solid lipid nanoparticles for prolonged systemic circulation, passive brain targeting and improved in vitro cytotoxicity against C6 glioma cell lines. *RSC Adv.* **2016**, *6*, 50336–50348. [CrossRef]
66. Wan, S.; Zhang, L.; Quan, Y.; Wei, K. Resveratrol-loaded PLGA nanoparticles: Enhanced stability, solubility and bioactivity of resveratrol for non-alcoholic fatty liver disease therapy. *R. Soc. Open Sci.* **2018**, *5*, 181457. [CrossRef] [PubMed]
67. Swamy, M.K.; Sinniah, U.R. Patchouli (*Pogostemon cablin* Benth.): Botany, agrotechnology and biotechnological aspects. *Ind. Crops Prod.* **2016**, *87*, 161–176. [CrossRef]
68. Mohanty, S.K.; Swamy, M.K.; Sinniah, U.R.; Anuradha, M. *Leptadenia reticulata* (Retz.) Wight & Arn. (Jivanti): Botanical, agronomical, phytochemical, pharmacological, and biotechnological aspects. *Molecules* **2017**, *22*, 1019. [CrossRef]
69. Rodrigues, T.; Reker, D.; Schneider, P.; Schneider, G. Counting on natural products for drug design. *Nat. Chem.* **2016**, *8*, 531. [CrossRef]
70. Siddiqui, A.A.; Iram, F.; Siddiqui, S.; Sahu, K. Role of natural products in drug discovery process. *Int. J. Drug Dev. Res.* **2014**, *6*, 172–204.
71. Beutler, J.A. Natural products as a foundation for drug discovery. *Curr. Prot. Pharmacol.* **2009**, *46*, 9–11. [CrossRef]
72. Thilakarathna, S.H.; Rupasinghe, H. Flavonoid bioavailability and attempts for bioavailability enhancement. *Nutrients* **2013**, *5*, 3367–3387. [CrossRef]

73. Bonifácio, B.V.; da Silva, P.B.; dos Santos Ramos, M.A.; Negri, K.M.S.; Bauab, T.M.; Chorilli, M. Nanotechnology-based drug delivery systems and herbal medicines: A review. *Int. J. Nanomed.* **2014**, *9*, 1. [CrossRef]
74. Watkins, R.; Wu, L.; Zhang, C.; Davis, R.M.; Xu, B. Natural product-based nanomedicine: Recent advances and issues. *Int. J. Nanomed.* **2015**, *10*, 6055. [CrossRef]
75. Perez, A.T.; Domenech, G.H.; Frankel, C.; Vogel, C.L. Pegylated liposomal doxorubicin (Doxil®) for metastatic breast cancer: The Cancer Research Network, Inc., experience. *Cancer Investig.* **2002**, *20*, 22–29. [CrossRef] [PubMed]
76. Tsai, Y.M.; Chang-Liao, W.L.; Chien, C.F.; Lin, L.C.; Tsai, T.H. Effects of polymer molecular weight on relative oral bioavailability of curcumin. *Int. J. Nanomed.* **2012**, *7*, 2957–2966. [CrossRef] [PubMed]
77. Nair, H.B.; Sung, B.; Yadav, V.R.; Kannappan, R.; Chaturvedi, M.M.; Aggarwal, B.B. Delivery, of anti-inflammatory nutraceuticals by nanoparticles for the prevention and treatment of Cancer. *Biochem. Pharmacol.* **2010**, *80*, 1833–1843. [CrossRef]
78. Jang, M.; Cai, L.; Udeani, G.O.; Slowing, K.V.; Thomas, C.F.; Beecher, C.W.; Fong, H.H.; Farnsworth, N.R.; Kinghorn, A.D.; Mehta, R.G.; et al. Cancer chemopreventive activity of resveratrol, a natural product derived from grapes. *Science* **1997**, *275*, 218–220. [CrossRef]
79. Banerjee, S.; Bueso-Ramos, C.; Aggarwal, B.B. Suppression of 7, 12-dimethylbenz (a) anthracene-induced mammary carcinogenesis in rats by resveratrol: Role of nuclear factor-κB, cyclooxygenase 2, and matrix metalloprotease 9. *Cancer Res.* **2002**, *62*, 4945–4954.
80. Aggarwal, B.B.; Takada, Y.; Oommen, O.V. From chemoprevention to chemotherapy: Common targets and common goals. *Expert Opin. Investig. Drugs* **2004**, *13*, 1327–1338. [CrossRef]
81. Nguyen, C.; Savouret, J.F.; Widerak, M.; Corvol, M.T.; Rannou, F. Resveratrol, potential therapeutic interest in joint disorders: A critical narrative review. *Nutrients* **2017**, *9*, 45. [CrossRef]
82. Zhang, J.; Song, X.; Cao, W.; Lu, J.; Wang, X.; Wang, G.; Wang, Z.; Chen, X. Autophagy and mitochondrial dysfunction in adjuvant-arthritis rats treatment with resveratrol. *Sci. Rep.* **2016**, *6*, 32928. [CrossRef]
83. Bhattarai, G.; Poudel, S.B.; Kook, S.-H.; Lee, J.-G. Resveratrol prevents alveolar bone loss in an experimental rat model of periodontitis. *Acta Biomater.* **2016**, *21*, 398–408. [CrossRef]
84. Wang, Z.M.; Chen, Y.C.; Wang, D.P. Resveratrol, a natural antioxidant, protects monosodium iodoacetate- induced osteoarthritic pain in rats. *Biomed. Pharmacother.* **2016**, *83*, 763–770. [CrossRef]
85. Wu, G.; Wang, L.; Li, H.; Ke, Y.; Yao, Y. Function of sustained released resveratrol on IL-1β-induced hBMSC MMP13 secretion inhibition and chondrogenic differentiation promotion. *J. Biomater. Appl.* **2016**, *30*, 930–939. [CrossRef] [PubMed]
86. Ikeda, K.; Torigoe, T.; Matsumoto, Y.; Fujita, T.; Sato, N.; Yotsuyanagi, T. Resveratrol inhibits fibrogenesis and induces apoptosis in keloid fibroblasts. *Wound Repair Regen.* **2013**, *21*, 616–623. [CrossRef] [PubMed]
87. Pastore, S.; Lulli, D.; Fidanza, P.; Potapovich, A.I.; Kostyuk, V.; De Luca, C.; Mikhal'Chik, E.; Korkina, L.G. Plant Polyphenols Regulate Chemokine Expression and Tissue Repair in Human Keratinocytes Through Interaction with Cytoplasmic and Nuclear Components of Epidermal Growth Factor Receptor System. *Antioxid. Redox Signal.* **2012**, *16*, 314–328. [CrossRef] [PubMed]
88. Wang, H.; Zhou, H.; Zou, Y.; Liu, Q.; Guo, C.; Gao, G.; Shao, C.; Gong, Y. Resveratrol modulates angiogenesis through the GSK3β/β-catenin/TCF-dependent pathway in human endothelial cells. *Biochem. Pharmacol.* **2010**, *80*, 1386–1395. [CrossRef] [PubMed]
89. Zhou, G.; Han, X.; Wu, Z.; Shi, Q.; Bao, X. Rosiglitazone accelerates wound healing by improving endothelial precursor cell function and angiogenesis in db/db mice. *PeerJ* **2019**, *7*, e7815. [CrossRef] [PubMed]
90. Gokce, E.H.; Tanrıverdi, S.T.; Eroglu, I.; Tsapis, N.; Gokce, G.; Tekmen, I.; Fattal, E.; Ozer, O. Wound healing effects of collagen-laminin dermal matrix impregnated with resveratrol loaded hyaluronic acid-DPPC microparticles in diabetic rats. *Eur. J. Pharm. Biopharm.* **2017**, *119*, 17–27. [CrossRef] [PubMed]
91. Yurdagul, A.; Kleinedler, J.J.; McInnis, M.C.; Khandelwal, A.R.; Spence, A.L.; Orr, A.W.; Dugas, T.R. Resveratrol promotes endothelial cell wound healing under laminar shear stress through an estrogen receptor-α-dependent pathway. *Am. J. Physiol. Circ. Physiol.* **2014**, *306*, H797–H806. [CrossRef]
92. Yaman, I.; Derici, H.; Kara, C.; Kamer, E.; Diniz, G.; Ortac, R.; Sayin, O. Effects of resveratrol on incisional wound healing in rats. *Surg. Today* **2013**, *43*, 1433–1438. [CrossRef]
93. Brem, H.; Kodra, A.; Golinko, M.S.; Entero, H.; Stojadinovic, O.; Wang, V.M.; Sheahan, C.M.; Weinberg, A.D.; Woo, S.L.; Ehrlich, H.P.; et al. Mechanism of Sustained Release of Vascular Endothelial Growth Factor in Accelerating Experimental Diabetic Healing. *J. Investig. Dermatol.* **2009**, *129*, 2275–2287. [CrossRef]
94. Çetinkalp, Ş.; Gökçe, E.H.; Şimşir, I.; Tanrıverdi, S.T.; Doğan, F.; Avcı, Ç.B.; Eroğlu, I.; Utku, T.; Gündüz, C.; Özer, Ö. Comparative Evaluation of Clinical Efficacy and Safety of Collagen Laminin–Based Dermal Matrix Combined with Resveratrol Microparticles (Dermalix) and Standard Wound Care for Diabetic Foot Ulcers. *Int. J. Low. Extrem. Wounds* **2021**, *20*, 217–226. [CrossRef] [PubMed]
95. Yager, D.R.; Zhang, L.-Y.; Liang, H.-X.; Diegelmann, R.F.; Cohen, I.K. Wound Fluids from Human Pressure Ulcers Contain Elevated Matrix Metalloproteinase Levels and Activity Compared to Surgical Wound Fluids. *J. Investig. Dermatol.* **1996**, *107*, 743–748. [CrossRef] [PubMed]
96. Tarnuzzer, R.W.; Schultz, G.S. Biochemical analysis of acute and chronic wound environments. *Wound Repair Regen.* **1996**, *4*, 321–325. [CrossRef] [PubMed]
97. Khodarahmian, M.; Amidi, F.; Moini, A.; Kashani, L.; Salahi, E.; Danaii-Mehrabad, S.; Nashtaei, M.S.; Mojtahedi, M.F.; Esfandyari, S.; Sobhani, A. A randomized exploratory trial to assess the effects of resveratrol on VEGF and TNF-α 2 expression in endometriosis women. *J. Reprod. Immunol.* **2021**, *143*, 103248. [CrossRef] [PubMed]

98. Bo, S.; Ciccone, G.; Castiglione, A.; Gambino, R.; De Michieli, F.; Villois, P.; Durazzo, M.; Cavallo-Perin, P.; Cassader, M. Anti-Inflammatory and Antioxidant Effects of Resveratrol in Healthy Smokers a Randomized, Double-Blind, Placebo-Controlled, Cross-Over Trial. *Curr. Med. Chem.* **2013**, *20*, 1323–1331. [CrossRef] [PubMed]
99. Tomé-Carneiro, J.; Gonzálvez, M.; Larrosa, M.; Yáñez-Gascón, M.J.; García-Almagro, F.J.; Ruiz-Ros, J.A.; Tomas-Barberan, F.; Conesa, M.T.G.; Espín, J.C. Grape Resveratrol Increases Serum Adiponectin and Downregulates Inflammatory Genes in Peripheral Blood Mononuclear Cells: A Triple-Blind, Placebo-Controlled, One-Year Clinical Trial in Patients with Stable Coronary Artery Disease. *Cardiovasc. Drugs Ther.* **2012**, *27*, 37–48. [CrossRef]
100. Khojah, H.M.; Ahmed, S.; Abdel-Rahman, M.S.; Elhakeim, E.H. Resveratrol as an effective adjuvant therapy in the management of rheumatoid arthritis: A clinical study. *Clin. Rheumatol.* **2018**, *37*, 2035–2042. [CrossRef]
101. Lin, L.X.; Wang, P.; Wang, Y.T.; Huang, Y.; Jiang, L.; Wang, X.M. Aloe Vera and Vitis vinifera improve wound healing in an in vitro rat burn wound model. *Mol. Med. Rep.* **2016**, *13*, 1070–1076. [CrossRef]
102. Eroğlu, I.; Gökçe, E.H.; Tsapis, N.; Tanrıverdi, S.T.; Gökçe, G.; Fattal, E.; Özer, Ö. Evaluation of Characteristics and in vitro antioxidant properties of RSV loaded hyaluronic acid-DPPC microparticles as a wound healing system. *Coll. Surf. B Biointerfaces* **2015**, *126*, 50–57. [CrossRef]
103. Kaleci, B.; Koyuturk, M. Efficacy of resveratrol in wound healing process by reducing oxiudative stress and promoting fibroblast cell proliferation and migration. *Dermatol Ther.* **2022**, *33*, e14357. [CrossRef]
104. Poornima, B.; Korrapati, P.S. Fabrication of chitosan-polycaprolactone composite nanofibrous scaffold for simultaneous delivery of ferulic acid and resveratrol. *Carbohydr. Polym.* **2017**, *157*, 1741–1749. [CrossRef] [PubMed]
105. Huo, X.; Zhang, T.; Meng, Q.; Li, C.; You, B. Resveratrol Effects on a Diabetic Rat Model with Coronary Heart Disease. *Med. Sci. Monit.* **2019**, *25*, 540–546. [CrossRef]
106. Abdelgawad, I.Y.; Grant, M.K.O.; Zordoky, B.N. Leveraging the Cardio-Protective and Anticancer Properties of Resveratrol in Cardio-Oncology. *Nutrients* **2019**, *11*, 627. [CrossRef] [PubMed]
107. Calabrese, E.J.; Mattson, M.P.; Calabrese, V. Resveratrol commonly displays hormesis: Occurrence and biomedical significance. *Hum. Exp. Toxicol.* **2010**, *29*, 980–1015. [CrossRef] [PubMed]
108. Chow, H.H.; Garland, L.L.; Hsu, C.H.; Vining, D.R.; Chew, W.M.; Miller, J.A.; Perloff, M.; Crowell, J.A.; Alberts, D.S. Resveratrol modulates drug- and carcinogen-metabolizing enzymes in a healthy volunteer study. *Cancer Prev. Res.* **2010**, *3*, 1168–1175. [CrossRef]
109. De Leo, A.; Arena, G.; Lacanna, E.; Oliviero, G.; Colavita, F.; Mattia, E. Resveratrol inhibits Epstein Barr Virus lytic cycle in Burkitt's lymphoma cells by affecting multiple molecular targets. *Antivir. Res.* **2012**, *96*, 196–202. [CrossRef]
110. Palomera-Ávalos, V.; Griñán-Ferré, C.; Izquierdo, V.; Camins, A.; Sanfeliu, C.; Canudas, A.M.; Pallàs, M. Resveratrol modulates response against acute inflammatory stimuli in aged mouse brain. *Exp. Gerontol.* **2018**, *102*, 3–11. [CrossRef]
111. Shevelev, A.B.; Isakova, E.P.; Trubnikova, E.V.; La Porta, N.; Martens, S.; Medvedev, O.A.; Trubnikov, D.V.; Akbaev, R.M.; Biryukova, Y.K.; Zylkova, M.V.; et al. A study of antimicrobial activity of polyphenols derived from wood. *Bull. Russ. State Med. Univ.* **2018**, *7*, 46–49. [CrossRef]
112. Shawon, J.; Akter, Z.; Hossen, M.M.; Akter, Y.; Sayeed, A.; Junaid, M.; Afrose, S.S.; Khan, M.A. Current Landscape of Natural Products against Coronaviruses: Perspectives in COVID-19 Treatment and Anti-viral Mechanism. *Curr. Pharm. Des.* **2020**, *26*, 5241–5260. [CrossRef]
113. Gautam, S.; Gautam, A.; Chhetri, S.; Bhattarai, U. Immunity Against COVID-19: Potential Role of Ayush Kwath. *J. Ayurveda Integr. Med.* **2020**, *13*, 100350. [CrossRef]
114. Zhao, X.; Xu, J.; Song, X.; Jia, R.; Yin, Z.; Cheng, A.; Jia, R.; Zou, Y.; Li, L.; Yin, L.; et al. Antiviral effect of resveratrol in ducklings infected with virulent duck enteritis virus. *Antivir. Res.* **2016**, *130*, 93–100. [CrossRef] [PubMed]
115. Lin, S.C.; Ho, C.T.; Chuo, W.H.; Li, S.; Wang, T.T.; Lin, C.C. Effective inhibition of MERS-CoV infection by resveratrol. *BMC Infect. Dis.* **2017**, *17*, 144. [CrossRef] [PubMed]

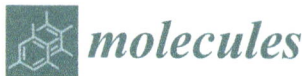

Article

Protective Effect of Flavonoids against Methylglyoxal-Induced Oxidative Stress in PC-12 Neuroblastoma Cells and Its Structure–Activity Relationships

Danyang Zhang [1], Xia Li [1], Xiaoshi He [1], Yan Xing [1], Bo Jiang [1], Zhilong Xiu [1], Yongming Bao [1,2,*] and Yuesheng Dong [1,*]

[1] School of Bioengineering, Dalian University of Technology, Dalian 116024, China
[2] School of Ocean Science and Technology, Dalian University of Technology, Panjin 124221, China
* Correspondence: biosci@dlut.edu.cn (Y.B.); yshdong@dlut.edu.cn (Y.D.)

Abstract: Methylglyoxal-induced oxidative stress and cytotoxicity are the main factors causing neuronal death-related, diabetically induced memory impairment. Antioxidant and anti-apoptotic therapy are potential intervention strategies. In this study, 25 flavonoids with different substructures were assayed for protecting PC-12 cells from methylglyoxal-induced damage. A structure–activity relationship (SAR) analysis indicated that the absence of the double bond at C-2 and C-3, substitutions of the gallate group at the 3 position, the pyrogallol group at the B-ring, and the *R* configuration of the 3 position enhanced the protection of flavan-3-ols, and a hydroxyl substitution at the 4′ and meta-positions were important for the protection of flavonol. These SARs were further confirmed by molecular docking using the active site of the Keap1–Nrf2 complex as the receptor. The mechanistic study demonstrated that EGCG with the lowest EC_{50} protected the PC-12 cells from methylglyoxal-induced damage by reducing oxidative stress via the Nrf2/Keap1/HO-1 and Bcl-2/Bax signaling pathways. These results suggested that flavan-3-ols might be a potential dietary supplement for protection against diabetic encephalopathy.

Keywords: flavonoids; methylglyoxal; PC-12 cells; structure–activity relationship; oxidative stress; molecular docking

Citation: Zhang, D.; Li, X.; He, X.; Xing, Y.; Jiang, B.; Xiu, Z.; Bao, Y.; Dong, Y. Protective Effect of Flavonoids against Methylglyoxal-Induced Oxidative Stress in PC-12 Neuroblastoma Cells and Its Structure–Activity Relationships. *Molecules* 2022, 27, 7804. https://doi.org/10.3390/molecules27227804

Academic Editor: Andrea Ragusa

Received: 17 October 2022
Accepted: 9 November 2022
Published: 12 November 2022

Publisher's Note: MDPI stays neutral with regard to jurisdictional claims in published maps and institutional affiliations.

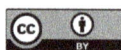

Copyright: © 2022 by the authors. Licensee MDPI, Basel, Switzerland. This article is an open access article distributed under the terms and conditions of the Creative Commons Attribution (CC BY) license (https://creativecommons.org/licenses/by/4.0/).

1. Introduction

Diabetic encephalopathy, a serious diabetic complication of a microvascular nature, is chiefly a consequence of central nervous system disease [1]. It is characterized by mild cognitive decline, which can progress to dementia in severe cases [2]. As reported in the literature, people with diabetes have a 60% higher risk of developing dementia [3]. Moreover, diabetic encephalopathy is tightly associated with long-term hyperglycemia in diabetic patients, owing to oxidative stress [4], inflammation [5], and an abnormal accumulation of advanced glycation end products (AGEs) [6]. Methylglyoxal (MG) is recognized as the most likely AGE precursor contributing to intracellular AGE formation [7].

In vivo, MG is derived from glucose metabolism, amino acid metabolism, fat metabolism, and, most importantly, the glycolysis pathway [8], with a low level under normal circumstances. However, an excessive MG level can be cytotoxic, leading to irreversible cell death [9] owing to an increase in oxidative stress [10]. As we know, it has already been reported that the concentration of MG is abnormally elevated in diabetics [11]. It is also implied that an over accumulation of MG caused by abnormal glucose metabolism is a major cause of diabetic encephalopathy [12]. Therefore, the intervention of oxidative stress is considered an effective strategy for preventing diabetic encephalopathy. Nuclear factor erythroid 2-related factor2 (Nrf2) is described as a master redox-related transcription factor, maintaining intracellular redox homeostasis [13]. When oxidative stress occurs, the binding of Nrf2 and Keap1 becomes unstable, and Nrf2 is released, transferring from the cytoplasm to the nucleus. This, in turn, can activate the expression of downstream antioxidant enzymes, including HO-1, a kind of phase II enzyme [14]. It was verified that the expression of Nrf2 decreased and that of Keap1 increased in HLECs after a treatment of MG [9]. As a result, the damage induced by MG can be alleviated by interventions in the Nrf2/Keap1 pathway.

Recently, it has been accepted that dietary supplementation has become a noteworthy intervention for improving glucose metabolism disorders and cognitive impairment. Flavonoids, a group of phenolic compounds, can be found in many fruits and vegetables, such as apples, scutellaria, celery, and so on [15], which are composed of two aromatic rings (A and B) connected to each other through a central three-carbon chain, generally with C6–C3–C6 as the basic skeleton. Increasing evidence has highlighted that flavonoids have abundant properties, including those anti-diabetic [15], anti-dementia [16], anti-tumor [17], anti-osteoporosis [18], anti-arteriosclerosis [19], antioxidant [15], and so on. The SAR of flavonoids has been studied in a cellular antioxidant activity assay using HepG2 cells [20]. The study clarified that a 3',4'-O-dihydroxyl group in the B-ring, a 2,3-double bond combined with a 4-keto group in the C-ring, and a 3-hydroxyl group enhanced antioxidant capacity to treat cancer. It was also reported that the SAR of grape seed procyanidins against H_2O_2-induced oxidative stress in PC-12 cells could be used to treat neurodegenerative disorders [21]. The authors claimed that there was a positive correlation between the procyanidins' polymerization degree and the protective effect against oxidative stress in PC-12 cells and that the presence of 3-galloylated groups increased the protective activity. However, procyanidins are a kind of flavan-3-ols polymer and the research on the SAR of the flavna-3-ols monomer and other flavonoids in diabetic encephalopathy is not comprehensive.

To the best of our knowledge, a systematic evaluation of the protection offered by flavonoids with different substructures against damage induced by MG in nerve cells has not been reported, and the SAR between the flavonoids and the protective activities against the toxicity of MG in neurons is also scarcely documented. Consequently, the design of dietary supplements for protection against diabetic encephalopathy is urgently required. It was indicated that hesperitin resisted oxidative stress via ER- and TrkA-mediated actions in PC-12 cells [22]. Prior research also showed that dihydromyricetin ameliorated oxidative stress via the AMPK/GLUT4 signaling pathway in MG-induced PC-12 cells [23].

In this study, the protective effects of different kinds of flavonoids against the damage induced by MG in PC-12 cells were determined. The SARs of these flavonoids were also analyzed and summarized. Furthermore, to understand the mechanism, the effects of the flavonoids with the highest activity on the signaling pathway related to oxidative stress were also investigated in the PC-12 cells.

2. Results

2.1. Cytotoxicity of Flavonoids to PC-12 Cells

In order to eliminate the effect of cytotoxicity in the activity assay of the flavonoids, the cytotoxicity test was initially performed using an MTT assay. The results showed that the flavonoid concentrations below 100 μM exhibited no cytotoxicity to PC-12 cells. The consequent protective activity was assayed and the concentration ranged below 100 μM for each flavonoid without apparent cytotoxicity to the PC-12 cells.

2.2. The Protective Activities and SAR Analysis of Different Flavonoids With Respect to the Damage Induced by MG

Concentrations from 0.25 to 4 mM of MG were added to PC-12 cells after they had incubated for 48 h and dose-responses of MG were detected by the MTT assay concerning the effect of MG on the damage to the PC-12 cells. Finally, the IC_{50} value of MG was selected as 0.5 mM after 48 h (Figure S1 in the Supplementary Material), which was chosen based on the PC-12 cells in order to examine the protective effect of the flavonoids in the following study. Curcumin was selected as the positive control (EC_{50} = 1.31 ± 0.42 μM) (Figure S2 in the Supplementary Material). A total of 25 flavonoids consisting of five types—5 flavan-3-ols, 5 flavonols, 2 flavanones, 8 flavones, and 5 isoflavones (Figure 1 and Figure S3 in the Supplementary Material)—were assayed to evaluate their protective effects on the cell viability of the PC-12 cells stimulated by MG using the MTT method. The activities were expressed as EC_{50} [24], and the data were summarized in Table 1. The compounds whose EC_{50} values were less than 100 µM were regarded as active compounds.

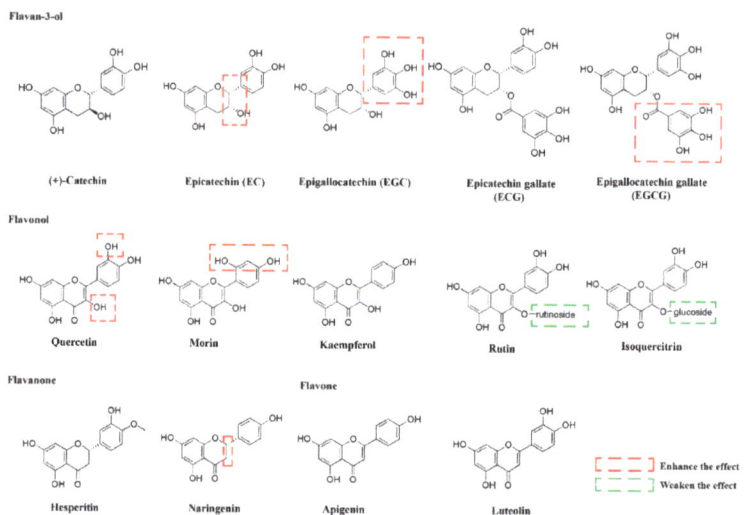

Figure 1. The main flavonoids tested in protective activities against MG-induced PC-12 cells.

Table 1. The protection activities and molecular-docking data of main flavonoids.

	Compound	EC$_{50}$ (µM)	Binding Energy (kJ/mol)	Number of H-Bonds
Flavan-3-ol				
	(+)-Catechin	>100	−24.811	3
	EC	52.34 ± 3.99	−35.313	3
	EGC	43.06 ± 1.18	−35.439	4
	ECG	34.52 ± 2.69	−39.790	5
	EGCG	11.98 ± 0.49	−40.041	8
Flavanone				
	Naringenin	13.35 ± 1.92	−35.271	3
	Hesperitin	48.14 ± 2.31	−34.058	3
Flavonol				
	Kaempferol	>100	−32.719	3
	Quercetin	28.83 ± 2.76	−34.351	4
	Morin	14.83 ± 1.70	−34.895	6
	Isoquercitrin	>100	−22.175	3
	Rutin	>100	−29.079	4
Flavone				
	Luteolin	>100	−33.932	3
	Apigenin	>100	−33.639	3

The values shown are the means ± standard deviation of triplicate assays.

The results indicated that the skeleton structure of the flavonoids had a crucial impact on their protective activities. Generally, most of the compounds in the flavan-3-ol subtypes exhibited the strongest protective activities, followed by the flavanone subtype, and the protective activity of most compounds under the flavonol subtype were weaker than the former two subtypes. In contrast, neither the compounds in the flavonoid subtype nor the isoflavone subtype showed protective activity.

For the subtype of the flavan-3-ols, EGCG and ECG showed stronger protective activities than those of EGC and EC (11.98 ± 0.49 µM vs. 43.06 ± 1.18 µM, and 34.52 ± 2.69 µM vs. 52.34 ± 3.99 µM), suggesting that the gallate group substitution enhanced the protective activity of the MG-treated PC-12 cells. Moreover, it was also crucial for the presence of the pyrogallol substitution on B-ring, since the protective effect of EC was weaker than EGC (52.34 ± 3.99 µM vs. 43.06 ± 1.18 µM) on the MG-induced PC-12 cells. Interestingly, it was found that the configuration of the 3 position in the flavan-3-ols played an important role in their protective activity. All the substitutions at the 3 position with an R configuration (EC, EGC, ECG, and EGCG) showed relatively strong protective activities; that is, no obvious protective activity was found for the (+) catechin, whose substitution at the 3 position was in the S configuration. A previous study also indicated that flavan-3-ols with the galloyl moiety substation and an R configuration at the 3 position had improved antioxidant activity in HepG2 tumor cells [20], suggesting that the substitution of the galloyl moiety and the R configuration at the 3 position are important for the protective activity of flavan-3-ols in different cell lines.

Regarding the flavanone subtype, both tested compounds showed protective activities. In addition, the naringenin showed relatively strong activities (EC$_{50}$ = 13.35 ± 1.92 µM), whereas no obvious activity was observed in apigenin, whose structure is almost identical with naringenin, wherein the only difference is the existence of a double bond between C-2 and C-3. These data were consistent with the result obtained for the flavan-3-ols subtype wherein the absence of a double bond at the C-2 and C-3 position was important to their protective activities. However, it was reported that naringenin did not show obvious activity in a cellular antioxidant activity (CAA) assay of HepG2 cells [20]. These data indicated that the influence of the double bond between C-2 and C-3 in flavanone on its cell protective activity is cell-line-specific. Of course, as the commercially available flavanone subtypes are limited, only two of them were tested for their protective activities. In the future, other SARs—besides the importance of the bond type between the C-2 and C-3—need to be summarized after the assaying of more flavanones with respect to their protective activities in the MG-treated PC-12 cells.

For the flavonol subtype, quercetin showed higher activities (EC$_{50}$ = 28.83 ± 2.76 µM) than luteolin (EC$_{50}$ > 100 µM). Meanwhile, the substitution of the hydroxyl group at the 3 position with a glycosyl group weakened flavonol's protective activities; for example, the substitutions of the hydroxyl group at the 3 position in quercetin with either glucosidase (isoquercitrin) or rutinosidase (rutin) nullified flavonol's protective activities. These results demonstrated the importance of the hydroxyl group substitution at the 3 position on the C-ring. The hydroxyl group substitution on the other position also influenced its protective activities: higher activities of quercetin (EC$_{50}$ = 28.83 ± 2.76 µM) than kaempferol (EC$_{50}$ > 100 µM) indicated that the 4'-hydroxyl group played an important part when the 3'-hydroxyl group was present. Moreover, it was clarified that meta-hydroxyl groups are stronger than the ortho-hydroxyl groups on the B-ring by comparing morin (EC$_{50}$ = 14.83 ± 1.70 µM) to quercetin (EC$_{50}$ = 28.83 ± 2.76 µM). However, quercetin showed stronger activity than morin in the CAA assay [20]; thus, its mechanism needs to be further explored.

2.3. Molecular Docking Study

To further explain the SARs of the flavonoids, in silico docking studies were performed using Autodock software. Consequently, it was suggested that the Keap1–Nrf2 complex was the target protein that the drug interacted with in the antioxidative signaling pathway [25]; therefore, the Keap1–Nrf2 complex (PDB ID: 2FLU [25]) was selected as the receptor in the docking study. For the subtype of the flavan-3-ols, the binding energy and the hydrogen bonds of the major flavonoids with the complex were calculated and summarized in Table 1. For the binding energy, EGCG showed the lowest binding energy

(−40.041 kJ/mol), followed by ECG, EGC, and EC, and (+)-Catechin showed the highest binding energy. The protective activities and binding energy showed the same tendency, which supported the importance of the gallate and pyrogallol groups' substitution as well as the 3 position in the flavan-3-ols found in the SAR analysis. The results of the SAR analysis in the assay could also be confirmed by hydrogen bond data (Table 1). In the best conformation of EGCG (Figure 2A), a gallic acid substituent formed five of the eight hydrogen bonds (H-bond) with three amino acids in the binding pocket (Val 561, Arg 326, and Val 369), and the hydroxyl groups on the basic skeleton formed the rest of the three hydrogen bonds with the other three amino acids in the binding pocket (Val 467, Val 418, and Val 420). Similarly, compared with EGCG, EGC, whose structure lacked a gallic acid substituent, was predicted to only form four H-bonds between the hydroxyl groups in the 3 position and B ring and with Val 418, Leu 557, and Val 604, which demonstrated that the presence of a gallic acid substituent could increase the activities in question (Figure 2A). The actual EC_{50} and predicted binding energy are presented in Figure S4, and a good linear correlation ($R^2 = 0.7084$) was observed. The binding energy reflected the neuroprotective activity against MG-induced damage and provided information for further drug screening.

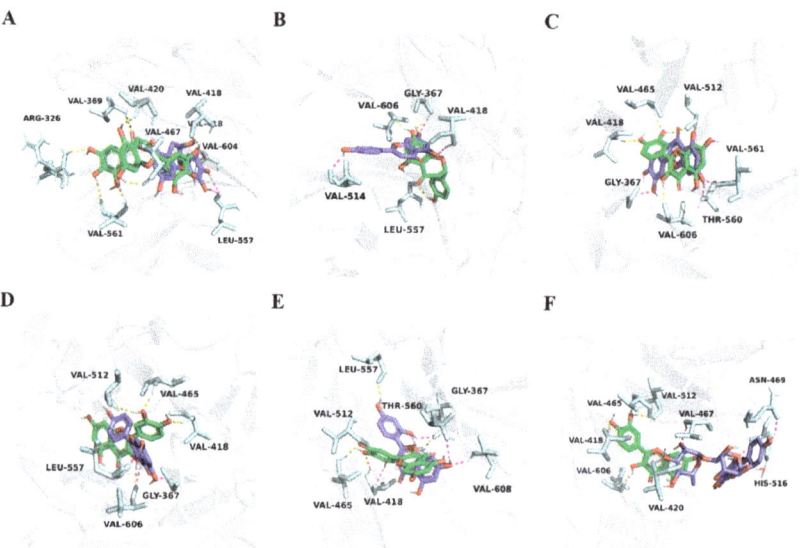

Figure 2. EGCG ((**A**) in green), EGC ((**A**) in purple), Naringenin ((**B**) in green), Apigenin ((**B**) in purple), Quercetin ((**C–F**) in green), Luteolin ((**C**) in purple), Kaempferol ((**D**) in purple), Morin ((**E**) in purple), and Rutin ((**F**) in purple) in the binding site of Keap1–Nrf2 complex. (PDB ID: 2FLU). The figure was generated using PyMol (http://pymol.sourceforge.net/) (accessed on 5 July 2022).

For the flavanone subtype, the binding energies of naringenin and apigenin were calculated as −35.271 kJ/mol and −33.639 kJ/mol, respectively, which also showed the same tendency with the assay. The H-bond data indicated that both the two compounds formed three H-bonds with the amino acids. Naringenin formed H-bonds with Gly 367, Val 606, and Leu 557 (Figure 2B), while apigenin formed H-bonds with Val 514, Gly 367, and Val 418(Figure 2B). It was supposed that a single bond in naringenin could be twisted, thus alternating the docked position, which affected the binding energy.

For the flavonol subtype, quercetin showed a relatively lower binding energy of −34.351 kJ/mol, forming four H-bonds between hydroxyl groups and amino acid residue; for instance, the 3′-hydroxyl group formed two hydrogen bonds with Val 465 and Val 512, the 3-hydroxyl group formed one hydrogen bond with Val 606, and another hydrogen bond formed between the 4′- hydroxyl group and Val 418 (Figure 2C). On the contrary, both luteolin (Figure 2C) and kaempferol (Figure 2D), which lack the 3-hydroxyl and 3′-hydroxyl groups, respectively, only formed three H-bonds and, consequently, showed higher binding energy. Moreover, it was calculated that morin had a lower binding energy than quercetin, namely, −34.895 kJ/mol, which might be because morin formed two key H-bonds between the 2′- hydroxyl group with Val 606 and Gly 367 (Figure 2E). On the other hand, compared with quercetin, the docking data indicated that the binding energies were higher in rutin (Figure 2F) and isoquercitrin, which might be due to the glycoside group substitution that blocked the entry of the compounds into the binding pocket. All these docking results were consistent with the assay data, and further confirmed the importance of the substitution of hydroxyl groups in the 2′, 3′, and 3 positions in the flavonol subtype.

In this study, the use of MG-induced PC-12 cells through an in vitro method were established to test the neuroprotective activity of the flavonoids, and a silicon molecular-docking method using the Keap1–Nrf2 complex as the receptor was used to further verify the SAR analysis. The in vitro assay and the silicon showed almost the same tendency. These results suggested that the docking of the test compounds with the Keap1–Nrf2 complex prior to the in vitro assay might constitute an alternative method for the neuroprotective assay, which could lower costs and greatly increase efficiency. On the other hand, only 25 flavonoids were tested in our study; thus, more flavonoids need to be tested to verify the results of the SAR analysis.

2.4. The Mechanism of EGCG on MG-Induced Oxidative Stress and Apoptosis in PC-12 Neuroblastoma Cells

Previous studies and our docking experiments demonstrated that the Nrf2-Keap1 complex and antioxidants play an important role in the protective activities of the flavonoids against the nerve cell damage induced by MG. Thus, the mechanism of the flavonoids against MG-induced oxidative stress in PC-12 neuroblastoma cells was studied through a Western blot analysis of the Nrf2/Keap1/HO-1 signaling pathway. As it was shown, after the MG treatment, the expression of HO-1 decreased, while the expression of Keap1 noticeably increased. However, EGCG significantly promoted the expression of HO-1 and inhibited the expression of Keap1 in a dose-dependent manner (Figure 3A–D). Meanwhile, the results showed that EGCG induced the nuclear translocation of Nrf2 (Figure 3E,F). This suggested that the intervention of the Nrf2/Keap1/HO-1 pathway, which is closely related to oxidative stress, is one of the key mechanisms of EGCG-mediated neuroprotection against MG-induced PC-12 cells.

Oxidative stress can cause neuronal apoptosis [26]. To investigate the effect of EGCG on the MG-induced PC-12 cells' apoptosis, PC-12 cells were co-cultured with EGCG in an MG-containing medium. The flow cytometry results showed that MG-induced PC-12 cells' apoptosis was markedly rescued by EGCG (Figure 4A). Moreover, the Bcl-2 family members are also of importance in oxidative stress-mediated neuronal death, especially the ratio of Bcl-2 to Bax [7,27]. It is the crucial marker of differentiating anti- or pro-apoptotic effects. Thus, the effects of EGCG on Bcl-2 and Bax were also investigated. The results showed that, after being treated with MG for 48h, the expression of Bax increased and that of Bcl-2 decreased. Moreover, the quantitative analysis implied that EGCG increased the ratio of Bcl-2 to Bax in a dose-dependent manner (Figure 4B,C). This was a strong indication that the decrease in the ratio of Bax and Bcl-2 caused by EGCG contributed to the prevention of MG-induced cell death.

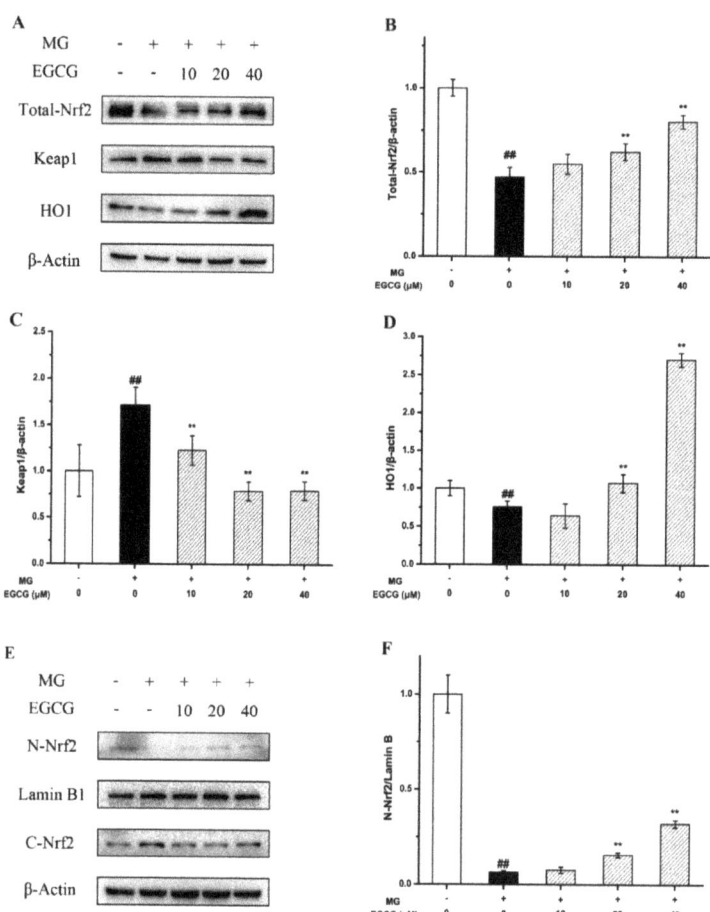

Figure 3. Effects of EGCG on MG-induced PC-12 cells of the Nrf2/Keap1/HO-1 pathway. (**A–D**) Western blot results and statistical analysis of the expression levels of Nrf2, Keap1, and HO1. (**E,F**) Western blot results and statistical analysis of the expression levels of nuclear Nrf2. Data shown are the mean ± SD of three independent experiments. ## $p < 0.01$ compared with the control. ** $p < 0.01$ compared with the MG group.

Oxidative stress, caused by hyperglycemia and accelerating neuronal apoptosis, is also a major event in neurodegenerative disorders, which is usually a noticeable cause of diabetic complications [28]. Quercetin has been reported to reduce oxidative stress levels, activate SIRT1, and inhibit ER pathways from potentiating cognitive dysfunction [29]. Morin exhibited neuroprotective effects via the TrkB/Akt pathway against diabetes-mediated oxidative stress and apoptosis in neuronal cells. Therefore, an intervention addressing oxidative stress and neuronal apoptosis [30] is considered an essential strategy to prevent diabetic encephalopathy.

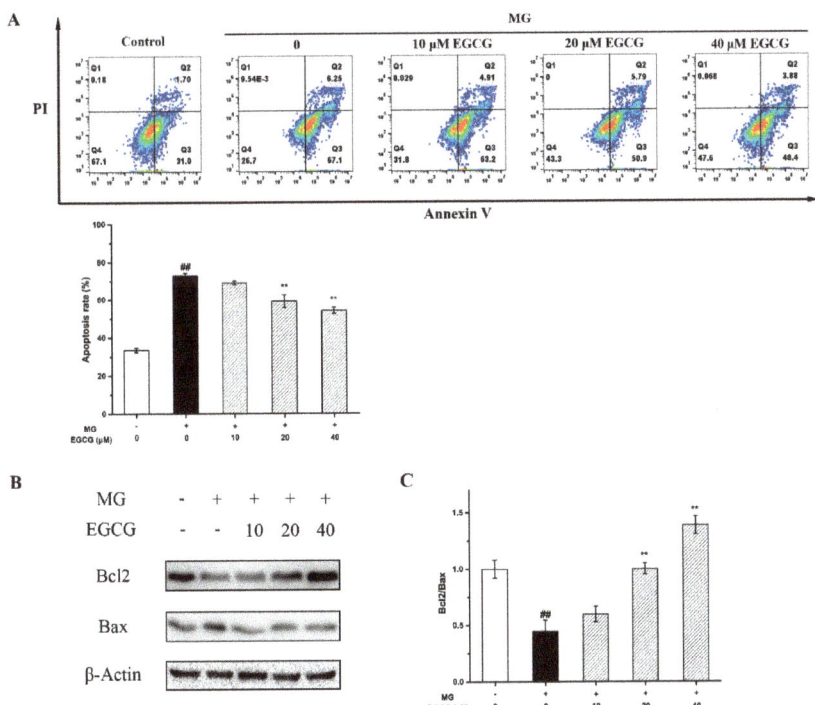

Figure 4. Effects of EGCG on MG-induced PC-12 cells' apoptosis. (**A**) Analysis of cell apoptosis by flow cytometry. (**B**) Western blot results of the expression levels of Bcl2 and Bax. (**C**) Statistical analysis of the expression levels of the ratio of Bcl2 and Bax. Data shown are the mean ± SD of three independent experiments. ## $p < 0.01$ compared with the control.** $p < 0.01$ compared with the MG group.

3. Materials and Methods

3.1. Reagents and Antibodies

All flavonoids (≥98% Purity) were purchased from Sichuan Weikeqi Biological Technology (Chengdu, China), and were dissolved at a concentration of 100 mM in DMSO as a stock solution (stored at −20 °C). The solution was then further diluted in cell culture medium to create working concentrations. Methylglyoxal was obtained from Aladdin. Antibodies against Bcl-2, Bax, HO-1, β-actin, and Lamin B1 were purchased from Proteintech (Wuhan, China). Antibodies against Nrf2 and Keap1 were purchased from Beyotime Biotechnology (Beijing, China). The secondary anti-rabbit or anti-mouse HRP-conjugated antibodies were purchased from Proteintech (Wuhan, China).

3.2. Cell Culture and Treatment

Rat pheochromocytoma PC-12 cells were provided by Chinese Academy of Sciences Cell Bank (Shanghai, China) and cultured in RPMI 1640 supplemented with 10% fetal bovine serum (FBS), 100 g/mL streptomycin, and 100 IU/mL penicillin in a humidified 5% CO_2 atmosphere at 37 °C. Cells were co-cultured with 0.5 mM MG and flavonoids for 48 h.

3.3. Analysis of Cell Viability

The proliferative activity of flavonoids on PC-12 cells was determined by 3-(4, 5-Dimethyl-2-thiazolyl)-2, 5-diphenyl-2H-tetrazolium bromide (MTT) assay. Cells were cultured in 96-well plates with 1×10^4 cells per well for overnight incubation and were treated with flavonoids co-cultured with methylglyoxal for 48 h. Then, the old medium was removed and the residual medium with drugs was washed away using sodium phosphate buffer (PBS). Afterwards, 100 μL of MTT solution diluted in fresh medium was added per well and the cells were incubated at 37 °C for another 4 h. After removal of the medium, 100 μL DMSO was added per well to dissolve the formazan crystals. When fully dissolved, the absorbance at 570 nm was measured by a microplate reader (Thermo Fisher Scientific, Waltham, MA, USA) and absorbance at 630 nm as reference.

3.4. Western Blot Analysis

Cells were lysed in RIPA buffer with protease inhibitor cocktail (MedChemExpress) after the treatment with MG and EGCG. Protein concentration was determined by BCA protein assay kit (Solarbio, Beijing, China). Same amounts of proteins were separated by SDS-polyacrylamide gel electrophoresis and transferred onto PVDF membranes (Merck Millipore, Darmstadt, Germany). The membranes were blocked with 5% skim milk for 2 h, followed by overnight incubation at 4 °C with primary antibodies Nrf2, Keap1, HO1, Bcl-2, Bax, β-actin, and Lamin B1. The membranes were washed with TBST three times, and then incubated with secondary antibodies (1:2000 dilution) for 1 h at room temperature. Finally, the bands were visualized using an ECL kit (Solarbio, China).

3.5. Molecular Docking

Molecular docking was performed to predict the binding sites and efficacy between Keap1–Nrf2 complex and EGCG using AutodockTools1.5.6. The crystal structure of Keap1–Nrf2 complex (PDB: 2FLU) was downloaded from the Protein Data Bank (www.rcsb.org, accessed on 16 October 2022). Before docking, water molecules were removed from protein file 2FLU. A grid box size of 166 × 140 × 134 points with a spacing of 0.431 Å between grid points was generated to cover almost the entire favorable protein binding site. The X, Y, and Z centers were 16.401, 16.672, and 7.238, respectively. In addition, the settings are as follows: maximum energy evaluation number = 25,000,000; number of generations = 27,000; mutation rate = 0.02.

3.6. Flow Cytometry

Cell apoptosis was detected by flow cytometry (BD Accuri C6, USA), wherein PC-12 cells were placed in 60mm plates and stained with PI and Annexin V-fluorescein isothiocyanate (FITC) according to manufacturer's protocols (Elabscience Annexin V-FITC/PI Apoptosis Kit). The apoptotic PC-12 cells were analyzed with FlowJo_V10.8.1.

3.7. Statistical Analysis

All experiments were performed three times. Data are presented as mean ± standard deviation (SD). SPSS 22.0 software was used for statistical analysis, and the significant difference was determined by one-way analysis of variance (ANOVA). $p < 0.05$ was considered statistically significant.

4. Conclusions

In conclusion, 25 flavonoids were evaluated for their protective activity of MG-induced PC-12 cells, and the SARs analyses obtained from the assay and molecular docking data indicated that gallate and pyrogallol groups, the configuration of the 3 position in flavan-3-ol, and some positions of the hydroxyl group's substitution in flavonol were crucial for their activities. The mechanistic study demonstrated that EGCG, the most active compound among the test flavonoids, showed neuroprotective effects that were mediated by antioxidant and anti-apoptotic activities induced via the Nrf2/Keap1/HO-1 and Bcl-2/Bax pathways. Our studies may provide a method for rapidly screening neuroprotective antioxidants, which would contribute to the development of diabetic encephalopathy treatments.

Supplementary Materials: The following supporting information can be downloaded at: https://www.mdpi.com/article/10.3390/molecules27227804/s1, Figure S1: Cell viability of PC-12 cells treated by MG. * $p < 0.05$ and ** $p < 0.01$ compared with the control; Figure S2: Cell viability of MG-induced PC-12 cells treated by curcumin. * $p < 0.05$ and ** $p < 0.01$ compared with the MG group; Figure S3: Other flavonoids tested in protective activities on MG-induced PC12 cells; Figure S4: The linear correlation between binding energy of main flavan 3-ols (EC, EGC, ECG, EGCG) and the EC_{50} for MG-induced PC-12 cells.

Author Contributions: Conceptualization, Y.D. and Y.B.; methodology, D.Z. and Y.X.; validation, X.L. and X.H.; investigation, D.Z.; resources, Y.B. and B.J.; writing—original draft preparation, D.Z.; writing—review and editing, Y.D.; supervision, Z.X.; project administration, Y.D.; funding acquisition, Y.D. All authors have read and agreed to the published version of the manuscript.

Funding: This research was funded by Fundamental Research Funds for the Central Universities (No. DUT21ZD208, DUT22YG203 and DUT22YG129).

Institutional Review Board Statement: Not applicable.

Informed Consent Statement: Not applicable.

Data Availability Statement: Not applicable.

Conflicts of Interest: The authors declare no conflict of interest.

References

1. Northam, E.A.; Rankins, D.; Lin, A.; Wellard, R.M.; Pell, G.S.; Finch, S.J.; Werther, G.A.; Cameron, F.J. Central Nervous System Function in Youth with Type 1 Diabetes 12 Years After Disease Onset. *Diabetes Care* **2009**, *32*, 445–450. [CrossRef] [PubMed]
2. Kuhad, A.; Chopra, K. Curcumin attenuates diabetic encephalopathy in rats: Behavioral and biochemical evidences. *Eur. J. Pharmacol.* **2007**, *576*, 34–42. [CrossRef] [PubMed]
3. Chatterjee, S.; Peters, S.; Woodward, M.; Arango, S.M.; Huxley, R.R. Type 2 Diabetes as a Risk Factor for Dementia in Women Compared with Men: A Pooled Analysis of 2.3 Million People Comprising More Than 100,000 Cases of Dementia. *Diabetes Care* **2016**, *39*, 300–307. [CrossRef] [PubMed]
4. Liu, D.; Chan, S.L.; de Souza-Pinto, N.C.; Slevin, J.R.; Wersto, R.P.; Zhan, M.; Mustafa, K.; de Cabo, R.; Mattson, M.P. Mitochondrial UCP4 mediates an adaptive shift in energy metabolism and increases the resistance of neurons to metabolic and oxidative stress. *Neuromol. Med.* **2006**, *8*, 389–413. [CrossRef]
5. Kierdorf, K.; Wang, Y.; Neumann, H. Immune-mediated CNS damage. *Results Probl. Cell Differ.* **2009**, *51*, 173–196.
6. Sugimoto, K.; Nishizawa, Y.; Horiuchi, S.; Yagihashi, S. Localization in human diabetic peripheral nerve of Nε-carboxymethyllysine-protein adducts, an advanced glycation endproduct. *Diabetologia* **1997**, *40*, 1380–1387. [CrossRef] [PubMed]
7. Arriba, S.; Stuchbury, G.; Yarin, J.; Burnell, J.; Münch, G. Methylglyoxal impairs glucose metabolism and leads to energy depletion in neuronal cells–protection by carbonyl scavengers. *Neurobiol. Aging* **2007**, *28*, 1044–1050. [CrossRef]
8. Maessen, D.E.M.; Stehouwer, C.D.A.; Schalkwijk, C.G. The role of methylglyoxal and the glyoxalase system in diabetes and other age-related diseases. *Clin. Sci.* **2015**, *128*, 839–861. [CrossRef]
9. Palsamy, P.; Bidasee, K.R.; Ayaki, M.; Augusteyn, R.C.; Chan, J.Y.; Shinohara, T. Methylglyoxal induces endoplasmic reticulum stress and DNA demethylation in the Keap1 promoter of human lens epithelial cells and age-related cataracts. *Free Radic. Biol. Med.* **2014**, *72*, 134–148. [CrossRef]
10. Ota, K.; Nakamura, J.; Li, W.; Kozakae, M.; Watarai, A.; Nakamura, N.; Yasuda, Y.; Nakashima, E.; Naruse, K.; Watabe, K.; et al. Metformin prevents methylglyoxal-induced apoptosis of mouse Schwann cells. *Biochem. Biophys. Res. Commun.* **2007**, *357*, 270–275. [CrossRef] [PubMed]
11. Thornalley, P.J.; Langborg, A.; Minhas, H.S. Formation of glyoxal, methylglyoxal and 3-deoxyglucosone in the glycation of proteins by glucose. *Biochem. J.* **1999**, *344*, 109–116. [CrossRef]
12. Liu, P.; Yin, Z.; Chen, M.; Huang, C.; Wu, Z.; Huang, J.; Ou, S.; Zheng, J. Cytotoxicity of adducts formed between quercetin and methylglyoxal in PC-12 cells. *Food Chem.* **2021**, *352*, 129424. [CrossRef] [PubMed]
13. Mmk, A.; Smh, B.; Ams, C.; Ay, A. Ameliorate impacts of scopoletin against vancomycin-induced intoxication in rat model through modulation of Keap1-Nrf2/HO-1 and IκBα-P65 NF-κB/P38 MAPK signaling pathways: Molecular study, molecular docking evidence and network pharmacology analysis. *Int. Immunopharmacol.* **2021**, *102*, 108382.
14. Su, J.; Yen, J.; Li, S.; Weng, C.; Lin, M.; Ho, C.; Wu, M. 3′,4′-Didemethylnobiletin induces phase II detoxification gene expression and modulates PI3K/Akt signaling in PC12 cells. *Free. Radic. Biol. Med.* **2012**, *52*, 126–141. [CrossRef] [PubMed]
15. Hoyer, S. Oxidative metabolism deficiencies in brains of patients with Alzheimer's disease. *Acta Neurol. Scand.* **2015**, *94*, 18–24. [CrossRef]
16. Spencer, J.P.E.; Vafeiadou, K.; Williams, R.J.; Vauzour, D. Neuroinflammation: Modulation by flavonoids and mechanisms of action. *Mol. Asp. Med.* **2012**, *33*, 83–97. [CrossRef]

17. Ponte, L.; Pavan, I.; Mancini, M.; Silva, L.D.; Morelli, A.; Severino, M.; Bezerra, R.; Simabuco, F. The Hallmarks of Flavonoids in Cancer. *Molecules* **2021**, *26*, 2029. [CrossRef]
18. Xie, C.L.; Park, K.H.; Kang, S.S.; Cho, K.M.; Lee, D.H. Isoflavone-enriched soybean leaves attenuate ovariectomy-induced osteoporosis in rats by anti-inflammatory activity. *J. Sci. Food Agric.* **2020**, *101*, 1499–1506. [CrossRef] [PubMed]
19. Xue, X.; Deng, Y.; Wang, J.; Zhou, M.; Liao, L.; Wang, C.; Peng, C.; Li, Y. Hydroxysafflor yellow A, a natural compound from Carthamus tinctorius L with good effect of alleviating atherosclerosis. *Phytomedicine* **2021**, *91*, 153694. [CrossRef]
20. Wolfe, K.L.; Liu, R.H. Structure-activity relationships of flavonoids in the cellular antioxidant activity assay. *J. Agric. Food Chem.* **2008**, *56*, 8404–8411. [CrossRef] [PubMed]
21. Luo, L.X.; Bai, R.F.; Zhao, Y.Q.; Li, J.; Wei, Z.M. Protective Effect of Grape Seed Procyanidins against H_2O_2-Induced Oxidative Stress in PC-12 Neuroblastoma Cells: Structure-Activity Relationships. *J. Food Sci.* **2018**, *83*, 2622–2628. [CrossRef]
22. Hwang, S.L.; Yen, G.C. Effect of Hesperetin against Oxidative Stress via ER- and TrkA-Mediated Actions in PC12 Cells. *J. Agric. Food Chem.* **2011**, *59*, 5779–5785. [CrossRef] [PubMed]
23. Jiang, B.; Liang, L.; Pan, H.; Hu, K.; Xiao, P. Dihydromyricetin ameliorates the oxidative stress response induced by methylglyoxal via the AMPK/GLUT4 signaling pathway in PC12 cells. *Brain Res. Bull.* **2014**, *109*, 117–126. [CrossRef] [PubMed]
24. Zhang, R.R.; Hu, R.D.; Lu, X.Y.; Ding, X.Y.; Zhang, S.J. Polyphenols from the flower of Hibiscus syriacus Linn ameliorate neuroinflammation in LPS-treated SH-SY5Y cell. *Biomed. Pharmacother.* **2020**, *130*, 110517. [CrossRef] [PubMed]
25. Jnoff, E.; Albrecht, C.; Barker, J.J.; Barker, O.; Beaumont, E.; Bromidge, S.; Brookfield, F.; Brooks, M.; Bubert, C.; Ceska, T. Inside Cover: Binding Mode and Structure-Activity Relationships around Direct Inhibitors of the Nrf2-Keap1 Complex. *ChemMedChem* **2014**, *9*, 674. [CrossRef]
26. Chen, Z.; Zhong, C. Oxidative stress in Alzheimer's disease. *Neurosci. Bull.* **2014**, *30*, 271–281. [CrossRef]
27. Song, J.H.; Shin, M.; Hwang, G.S.; Oh, S.T.; Hwang, J.J.; Kang, K.S. Chebulinic acid attenuates glutamate-induced HT22 cell death by inhibiting oxidative stress, calcium influx and MAPKs phosphorylation. *Bioorganic Med. Chem. Lett.* **2018**, *28*, 249–253. [CrossRef]
28. Xu, Y.; Hua, Z.; Zhu, Q. The Impact of Microbiota-Gut-Brain Axis on Diabetic Cognition Impairment. *Front. Aging Neurosci.* **2017**, *9*, 106. [CrossRef]
29. Hu, T.; Shi, J.J.; Fang, J.; Wang, Q.; Chen, Y.B.; Zhang, S.J. Quercetin ameliorates diabetic encephalopathy through SIRT1/ER stress pathway in db/db mice. *Aging* **2020**, *12*, 7015–7029. [CrossRef]
30. Shyma, R.L.; Mini, S. Neuroprotective effect of Morin via TrkB/Akt pathway against diabetes mediated oxidative stress and apoptosis in neuronal cells. *Toxicol. Mech. Methods* **2022**, *32*, 695–704. [CrossRef]

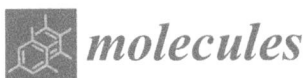

Article

Therapeutic Effects of Gallic Acid in Regulating Senescence and Diabetes; an In Vitro Study

Mahban Rahimifard [1], Maryam Baeeri [1,*], Haji Bahadar [2], Shermineh Moini-Nodeh [1], Madiha Khalid [1], Hamed Haghi-Aminjan [3], Hossein Mohammadian [1,4] and Mohammad Abdollahi [1,4,*]

1. Toxicology and Diseases Group, Pharmaceutical Sciences Research Center (PSRC), The Institute of Pharmaceutical Sciences (TIPS), Tehran University of Medical Sciences, Tehran 1417613151, Iran; mahban.rahimifard@gmail.com (M.R.); sherminehmoeini@gmail.com (S.M.-N.); madihakhalid777@gmail.com (M.K.); mr.hosein73@gmail.com (H.M.)
2. Institute of Paramedical Sciences, Khyber Medical University, Peshawar 25120, Pakistan; hajipharmacist@gmail.com
3. Pharmaceutical Sciences Research Center, Ardabil University of Medical Sciences, Ardabil 5618953141, Iran; hamedhaghi.a@gmail.com
4. Department of Toxicology and Pharmacology, School of Pharmacy, Tehran University of Medical Sciences, Tehran 1417614411, Iran
* Correspondence: m-baeeri@tums.ac.ir (M.B.); mohammad@TUMS.Ac.Ir (M.A.)

Academic Editors: Andrea Ragusa and Luciano Saso
Received: 22 October 2020; Accepted: 9 December 2020; Published: 11 December 2020

Abstract: Gallic acid (GA), a plant-derived ubiquitous secondary polyphenol metabolite, can be a useful dietary supplement. This in vitro study's primary purpose was to assess the anti-aging properties of GA using rat embryonic fibroblast (REF) cells, antidiabetic effects via pancreatic islet cells, and finally, elucidating the molecular mechanisms of this natural compound. REF and islet cells were isolated from fetuses and pancreas of rats, respectively. Then, several senescence-associated molecular and biochemical parameters, along with antidiabetic markers, were investigated. GA caused a significant decrease in the β-galactosidase activity and reduced inflammatory cytokines and oxidative stress markers in REF cells. GA reduced the G0/G1 phase in senescent REF cells that led cells to G2/M. Besides, GA improved the function of the β cells. Flow cytometry and spectrophotometric analysis showed that it reduces apoptosis via inhibiting caspase-9 activity. Taken together, based on the present findings, this polyphenol metabolite at low doses regulates different pathways of senescence and diabetes through its antioxidative stress potential and modulation of mitochondrial complexes activities.

Keywords: antioxidant; diabetes; gallic acid; polyphenol; secondary metabolite; senescence

1. Introduction

Reactive oxygen species (ROS) are oxygen-containing chemically reactive species, such as superoxide, peroxide, and hydroxyl radicals. The dismutation of superoxide generates hydrogen peroxide (H_2O_2), which reduces the generation of hydroxyl radical and hydroxide ions. The generation of such free radicals induces oxidative stress that leads to DNA, lipid, and protein damages [1]. ROS are typically generated during the ordinary course of cellular functions such as mitochondrial respiration. Thus, the mitochondrial organelle is a leading ROS generation site and the primary target of such free radicals. ROS is also generated in the body through exposure to chemicals, chemotherapeutic agents, toxins, and toxicants, environmentally [2–4].

Moreover, the inflammatory cytokines and cytosolic enzymes contribute to ROS generation [5]. One of the main long-term consequences of increasing ROS generation in the body is aging. Aging is a morphological and physiological deterioration and changes occurring in the body with time. Several factors, including the generation of free radicals, are responsible for aging. Despite several advancements in this area, the exact molecular mechanism responsible for the aging process remains unclear [6]. According to the free radical theory of aging described by Denham Harman, free radicals, especially ROS, play an essential role in all steps of aging [7]. According to the free radical theory of aging, ROS's continuous production induces oxidative damage to macromolecules, disrupts physiological functions, and shortens the life span [8,9]. In the meantime, the generation of ROS is linked with the pathogenesis of chronic diseases such as cancer, atherosclerosis, inflammatory disorders, etc. Oxidative damage induced by the ROS disrupts the normal beta cells' function, causes insulin resistance, and impairs glucose tolerance, leading to type 2 diabetes mellitus (T2DM) [10]. Studies have shown an increase in oxidative stress biomarkers in the pancreas of diabetic patients [11,12]. Likewise, ROS-mediated oxidative stress injury is the primary risk factor in the inception and progression of type 1 diabetes mellitus (T1DM) [13]. Several studies have been accomplished to evaluate an efficient and therapeutically safe antioxidant against ROS. Only a few natural and synthetic antioxidants have been developed as medicine due to their therapeutic efficacy with minimal side effects [14].

Gallic acid (GA), or 3,4,5-trihydroxy benzoic acid, is a plant-derived polyphenolic compound. It has demonstrated antidiabetic function in an animal model [14]. GA is abundantly present in different berries, fruits, and grapes as endogenous plant phenol. Wine also contains GA [15]. Several animal studies have shown the antioxidant property and therapeutic activity of GA in reducing hyperglycemia after oral administration of GA to diabetic rats. The oxidative stress biomarkers and parameters were also significantly reduced [16–19]. GA can improve neurological dysfunction by acting directly on the nerve and glial cells [20]. Also, it boosts the natural antioxidant machinery of the body against ROS. Therefore, the ROS-mediated aging process is slowed down or even averted. Besides, new GA features, such as inhibition of aldose reductase, have been reported [21]. Although GA is believed to have a low risk of side effects, doses greater than 1.02 mg/kg might have teratogenic properties and pose a threat to the fetus in pregnant women [22]. So, choosing the best concentration and dose for GA is an essential concern in the studies.

The purpose of this in vitro study is to evaluate the attenuating property of GA in H_2O_2-induced aging using the rat's embryonic fibroblast (REF) cells. The level of oxidative stress biomarkers was measured to determine the protective effect of GA in the isolated pancreatic islet cells. Furthermore, the optimum dose of GA is determined, i.e., required for the survival and function of pancreatic islet cells in an ex vivo model. StatsDirect 3.3.4 was used to calculate the statistics.

2. Results

2.1. Identification of Half Maximal Effective Voncentration (EC_{50}) of Gallic Acid

The 3-(4,5-Dimethylthiazol-2-yl)-2,5-diphenyltetrazolium bromide (MTT) assay showed that the concentration of GA resulted in a 150% viability of cells compared to the control group (Figure 1). All concentrations of GA were found safe without any toxic effect. The 1000 µM of GA demonstrated a significant increase in the REF cell viability with $p < 0.001$ (Figure 1A). In contrast, 100 and 1000 µM of GA represented a significant increase in pancreatic islet cells' viability, with $p < 0.05$ and $p < 0.001$, respectively (Figure 1B). EC_{50} values of GA found 554.25 and 400 µM for REF and pancreatic islet cells, respectively.

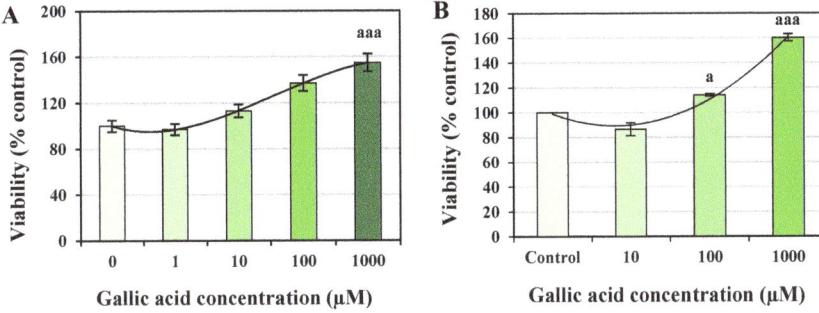

Figure 1. Effect of different concentrations of gallic acid (GA) on the viability of rat's embryonic fibroblast (REF) (**A**) and pancreatic islet cells (**B**). The MTT assay was performed after 24 h of exposure to determine the EC_{50} of GA. The EC_{50} of GA on REF and pancreatic islet cells was calculated as 554.25 and 400 µM, respectively. Data are presented as the mean ± standard error of measurements performed on six groups, with three independent replicates; [a] $p < 0.05$; [aaa] $p < 0.001$.

2.2. Anti-Ageing Effect of GA

(a) β-galactosidase concentration: REF cells treated with H_2O_2 represented a significant increase in β-galactosidase concentration compared to the control group ($p < 0.001$). In contrast, GA and H_2O_2 + GA treatment of REF cells showed a significant reduction in the β-galactosidase concentration compared to the H_2O_2 group ($p < 0.001$, Figure 2).

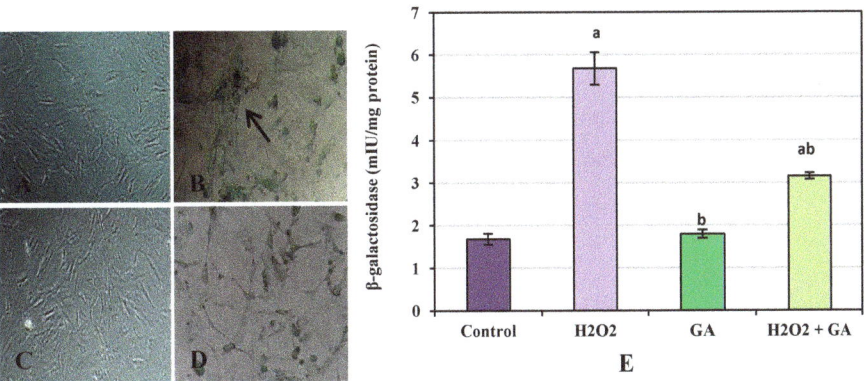

Figure 2. β-galactosidase assay in rat embryonic fibroblast cells (200× magnification). Control (**A**), H_2O_2 (**B**), Gallic acid (**C**), H_2O_2 + Gallic acid (**D**). Quantitative data of β-galactosidase assay are shown in graph (**E**). Data are presented as the mean ± standard error of measurements performed on six groups, with three independent replicates. [a] Significant difference from control ($p < 0.001$), [b] significant difference from H_2O_2 ($p < 0.001$). Arrow indicates senescent cells.

(b) Cell cycle analysis: The cell cycle distribution of REF cells was determined after treatment of GA and H_2O_2 alone and in combinations. The status of REF cells in three phases of the cell cycle, including G0/G1, S, and G2/M, was interpreted (Figure 3). The population of control REF cells in G0/G1, S, and G2/M phases was 78.75% ± 1.97%, 5.10% ± 0.24%, and 16.15% ± 0.75%, respectively. Comparative to the control group, a significant rise in G0/G1 arrest was detected in the H_2O_2 group ($p < 0.01$). Interestingly, in comparison to the H_2O_2 group, a significant enhancement in G2/M arrest was observed in GA (20.54%; $p < 0.001$) and H_2O_2 + GA (12.50%; $p < 0.001$) groups.

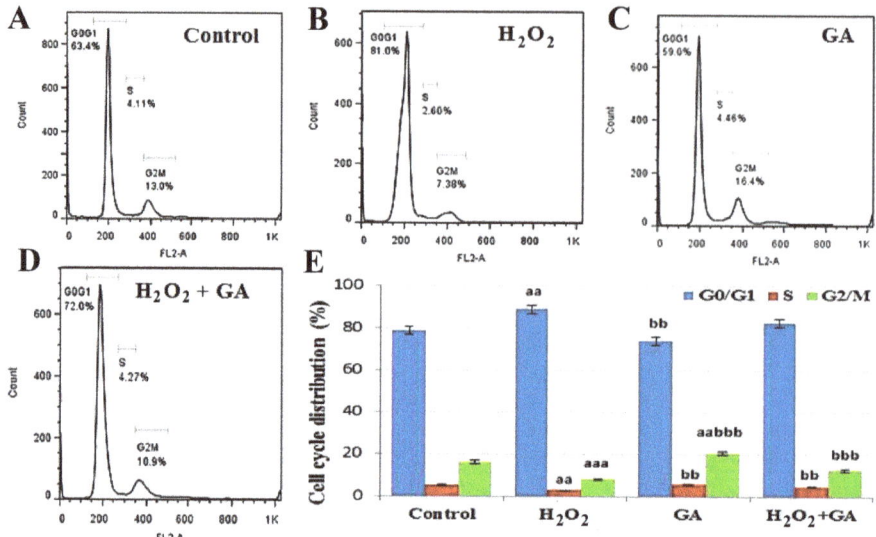

Figure 3. Cell cycle distribution is shown in the presence of control (**A**), H$_2$O$_2$ (**B**), gallic acid (GA) (**C**), and H$_2$O$_2$ + GA (**D**). The percentage of cells in different phases is shown in graph (**E**). Data are presented as the mean ± standard error of measurements performed on six groups, with three independent replicates. Significant difference from control ([aa] $p < 0.01$, [aaa] $p < 0.001$), significant difference from H$_2$O$_2$ ([bb] $p < 0.01$, [bbb] $p < 0.001$).

(c) Mitochondrial activity: As shown in Table 1, in REF cells exposed to H$_2$O$_2$, the mitochondrial complexes I, II, and IV activities were reduced ($p < 0.001$). On the other hand, treating REF cells with GA showed a significant enhancement in mitochondrial complexes activity compared to the H$_2$O$_2$ group ($p < 0.001$). Furthermore, exposure to H$_2$O$_2$ + GA significantly enhanced the level of mitochondrial complexes I, II, and IV ($p < 0.01$, $p < 0.001$, and $p < 0.05$, respectively).

Table 1. Effects of gallic acid on the mitochondrial complexes' activity of REF cells.

Mitochondrial Complexes	Control (Mean ± SE)	H$_2$O$_2$ (Mean ± SE)	Gallic Acid (Mean ± SE)	H$_2$O$_2$ + Gallic Acid (Mean ± SE)
Complex I	36.34 ± 0.72	20.53 ± 0.83 [aaa]	32.09 ± 1.09 [bbb]	27.65 ± 1.34 [aabb]
Complex II	83.05 ± 2.30 [aaa]	50.70 ± 1.57 [bbb]	78.07 ± 1.20 [bbb]	67.90 ± 1.28 [aaabbb]
Complex IV	1.48 ± 0.11	0.71 ± 0.04 [aaa]	1.53 ± 0.05 [bbb]	1.04 ± 0.04 [aaa]

Data are presented as the mean ± standard error (SE) of measurements performed on six groups, with three independent replicates. Significant difference from control ([aa] $p < 0.01$, [aaa] $p < 0.001$), significant difference from H$_2$O$_2$ ([bb] $p < 0.01$, [bbb] $p < 0.001$).

2.3. Antioxidant Effect of GA

In the case of pancreatic islet cells, a reduction in both ROS and lipid peroxidation (LPO) levels was observed after GA treatment compared to the control group ($p < 0.001$). GA treatment showed a considerable increment in both Ferric reducing antioxidant power (FRAP) and thiol levels. A significant rise in FRAP levels in GA vs. control groups, i.e., 106.83 vs. 56.60 mM ($p < 0.001$) was observed. Likewise, a considerable increase in thiol levels in GA vs. control groups, i.e., 5 vs. 3 µM ($p < 0.001$) was observed (Table 2). There was an increase in both LPO and ROS levels after H$_2$O$_2$ treatment in REF cells compared to the control group, i.e., $p < 0.001$ and $p < 0.01$, respectively. Furthermore, GA significantly attenuated H$_2$O$_2$ and reduced ROS and LPO in REF cells. Likewise, GA + H$_2$O$_2$

treatment significantly increased FRAP and thiol levels compared to H_2O_2, i.e., $p < 0.001$ and $p < 0.05$, respectively (Table 2).

Table 2. Effects of gallic acid on oxidative stress markers of rat's embryonic fibroblast and pancreatic islet cells.

	Oxidative Stress Markers	Pancreatic Islet Cells		Embryonic Fibroblast Cells			
		Control (Mean ± SE)	GA (Mean ± SE)	Control (Mean ± SE)	H_2O_2 (Mean ± SE)	GA (Mean ± SE)	GA + H_2O_2 (Mean ± SE)
1	ROS (mole/min.mg protein)	679.50 ± 41.54	99.10 ± 3.13 [aaa]	1.94 ± 0.18	4.03 ± 0.23 [aaa]	1.85 ± 0.09 [bbb]	2.54 ± 0.06 [bbb]
2	LPO (µM)	1.43 ± 0.01	1.22 ± 0.01 [aaa]	109.99 ± 4.24	178.80 ± 4.76 [aaa]	91.00 ± 4.17 [abbb]	132.80 ± 2.33 [aabbb]
3	FRAP (mM)	56.60 ± 0.73	106.83 ± 1.09 [aaa]	160.84 ± 1.96	87.79 ± 2.70 [aaa]	155.84 ± 4.17 [bbb]	113.79 ± 1.86 [aaabb]
4	Thiol (µmole/mg protein)	3.00 ± 0.07	5.00 ± 0.11 [aaa]	60.39 ± 3.12	35.96 ± 3.01 [aa]	65.98 ± 8.40 [b]	54.28 ± 3.84 [b]

Abbreviations: FRAP: ferric reducing antioxidant power; LPO: lipid peroxidation; ROS: reactive oxygen species. Data are presented as the mean ± standard error of measurements performed on six groups, with three independent replicates. Significant difference from control ([a] $p < 0.05$, [aa] $p < 0.01$, and [aaa] $p < 0.001$), significant difference from H_2O_2 ([b] $p < 0.05$, [bb] $p < 0.01$, and [bbb] $p < 0.001$).

2.4. Anti-Inflammatory Effect of GA

A higher tumor necrosis factor α (TNFα) was observed when REF cells were exposed to H_2O_2 ($p < 0.001$). While in comparison to H_2O_2, there was a significant decrease in the level of TNFα of GA ($p < 0.001$) and H_2O_2 + GA ($p < 0.001$) groups. Similarly, a higher amount of interleukin (IL)-1β and IL-6 were observed when REF cells were exposed to H_2O_2 ($p < 0.001$)—while in comparison to H_2O_2, a considerable decrease in the level of IL-1β of GA ($p < 0.01$) and H_2O_2 + GA ($p < 0.01$) groups was observed. In the case of nuclear factor kappa-light-chain-enhancer of activated B cells (NFκB), there was a significant increase in the H_2O_2 ($p < 0.001$) compared to control, while in comparison to H_2O_2, a considerable decrease in the level of NFκB of GA ($p < 0.001$) and H_2O_2 + GA ($p < 0.01$) groups was observed (Table 3).

Table 3. Effects of gallic acid on inflammatory markers of rat's embryonic fibroblast cells.

	Inflammatory Markers	Control (Mean ± SE)	H_2O_2 (Mean ± SE)	Gallic Acid (Mean ± SE)	H_2O_2 + Gallic Acid (Mean ± SE)
1	TNFα	98.92 ± 2.16	147.46 ± 0.95 [aaa]	109.39 ± 5.10 [bbb]	125.42 ± 3.45 [aaabbb]
2	IL-1β	80.81 ± 3.91	163.05 ± 14.46 [aaa]	106.15 ± 4.28 [bb]	130.86 ± 9.41 [bb]
3	IL-6	170.40 ± 6.22	364.98 ± 6.06 [aaa]	165.77 ± 4.63 [bbb]	273.99 ± 14.48 [aaabbb]
4	NFκB	20.01 ± 0.70	46.18 ± 1.35 [aaa]	20.16 ± 0.95 [bbb]	26.78 ± 1.35 [aabbb]

Abbreviations: IL: interleukin; NFκB: nuclear factor kappa-light-chain-enhancer of activated B cells; TNFα: tumor necrosis factor α. Data are presented as the mean ± standard error of measurements performed on six groups, with three independent replicates. Significant difference from control ([aa] $p < 0.01$ and [aaa] $p < 0.001$), significant difference from H_2O_2 ([bb] $p < 0.01$ and [bbb] $p < 0.001$).

2.5. Antidiabetic Effect of GA

The amount of insulin secretion was calculated in both basal (2.8 mM) and stimulated (16.7 mM) phases. A significant increase in insulin secretion was observed in the basal phase when the cells were treated with GA. The increment in control vs. GA group was from 2.2 ± 0.11 to 7.3 ± 0.11 mU/mg protein/h ($p < 0.001$). In contrast, a significant decrease in insulin secretion was observed in the stimulated phase when the cells were treated with GA. The decrement in the control vs. GA group was from 22.10 ± 0.36 to 18.10 ± 0.80 mU/mg protein/h ($p < 0.01$) (Figure 4).

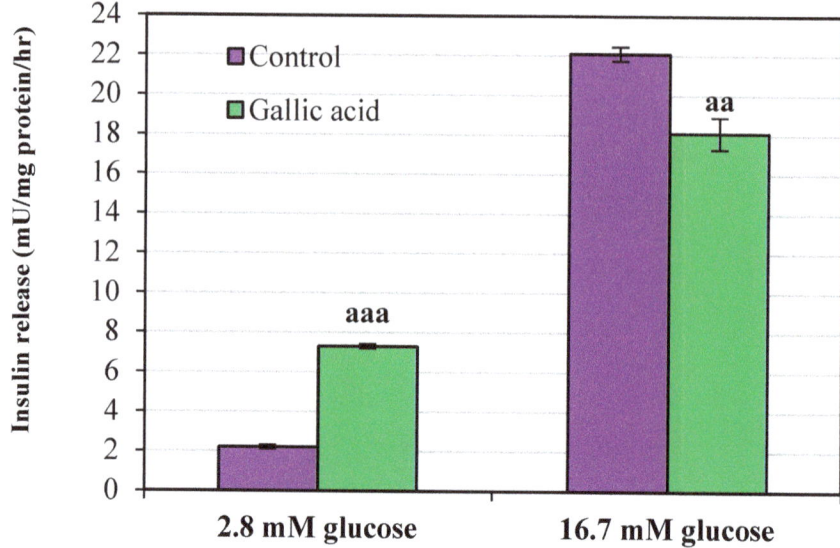

Figure 4. Effect of gallic acid on the level of insulin secretion on rat's pancreatic islets cells after 24 h. Pancreatic islet cells incubated for 1 h in the presence of 2.8 mM (basal phase) and 16.7 mM (stimulated phase) glucose concentrations. Data are presented as the mean ± standard error of measurements performed on six groups, with three independent replicates. Significant difference from control ([aa] $p < 0.01$, [aaa] $p < 0.001$).

2.6. Antiapoptotic Effect of GA

(a) Acridine orange (AO) and ethidium bromide (EB) double staining: The absorption of AO and EB shows the number of viable cells and necrotic cells, respectively. A significant decrease in the number of viable cells in the controls (49.50%) vs. GA (64.82%) ($p < 0.01$) group was observed. Similarly, a significant decrease in the number of necrotic cells in the GA vs. control ($p < 0.01$) group was observed (Figure 5A,B).

(b) Flow cytometry assay: The flow cytometry assay has shown a significant increase in the percentage of live cells in the GA (78.2%) vs. the control (71.1%) group ($p < 0.05$). In comparison, the number of necrotic cells was significantly decreased in GA (3.73%) vs. the control group (20.5%) ($p < 0.01$) (Figure 5B). Figure 5C shows the higher percentage of late apoptotic cells, i.e., 16.8%, in the GA group than the control group, i.e., 7.73%. While a higher rate of necrotic cells, i.e., 20.5% in the control group, was observed compared to the GA group, i.e., 3.73%. Similarly, the vertical bar graph of Figure 5D shows a significant increase in the number of live cells in the GA vs. control group, i.e., 78.2% vs. 71.1%, while the number of necrotic cells in the early apoptosis phase was found to decrease in the GA vs. control group, i.e., 0.62% vs. 1.3%.

(c) Caspase-3 and 9 activities: In comparison to control groups, a decrease in the caspase-3 and 9 activities was observed in the GA groups. The activity of caspase-3 and 9 was reduced to 85% ($p < 0.05$) and 46.4% ($p < 0.001$), respectively. A more noticeable decline in the activity was observed with the caspase-9 (Figure 5E).

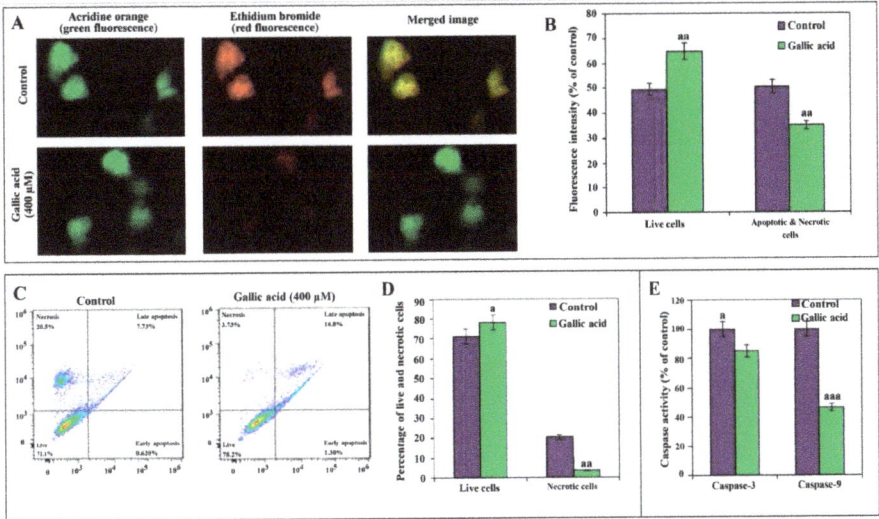

Figure 5. Apoptosis in pancreatic islet cells exposed to gallic acid (GA) demonstrated by Fluorescence microscopy images of cells (40× magnification) stained with acridine orange (AO) and ethidium bromide (EB) after 400 µM GA exposure. Pancreatic islet cells stained with acridine orange (green fluorescence), ethidium bromide (red fluorescence), and merged image (yellow/green fluorescence) (**A**). The percentage of viable, apoptotic, and necrotic cells from the staining data is also graphically shown (**B**). Contour diagrams of flow cytometry presents live, early/late apoptotic, and necrotic cells (**C**), and the percentage of live and necrotic cells from flow cytometry data is also graphically shown (**D**). Effect of 24 h exposure of 400 µM GA on the level of caspase-3/9 activities is shown in the last graph (**E**). Data are presented as the mean ± standard error of measurements performed on six groups, with three independent replicates. Significant difference from control ([a] $p < 0.05$, [aa] $p < 0.01$ and [aaa] $p < 0.001$).

3. Discussion

Fibroblasts are among attractive research models for in vitro studies due to their potential role in tissue repair, organ development, and wound healing [23,24]. However, oxidative stress slows down the normal function of many tissues and cells, including fibroblasts. The purpose of this study was to evaluate the protective activity of GA against H_2O_2-induced ROS-mediated aging in REF cells and to evaluate the GA-mediated improvement in the function of pancreatic islet cells.

Cellular senescence is a major cause of aging. It is characterized by numerous biochemical changes, such as the increased activity of β-galactosidase [25]. It is well known that the exposure of H_2O_2 induces higher β-galactosidase activity that allows an in vitro identification of senescent cells [26]. Similarly, in this study, a significant increase in the β-galactosidase activity was observed when the REF cells were exposed to H_2O_2. However, the treatment of cells with a combination of GA + H_2O_2 demonstrated a significant reduction in β-galactosidase activity ($p < 0.05$). Such a decrease in the β-galactosidase activity supports the protective anti-aging potential of GA. A few studies have shown a beneficial role of GA in limiting the activity of redox-sensitive transcription factors.

Controlling cellular senescence in the G1 phase of the cell cycle is the main target for regulating the aging process [27,28]. Studies have shown the negative impact of H_2O_2-mediated cellular senescence on the P53 transcription factor, P21, P16, Rb protein [27]. Furthermore, DNA damage and shortening of telomeres are critical in the distribution and cell cycle arrest in the G1 phase [28,29]. Similar to the previous studies, our study demonstrated H_2O_2-mediated cell cycle arrest G1 phase of REF cells. Furthermore, in comparison to H_2O_2, GA treatment confirmed cell cycle arrest in the G2/M phase ($p < 0.01$). In line with the obtained results, Ou et al. showed that GA causes cell cycle arrest at the G2/M phase in the human bladder transitional carcinoma cell line through checkpoint kinase 2 (Chk2)-mediated phosphorylation of Cdc25C [30].

Generally, superoxides are deactivated by superoxide dismutase and glutathione peroxidase. The deficiency of mitochondrial complex I resulted in increased superoxide production followed by subsequent induction of superoxide dismutase [31]. A study has shown an association of lower mitochondrial complexes with certain neurodegenerative diseases such as Parkinsonism [32]. This study has shown a significant increment in mitochondrial complexes I, II, and IV after GA treatment, suggesting the therapeutic potential of GA to counteract the oxidative stress by introducing various mitochondrial complexes. In 2018, another study indicated the therapeutic application of GA in mitochondria dysfunction-related diseases and GA was introduced as a new mitochondriotropic antioxidant [33].

Inflammation acts as a defensive response by cells after exposure to a toxic agent. The cell inflammatory response involves the secretion of various inflammatory cytokines [34,35]. Transcription factor NFκB regulates many cytokines' production, while its level is upregulated in certain chronic diseases [36,37]. In this study, GA-treated REF cells demonstrated a decreased concentration of NFκB ($p < 0.001$) and inflammatory cytokines, including TNFα ($p < 0.001$), IL-1β ($p < 0.01$), and IL-6 ($p < 0.001$), compared to the H_2O_2 group. The present results are similar to the previous ones suggesting the protective role of GA against inflammation via suppressing mast and cancer cells [38,39].

It was demonstrated that phenolic compounds significantly decline oxidative stress generated by neutrophil-mediated ROS [40]. Antioxidant enzymes such as superoxide dismutase and catalase suppress oxidative stress by controlling ROS's overproduction, such as superoxide anion and H_2O_2 [41]. Like other phenolic compounds, GA has also demonstrated a significantly increased expression and activity of antioxidant enzymes. In this study, the results of REF cells showed a significant decrease in the oxidative stress markers compared to the H_2O_2 group ($p < 0.001$). Also, GA significantly improved antioxidant capacity by enhancing FRAP and TTM levels in both REF and pancreatic islets cells after GA treatment.

Caspase-3 and 9 are the group of enzymes regulating inflammation and apoptosis. As a cancer-selective agent, GA in apoptosis of normal and cancer cells can act dually [42]. In this study, GA treatment demonstrated a significant reduction in the activities of both caspase-3 and 9 in the normal pancreatic islet cells, supporting the protective effects of GA against cellular apoptosis through decreasing caspase-3 and 9 activities. As mentioned above, the results were further confirmed by flow cytometry and AO/EB staining analysis. The GA-treated cells have shown a significant decrease in apoptotic cells and improved cell viability.

Studies on the effects of GA in diabetes show that this compound inhibits diet-induced hypertriglyceridemia and hyperglycemia and protects pancreatic β-cells. GA induces a nuclear transcription factor, which causes differentiation and insulin sensitivity in adipocytes, called peroxisome proliferator-activated receptor-γ (PPAR-γ). GA also enhances the cellular glucose uptake by stimulating the phosphatidylinositol 3-kinase (PI3K)/p-Akt signaling pathway and translocating GLUT1, GLUT2, and GLUT4 as insulin-stimulated glucose transporters [14]. Further study on type II diabetic rats' brain metabolism revealed that a diet high in GA could benefit type II diabetics [18]. More studies showed that GA in streptozotocin-induced type II diabetic rats has many benefits, including antioxidant, antihyperglycemic, and anti-lipid peroxidative properties [16,17]. In confirmation of previous studies, the present results also showed that GA can significantly increase insulin secretion in beta cells in the basal glucose concentration phase (2.8 mM glucose). Also, by decreasing apoptosis, it can protect the pancreatic islet cells.

This study has demonstrated the protective role of GA on the REF and rat pancreatic islets. Therefore, we found that GA at all studied concentrations attenuates oxidative stress and is safe. Moreover, GA reduces apoptosis, suppresses caspases activity, and improves insulin secretion, thus demonstrating antioxidant, antidiabetic, and antiapoptotic potential. Hence, GA is the right candidate for anti-aging in skincare products or a dietary supplement, warranting future human studies.

4. Materials and Methods

4.1. Chemicals

All chemicals were purchased from Sigma-Aldrich (GmbH, Munich, Germany) unless otherwise mentioned. Nuclear factor kappa-light-chain-enhancer of activated B cells (NFκB), interleukins (IL-6 and IL-1β), ELISA kits (BenderMed Systems Inc. Vienna, Austria), Senescence β-galactosidase staining kit (Cell Signaling Technology, Mississauga, ON, Canada), rat-specific β-galactosidase kit (Cusabio, Wuhan, China), rat-specific enzyme-linked immunosorbent insulin ELISA kit (Mercodia, Sweden), and ApoFlowEx® fluorescein isothiocyanate (FITC) kit (Exbio, Vestec, Czech Republic) were used in this study.

4.2. Isolation of Rats' Cells and Identification of Half-Maximal Effective Concentration (EC_{50}) of GA

Ethical approval for the animal study: This study is performed according to the NIMAD Ethics Committee Approval (IR.NIMAD.REC.1397.028). All ethical protocols related to the use of animals in research were carefully noted.

Isolation of rats' embryonic fibroblast (REF) cells: Rats were kept for induction of pregnancy. The isolation and culture of primary REF cells were done as per the standard protocol explained previously [23]. Pregnant rats were anesthetized with 50 mg/kg pentobarbital. The 12 to 12.5 days old embryos were washed with antibiotic-containing phosphate-buffered saline (PBS). Visceral mass such as uterine horns, placenta, heads, limbs, and gonads were detached. The tissues were mechanically chopped into fine pieces and enzymatically digested using 0.25% trypsin/ethylenediaminetetraacetic acid (EDTA) to isolate cells. Enzymatic activity was inhibited by Dulbecco's modified medium-high glucose (DMEM-HG), 10% fetal bovine serum (FBS), 1% penicillin-streptomycin, and 1% glutamate. Isolated cells were treated with an appropriate culture medium and pipetted to get a single cell suspension. The cells were cultured in T75 flasks until 75% to 80% confluency and sub-cultured at a ratio of 1:3. REFs were collected from three pregnant rats and were used at passages (P3) for this study.

Isolation of pancreatic islet cells: Pancreas was removed and washed using the Krebs buffer to remove the attached lymph nodes, blood vessels, and fat. Krebs buffer solution at pH 7 consists of 0.22 g/L $CaCl_2.2H_2O$, 2.38 g/L HEPES, 0.27 g/L KCl, 0.05 g/L $MgCl_2$, 8 g/L NaCl, 0.42 g/L NaH_2PO_4, and 0.5 g/L glucose.$1H_2O$. The pancreas was cut into small pieces over the ice, washed twice, and centrifuged at 3000× g for 60 s. They were exposed to collagenase enzyme solution (0.0025 g/5 mL Krebs buffer) at 37 °C to digest the attached tissues for about 10 min. Krebs buffer containing 0.5% bovine serum albumin (BSA) was then added to stop the digestion, and the pancreatic pieces were again centrifuged twice at 3000× g for 60 s. The pancreatic islet cells of approximately 100 to 150 µm were isolated using a sampler under a stereomicroscope. Standard RPMI-1640 culture medium comprising 5% FBS, 0.5% penicillin-streptomycin, and 8.3 mMol/L glucose was added to the isolated cells. The pancreatic islets at a density of 10 islets/200 µL culture medium were kept for 24 h at 37 °C under 5% CO_2 for further use [43]. For normalizing data obtained from different treated groups of islets, protein content was also measured.

MTT assay: The viability of REF and pancreatic islet cells were determined after different concentrations of GA treatment, i.e., 0, 1, 10, 100, and 1000 µM (in case of 1×10^4 REF cells/well in each group) and 10, 100, and 1000 µM (in case of 10 islet cells in each group). Cultured cells were treated with 20 µL MTT reagent, i.e., 0.5 mg/mL and 50 µL culture medium. After incubation at 37 °C and 5% CO_2 humidified atmosphere for 4 h, the formazan dye was made soluble by adding 150 µL dimethyl sulfoxide (DMSO) to each sample. Finally, the absorbance was determined at 570 nm using a microplate reader. The probit regression model was employed to estimate the EC_{50} of GA [44].

Study design: After determining the EC_{50} of GA, the REF cells were divided into the following four groups based on different exposure treatments, i.e., (a) 1×10^4 REF cells in DMEM-HG (Control), (b) REF cells exposed to 600 µM H_2O_2 for 2 h (H_2O_2), (c) REF cells in EC_{50} of GA (GA), and (d) REF cells with EC_{50} of GA + 600 µM H_2O_2 (GA + H_2O_2). A concentration of 600 µM H_2O_2 was observed as a potent inducer of cellular senescence [45]. Simultaneously, the pancreatic islet cells were divided into control and treatment groups with 10 pancreatic islets in each. The treatment group received EC_{50} of GA on pancreatic islet cells. All cells were incubated at 37 °C and 5% CO_2 humidified atmosphere.

4.3. Anti-Ageing Effect of Gallic Acid

Senescence-associated β-galactosidase (SABG) concentration: The β-galactosidase concentration in REF cells was determined using a rat-specific SA-βGAL kit. The well plates containing the REF cells at the density of 1×10^5 cells/well for samples (Control, H_2O_2, GA, and GA + H_2O_2 groups) and different concentrations of βGAL (1.56, 3.12, 6.25, 12.5, 25, 50, 100 mIU/mL) as standards were incubated at 37 °C for 2 h. The supernatant was removed, and 100 µL of biotin antibody was added to each well and set at 37 °C for another hour. After washing the cells by filling each well with 200 µL of wash buffer for a total of three washes, 100 µL of Avidin horseradish peroxidase (HRP) was added to each well, and plates were incubated at 37 °C for another hour. After aspiration, 90 µL of 3,3′,5,5′-tetramethylbenzidine (TMB) was added to the plates and set again for 30 min. The 50 µL of stop solution was then added, and the optical density was determined at 450 nm. Along with the quantitative assay, β-galactosidase was also investigated qualitatively. REF cells were washed, and then they were exposed to the fixative solution containing 2% glutaraldehyde and 20% formaldehyde in 10× PBS for about 15 min at room temperature. Next, cells were washed with PBS and then stained with b-galactosidase stain. The bluish-green color of senescent cells was observed under the light microscope (Olympus BX51, Tokyo, Japan) at 200× magnification [43].

Cell cycle analysis by propidium iodide staining: REF cells were seeded in 6 well plates at the density of 5×10^5 cells/well. The cells were exposed to 600 µM H_2O_2 and EC_{50} of GA alone or in combination for 24 h. After the incubation period, the REF cells were appropriately harvested, washed twice with PBS, and fixed in ice-cold 70% ethanol. After centrifuging at 10,000× g for 5 min, pellets were washed with ice-cold PBS and were redistributed in 200 µL (from 50 µg/mL stock solution) propidium iodide (PI) containing 20 µg/mL RNAse-A and incubated at 37 °C for 30 min. The cells were then washed with PBS, and cell cycle distribution at G0/G1, S, and G2/M phases was determined by a flow cytometer (Mindray, Shenzhen, China). The data were processed using FlowJo analysis software [46].

Activity assay of mitochondrial complexes: Density of 1×10^4 cells/well for each group was used for assessing mitochondrial complexes. (a) Mitochondrial complex I (NADH dehydrogenase): Activity of mitochondrial complex I was determined by measuring NADH's consumption, which is determined by the translocation of electrons initially to complex I and subsequently to an electron acceptor, such as synthetic ubiquinone. Electrons through NADH passed to mitochondrial complex I and were then accepted by synthetic ubiquinone. In this method, 100 to 200 µg/mL of total mitochondrial protein were added to a reaction mixture containing potassium phosphate buffer (25 mM; pH 7.4), 25% BSA, $MgCl_2$ (5 mM), decylubiquinone (2.8 mM), NADH (5.7 mM), antimycin-A (3.7 mM), and KCN (2 mM). The absorbance of NADH was performed spectrophotometrically at 340 nm. Soon after, the rotenone was added to the reaction mixture, and the rotenone-insensitive activity of NADH-cytochrome b oxidoreductase was evaluated. Finally, the rotenone-insensitive activity was subtracted from the total activity, and the overall net rate was determined. The obtained results of enzyme activity were expressed as nanomoles of NADH per minute per milligram of mitochondrial protein (nmol/min/mg protein) at 340 nm [47,48]. (b) Mitochondrial complex II (succinate dehydrogenase): The activity of succinate ubiquinone oxidoreductase was determined by measuring 2,6-dichlorophenolindophenol (DCPIP) reduction through colorimetric assay at 600 nm. In this assay, the mitochondria were incubated in potassium phosphate buffer, $MgCl_2$, and succinate. Then, antimycin A, rotenone, KCN, and DCPIP were added, and baseline was recorded for 3 min. The enzyme-dependent reduction of DCPIP was then measured for 3 to 5 min at 600 nm. The activity of mitochondrial complex II was calculated using a DCPIP standard curve. (c) Mitochondrial complex IV (cytochrome C oxidase): The cytochrome C was reduced by adding 60 µL of sodium hydrosulfite (10 mg/mL). Then, the mitochondrial protein and

Lubrol-PX in potassium phosphate buffer were added to further reduce the cytochrome C. The decrease in optical absorbance at 550 nm was recorded for 3 to 6 min. The results were presented as the natural logarithm of the absorbance and reported as the first-order rate constant, i.e., (k) min/mg of mitochondrial protein [49].

4.4. Antioxidant Effect of GA

Each group of cells, containing 1×10^4 REF cells or 10 islet cells for the pancreatic section, was homogenized with 100 μL phosphate buffer and was then centrifuged at 2375× g for 15 min. Next, the supernatant of the extractions was used for the following oxidative stress markers.

Lipid peroxidation measurement: The thiobarbituric acid (TBA) was used to determine lipid peroxidation in REF cells. Following homogenization, the REF cells were mixed with 800 μL trichloroacetic acid. After 30 min centrifuging at 3000× g, the 600 μL supernatant was removed, and cell deposition was combined with 150 μL TBA (1% w/v). The mixture was incubated in a boiling water bath for 15 min, followed by 400 μL n-butanol. Finally, the absorbance was recorded at 532 nm [50].

ROS assay: This involves converting a fluorescent dye, i.e., 2,7-dichlorofluorescein diacetate (DCFDA), to a non-fluorescent compound. Cellular esterase deacetylates, DCFDA, and ROS then oxidized the deacetylated compound into 2,7-dichlorofluorescein (DCF). Finally, the changes in the fluorescence intensity were detected by a microplate reader with excitation and emission spectra at 488 and 525 nm, respectively [51].

Ferric reducing antioxidant power (FRAP) assay: This is based on assessing antioxidant potential. The reduction of Fe^{3+}TPTZ (2,4,6-tris-(2-pyridyl)-s-triazine) complex to the ferrous form was determined at 593 nm [52].

Assay of total thiol molecules (TTM): This involves the addition of 0.6 mL Tris-EDTA buffer (Tris base 0.25 M, ethylene diamine tetraacetic acid 20 mM at pH 8.2) to 0.2 mL supernatant of the cell extraction, and 40 μL 5-5'-dithiobis-2-nitrobenzoic acid (10 mM in pure methanol). The final volume of 4 mL was made using pure methanol. This mixture was incubated at room temperature for 15 min and then centrifuged at 3000× g for 10 min. The supernatant's absorbance was measured at 412 nm, and results were presented in μmol/mg protein [2].

4.5. Anti-Inflammatory Effect of GA

Measurement of Inflammatory Cytokines (TNFα, IL-1β, and IL-6) and Transcription Factor (NFκB): Quantitative measurement of inflammatory cytokines and NFκB levels in the REF cells (at the density of 1×10^4 cells/well for each group) was performed using rat-specific inflammatory cytokine ELISA kits. In brief, the specific antibody was coated to the wells. Then, standards and all samples were added to the wells. After washing the wells, the enzyme streptavidin-HRP, which binds to the biotinylated antibody, was added. After the washing step and incubation time, the TMB substrate solution was added. Finally, the stop solution was added to change the color from blue to yellow. The absorbance of yellow color was detected at 450 nm.

4.6. Antidiabetic Effect of GA

Pancreatic islet cells, 10 islets in each group, were exposed to 100 μM GA for 24 h and incubated. After the incubation period, 1 mL Krebs medium was added, centrifuged at 3000× g for 1 min. The supernatant was removed, and the islet cells were incubated with 2.8 mM glucose for 30 min. The cells were then divided into two treatment groups with a basal and stimulant glucose dose, i.e., 2.8 and 16.7 mM, respectively. After an hour of exposure, the cells were centrifuged, and the supernatant was removed and analyzed for the insulin measurement according to the insulin kit manufacturer's protocol. The obtained data were normalized with protein concentration and were presented in mU/mg protein/h [53].

4.7. Antiapoptotic Effect of GA

(a) Acridine orange (AO) and ethidium bromide (EB) double staining: 10 pancreatic islets for each group were used to perform AO/EB staining. The antiapoptotic effect of GA was determined by identifying morphological apoptotic and necrotic cells through the use of DNA-binding AO and EB dyes. Viable and nonviable cells both emit green fluorescence after absorbing an intercalated AO in the DNA. However, only nonviable cells emit red fluorescence after absorbing an intercalated EB in the DNA. After treating pancreatic islet cells with GA for 24 h, the cells were washed and stained with a mixture of 100 µg/mL of AO and EB and kept at room temperature for 5 min. Finally, the fluorescence of stained cells was observed through fluorescence microscopy (Olympus BX51; Olympus Corporation, Tokyo, Japan) at a magnification of 40×, and the staining intensity was measured by ImageJ analysis software.

(b) Flow cytometry assay: This was used to determine the apoptotic vs. necrotic cells. The isolated pancreatic islet cells were treated with trypsin and then with BSA to stop the digestion. The suspended cells were washed twice with PBS, and dual staining was done using the ApoFlowEx® FITC kit. Cells with an approximated density of 3×10^5 cells/100 µL were incubated with 5 µL each of annexin V-FITC and PI at room temperature for 15 min. Then, the samples were analyzed with a flow cytometer (Mindray, Shenzhen, China).

(c) Measurement of caspase-3 and 9 activity: The activity of caspase-3 and 9 was determined via a colorimetric assay, as reported previously [44]. After adding the lysis buffer to the treated islet cells (10 in each group), they were incubated on ice for 10 min. The whole lysate was then incubated in a caspase buffer containing caspase-3 and 9 substrates (Ac-DEVD-pNA and Ac-LEHD-pNA). A short peptide substrate that contains a specific caspase recognition sequence was labeled with chromophore r-nitroaniline (pNA). The caspase enzyme caused a cleavage in the substrate, and pNA was released. The absorbance was measured at 405 nm, and the enzyme activity was reported as the % control, assumed as 100%.

4.8. Protein Content Measurement

For normalizing data obtained from the above tests, each group of islets or REF cells was homogenized in 1 mL of each test's related buffer. Then, 10 µL Bradford reagent was added to 100 µL of diluted samples, and after 5 min, the absorbance was read at 595 nm by the spectrophotometer. BSA was used as the standard.

4.9. Statistical Analysis

All experiments were repeated three times, with six groups for each condition. Results were recorded as Mean ± standard error (SE). One-way analysis of variance (ANOVA) and Tukey's tests were used to compare treatment and control groups. The differences were considered significant if $p < 0.05$.

5. Conclusions

This study has concluded GA with a potential of being an (a) anti-aging agent, through the reduced β-galactosidase activity and cell cycle arrest in G2/M phase, (b) antioxidant agent, via enhancing the level of mitochondrial complexes I, II, and IV, (c) anti-inflammatory agent, by decreasing levels of NFκB, TNFα, IL-1β, and IL-6, (d) antidiabetic agent, through increasing insulin secretion in pancreatic islet cells, and (e) antiapoptotic agent, by decreasing caspase-3 and 9 activities. The facts mentioned above suggest GA's therapeutic benefits for the formulations of anti-aging skincare products or dietary supplementations for metabolic disorders, e.g., diabetes, through parallel molecular mechanisms.

Author Contributions: The authors declare that all data were generated in-house and that no paper mill was used. Conception and design of the study: M.A., M.R., and M.B.; Acquisition of data: M.R., H.B., S.M.-N., H.H.-A., M.K., and H.M.; Analysis and/or interpretation of data: M.B., M.R., and H.B.; Drafting the manuscript: M.A., M.B., M.R., and H.B.; Revision and approval of the submitted version: M.B., M.A., M.R., H.B., S.M.-N., M.K., H.H.-A., and H.M. All authors have read and agreed to the published version of the manuscript.

Funding: Research reported in this publication was supported by Elite Researcher Grant Committee under award numbers 977125 and 943614 from the National Institutes for Medical Research Development (NIMAD), Tehran, Iran, received by the authors Maryam Baeeri and Mohammad Abdollahi.

Acknowledgments: Authors acknowledge TUMS and Iran National Science Foundation (INSF) for their general support.

Conflicts of Interest: The authors declare no conflict of interest.

References

1. Abdollahi, M.; Moridani, M.Y.; Aruoma, O.I.; Mostafalou, S. Oxidative stress in aging. *Oxidative Med. Cell. Longev.* **2014**, *2014*, 876834. [CrossRef] [PubMed]
2. Bahadar, H.; Maqbool, F.; Mostafalou, S.; Baeeri, M.; Rahimifard, M.; Navaei-Nigjeh, M.; Abdollahi, M. Assessment of benzene induced oxidative impairment in rat isolated pancreatic islets and effect on insulin secretion. *Environ. Toxicol. Pharmacol.* **2015**, *39*, 1161–1169. [CrossRef] [PubMed]
3. Choi, M.J.; Kim, B.K.; Park, K.Y.; Yokozawa, T.; Song, Y.O.; Cho, E.J. Anti-aging effects of Cyanidin under a stress-induced premature senescence cellular system. *Biol. Pharm. Bull.* **2010**, *33*, 421–426. [CrossRef] [PubMed]
4. Khalid, M.; Abdollahi, M. Epigenetic modifications associated with pathophysiological effects of lead exposure. *J. Environ. Sci. Heal. Part. C* **2019**, *37*, 235–287. [CrossRef]
5. Finkel, T.; Holbrook, N.J. Oxidants, oxidative stress and the biology of ageing. *Nat. Cell Biol.* **2000**, *408*, 239–247. [CrossRef]
6. Manayi, A.; Saeidnia, S.; Gohari, A.R.; Abdollahi, M. Methods for the discovery of new anti-aging products-targeted approaches. *Expert Opin. Drug Discov.* **2014**, *9*, 383–405. [CrossRef]
7. Cui, H.; Kong, Y.; Zhang, H. Oxidative stress, mitochondrial dysfunction, and aging. *J. Signal. Transduct.* **2011**, *2012*. [CrossRef]
8. The aging process. In *Proceedings of the PsycEXTRA Dataset*; American Psychological Association (APA): Washington, DC, USA, 2013; Volume 78, pp. 7124–7128.
9. Kregel, K.C.; Zhang, H.J. An integrated view of oxidative stress in aging: Basic mechanisms, functional effects, and pathological considerations. *Am. J. Physiol. Integr. Comp. Physiol.* **2007**, *292*, R18–R36. [CrossRef]
10. Gerber, P.A.; Rutter, G.A. The role of oxidative stress and hypoxia in pancreatic beta-cell dysfunction in Diabetes Mellitus. *Antioxid. Redox Signal.* **2017**, *26*, 501–518. [CrossRef]
11. Mohseni, S.M.S.S.; Larijani, B.; Abdollahi, M. Islet transplantation and antioxidant management: A comprehensive review. *World J. Gastroenterol.* **2009**, *15*, 1153–1161. [CrossRef]
12. Phillips, M.; Cataneo, R.N.; Cheema, T.; Greenberg, J. Increased breath biomarkers of oxidative stress in diabetes mellitus. *Clinica Chimica Acta* **2004**, *344*, 189–194. [CrossRef] [PubMed]
13. Domínguez, C.; Ruiz, E.; Gussinye, M.; Carrascosa, A. Oxidative stress at onset and in early stages of type 1 diabetes in children and adolescents. *Diabetes Care* **1998**, *21*, 1736–1742. [CrossRef] [PubMed]
14. Kahkeshani, N.; Farzaei, F.; Fotouhi, M.; Alavi, S.S.; Bahramsoltani, R.; Naseri, R.; Momtaz, S.; Abbasabadi, Z.; Rahimi, R.; Farzaei, M.H.; et al. Pharmacological effects of gallic acid in health and diseases: A mechanistic review. *Iran. J. Basic Med. Sci.* **2019**, *22*, 225–237. [CrossRef] [PubMed]
15. Ma, J.; Luo, X.-D.; Protiva, P.; Yang, H.; Ma, C.; Basile, M.J.; Weinstein, I.B.; Kennelly, E.J. Bioactive novel polyphenols from the fruit of Manilkara zapota (Sapodilla). *J. Nat. Prod.* **2003**, *66*, 983–986. [CrossRef] [PubMed]
16. Punithavathi, V.R.; Prince, P.S.M.; Kumar, M.R.; Selvakumari, C.J. Protective effects of gallic acid on hepatic lipid peroxide metabolism, glycoprotein components and lipids in streptozotocin-induced type II diabetic wistar rats. *J. Biochem. Mol. Toxicol.* **2011**, *25*, 68–76. [CrossRef] [PubMed]
17. Punithavathi, V.R.; Prince, P.S.M.; Kumar, R.; Selvakumari, J. Antihyperglycaemic, antilipid peroxidative and antioxidant effects of gallic acid on streptozotocin induced diabetic Wistar rats. *Eur. J. Pharmacol.* **2011**, *650*, 465–471. [CrossRef]
18. Prince, P.S.M.; Kumar, M.R.; Selvakumari, C.J. Effects of gallic acid on brain lipid peroxide and lipid metabolism in streptozotocin-induced diabetic Wistar rats. *J. Biochem. Mol. Toxicol.* **2010**, *25*, 101–107. [CrossRef]

19. Latha, R.C.R.; Daisy, P. Insulin-secretagogue, antihyperlipidemic and other protective effects of gallic acid isolated from *Terminalia bellerica* Roxb. in streptozotocin-induced diabetic rats. *Chem. Interact.* **2011**, *189*, 112–118. [CrossRef]
20. Moradi, S.Z.; Momtaz, S.; Bayrami, Z.; Farzaei, M.H.; Abdollahi, M. Nanoformulations of herbal extracts in treatment of neurodegenerative disorders. *Front. Bioeng. Biotechnol.* **2020**, *8*, 8. [CrossRef]
21. Balestri, F.; Poli, G.; Pineschi, C.; Moschini, R.; Cappiello, M.; Mura, U.; Tuccinardi, T.; Del-Corso, A. Aldose reductase differential inhibitors in green tea. *Biomolecules* **2020**, *10*, 1003. [CrossRef]
22. Hsieh, C.L.; Lin, C.-H.; Chen, K.-C.; Peng, C.-C.; Peng, R.Y. The Teratogenicity and the action mechanism of gallic acid relating with brain and cervical muscles. *PLoS ONE* **2015**, *10*, e0119516. [CrossRef] [PubMed]
23. Yusuf, B.; Gopurappilly, R.; Dadheech, N.; Gupta, S.; Bhonde, R.; Pal, R. Embryonic fibroblasts represent a connecting link between mesenchymal and embryonic stem cells. *Dev. Growth Differ.* **2013**, *55*, 330–340. [CrossRef] [PubMed]
24. Haniffa, M.A.; Collin, M.P.; Buckley, C.D.; Dazzi, F. Mesenchymal stem cells: The fibroblasts' new clothes? *Haematologica* **2008**, *94*, 258–263. [CrossRef] [PubMed]
25. Buachan, P.; Chularojmontri, L.; Wattanapitayakul, S.K. Selected activities of Citrus Maxima Merr. Fruits on human endothelial cells: Enhancing cell migration and delaying cellular aging. *Nutrients* **2014**, *6*, 1618–1634. [CrossRef] [PubMed]
26. Debacq-Chainiaux, F.; Erusalimsky, J.D.; Campisi, J.; Toussaint, O. Protocols to detect senescence-associated beta-galactosidase (SA-βgal) activity, a biomarker of senescent cells in culture and in vivo. *Nat. Protoc.* **2009**, *4*, 1798–1806. [CrossRef] [PubMed]
27. Chen, Q.M. Replicative senescence and oxidant-induced premature senescence: Beyond the control of cell cycle checkpoints. *Ann. N. Y. Acad. Sci.* **2006**, *908*, 111–125. [CrossRef] [PubMed]
28. Duan, J.; Zhang, Z.; Tong, T. Irreversible cellular senescence induced by prolonged exposure to H_2O_2 involves DNA-damage-and-repair genes and telomere shortening. *Int. J. Biochem. Cell Biol.* **2005**, *37*, 1407–1420. [CrossRef]
29. Furukawa, A.; Tada-Oikawa, S.; Kawanishi, S.; Oikawa, S. H_2O_2 accelerates cellular senescence by accumulation of acetylated p53 via decrease in the function of SIRT1 by NAD+ depletion. *Cell. Physiol. Biochem.* **2007**, *20*, 045–054. [CrossRef]
30. Ou, T.T.; Wang, C.J.; Lee, Y.S.; Wu, C.H.; Lee, H.J. Gallic acid induces G2/M phase cell cycle arrest via regulating 14-3-3β release from Cdc25C and Chk2 activation in human bladder transitional carcinoma cells. *Mol. Nutr. Food Res.* **2010**, *54*, 1781–1790. [CrossRef]
31. Pitkanen, S.; Robinson, B.H. Mitochondrial complex I deficiency leads to increased production of superoxide radicals and induction of superoxide dismutase. *J. Clin. Investig.* **1996**, *98*, 345–351. [CrossRef]
32. Haas, R.H.; Nasirian, F.; Nakano, K.; Ward, D.; Pay, M.; Hill, R.; Shults, C.W. Low platelet mitochondrial complex I and complex II/III activity in early untreated Parkinson's disease. *Ann. Neurol.* **1995**, *37*, 714–722. [CrossRef] [PubMed]
33. Teixeira, J.; Oliveira, C.; Cagide, F.; Amorim, R.; Garrido, J.; Borges, F.; Oliveira, P.J. Discovery of a new mitochondria permeability transition pore (mPTP) inhibitor based on gallic acid. *J. Enzym. Inhib. Med. Chem.* **2018**, *33*, 567–576. [CrossRef] [PubMed]
34. Sarkar, D.; Fisher, P.B. Molecular mechanisms of aging-associated inflammation. *Cancer Lett.* **2006**, *236*, 13–23. [CrossRef] [PubMed]
35. Mohammadirad, A.; Aghamohammadali-Sarraf, F.; Badiei, S.; Faraji, Z.; Hajiaghaee, R.; Baeeri, M.; Gholami, M.; Abdollahi, M. Anti-aging effects of some selected iranian folk medicinal herbs-biochemical evidences. *Iran. J. Basic Med. Sci.* **2013**, *16*, 1170–1180.
36. Haghi Aminjan, H.; Abtahi, S.R.; Hazrati, E.; Chamanara, M.; Jalili, M.; Paknejad, B. Targeting of oxidative stress and inflammation through ROS/NF-kappaB pathway in phosphine-induced hepatotoxicity mitigation. *Life Sci.* **2019**, *232*, 116607. [CrossRef]
37. Lee, H.A.; Hughes, D.A. Alpha-lipoic acid modulates NF-kappaB activity in human monocytic cells by direct interaction with DNA. *Exp. Gerontol.* **2002**, *37*, 401–410. [CrossRef]
38. Kim, S.-H.; Jun, C.-D.; Suk, K.; Choi, B.-J.; Lim, H.; Park, S.; Lee, S.H.; Shin, H.-Y.; Kim, D.-K.; Shin, T.-Y. Gallic acid inhibits histamine release and pro-inflammatory cytokine production in mast cells. *Toxicol. Sci.* **2006**, *91*, 123–131. [CrossRef]

39. Choi, K.-C.; Lee, Y.-H.; Jung, M.G.; Kwon, S.H.; Kim, M.-J.; Jun, W.J.; Lee, J.; Lee, J.M.; Yoon, H.-G. Gallic acid suppresses lipopolysaccharide-induced nuclear factor-κB signaling by preventing RelA acetylation in A549 lung cancer cells. *Mol. Cancer Res.* **2009**, *7*, 2011–2021. [CrossRef]
40. Tunin, L.M.; Borghi, F.B.; Nogueira, A.C.; Higachi, L.; Barbosa, D.S.; Baesso, M.L.; Hernandes, L.; Diniz, A.; Truiti, M.D.C.T. Employing photoacoustic spectroscopy in the evaluation of the skin permeation profile of emulsion containing antioxidant phenolic-rich extract of Melochia arenosa. *Pharm. Biol.* **2015**, *54*, 1–7. [CrossRef]
41. Kuczmannová, A.; Gál, P.; Varinská, L.; Treml, J.; Kováč, I.; Novotný, M.; Vasilenko, T.; Dall'Acqua, S.; Nagy, M.; Mučaji, P. *Agrimonia eupatoria* L. and *Cynara cardunculus* L. water infusions: Phenolic profile and comparison of antioxidant activities. *Molecules* **2015**, *20*, 20538–20550. [CrossRef]
42. Liu, Z.; Li, D.; Yu, L.; Niu, F. Gallic acid as a cancer-selective agent induces apoptosis in pancreatic cancer cells. *Chemotherapy* **2012**, *58*, 185–194. [CrossRef] [PubMed]
43. Rahimifard, M.; Navaei-Nigjeh, M.; Mahroui, N.; Mirzaei, S.; Siahpoosh, Z.; Pharm, D.; Nili-Ahmadabadi, A.; Mohammadirad, A.; Baeeri, M.; Hajiaghaie, R.; et al. Improvement in the function of isolated rat pancreatic islets through reduction of oxidative stress using traditional Iranian medicine. *Cell J.* **2014**, *16*, 147–163. [PubMed]
44. Rahimifard, M.; Navaei-Nigjeh, M.; Baeeri, M.; Maqbool, F.; Abdollahi, M. Multiple protective mechanisms of alpha-lipoic acid in oxidation, apoptosis and inflammation against hydrogen peroxide induced toxicity in human lymphocytes. *Mol. Cell. Biochem.* **2015**, *403*, 179–186. [CrossRef] [PubMed]
45. Chen, J.-H.; Ozanne, S.E.; Hales, C.N. Methods of cellular senescence induction using oxidative stress. *Adv. Struct. Safety Stud.* **2007**, *371*, 179–189. [CrossRef]
46. Baeeri, M.; Mohammadi-Nejad, S.; Rahimifard, M.; Navaei-Nigjeh, M.; Moeini-Nodeh, S.; Khorasani, R.; Abdollahi, M. Molecular and biochemical evidence on the protective role of ellagic acid and silybin against oxidative stress-induced cellular aging. *Mol. Cell. Biochem.* **2017**, *441*, 21–33. [CrossRef]
47. Sherwood, S.; Hirst, J. Investigation of the mechanism of proton translocation by NADH: Ubiquinone oxidoreductase (complex I) from bovine heart mitochondria: Does the enzyme operate by a Q-cycle mechanism? *Biochem. J.* **2006**, *400*, 541–550. [CrossRef]
48. William, S.; Immo, E.; Allison, W.; Scheffler, I. Methods in enzymology. In *Mitochondrial Function, Part A: Mitochondrial Electron Transport Complexes and Reactive Oxygen Species*; Elsevier Inc.: London, UK, 2009; pp. 174–179.
49. Smith, L. Spectrophotometric assay of cytochrome c oxidase. In *Methods of Biochemical Analysis*; Glick, D., Ed.; John Wiley & Sons, Inc.: Hoboken, NJ, USA, 1955; Volume 2, pp. 427–434. ISBN 978-0-471-30459-3.
50. Moeini-Nodeh, S.; Rahimifard, M.; Baeeri, M.; Abdollahi, M. Functional Improvement in rats' pancreatic islets using magnesium oxide nanoparticles through antiapoptotic and antioxidant pathways. *Biol. Trace Element Res.* **2016**, *175*, 146–155. [CrossRef]
51. Hodjat, M.; Baeeri, M.; Rezvanfar, M.A.; Rahimifard, M.; Gholami, M.; Abdollahi, M. On the mechanism of genotoxicity of ethephon on embryonic fibroblast cells. *Toxicol. Mech. Methods* **2017**, *27*, 173–180. [CrossRef]
52. Abdollahi, M.; Heydary, V.; Navaei-Nigjeh, M.; Rahimifard, M.; Mohammadirad, A.; Baeeri, M. Biochemical and molecular evidences on the protection by magnesium oxide nanoparticles of chlorpyrifos-induced apoptosis in human lymphocytes. *J. Res. Med. Sci.* **2015**, *20*, 1021–1031. [CrossRef]
53. Nobakht-Haghighi, N.; Rahimifard, M.; Baeeri, M.; Rezvanfar, M.A.; Nodeh, S.M.; Haghi-Aminjan, H.; Hamurtekin, E.; Abdollahi, M. Regulation of aging and oxidative stress pathways in aged pancreatic islets using alpha-lipoic acid. *Mol. Cell. Biochem.* **2018**, *449*, 267–276. [CrossRef]

Sample Availability: Samples of the compounds are not available from the authors.

Publisher's Note: MDPI stays neutral with regard to jurisdictional claims in published maps and institutional affiliations.

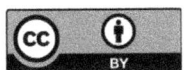

© 2020 by the authors. Licensee MDPI, Basel, Switzerland. This article is an open access article distributed under the terms and conditions of the Creative Commons Attribution (CC BY) license (http://creativecommons.org/licenses/by/4.0/).

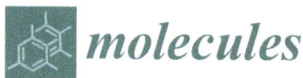

Article

Compound 275# Induces Mitochondria-Mediated Apoptosis and Autophagy Initiation in Colorectal Cancer Cells through an Accumulation of Intracellular ROS

Dong-Lin Yang [1,2], Yong Li [1], Shui-Qing Ma [1], Ya-Jun Zhang [1], Jiu-Hong Huang [1,2,*] and Liu-Jun He [1,*]

1 College of Pharmacy, National & Local Joint Engineering Research Center of Targeted and Innovative Therapeutics, Chongqing Key Laboratory of Kinase Modulators as Innovative Medicine, Chongqing University of Arts and Sciences, Chongqing 402160, China
2 College of Pharmaceutical Sciences and Chinese Medicine, Southwest University, Chongqing 400715, China
* Correspondence: huang_jiuhong@163.com (J.-H.H.); 15703083281@163.com (L.-J.H.)

Abstract: Colorectal cancer (CRC) is the most common intestinal malignancy, and nearly 70% of patients with this cancer develop metastatic disease. In the present study, we synthesized a novel compound, termed N-(3-(5,7-dimethylbenzo [d]oxazol-2-yl)phenyl)-5-nitrofuran-2-carboxamide (compound 275#), and found that it exhibits antiproliferative capability in suppressing the proliferation and growth of CRC cell lines. Furthermore, compound 275# triggered caspase 3-mediated intrinsic apoptosis of mitochondria and autophagy initiation. An investigation of the molecular mechanisms demonstrated that compound 275# induced intrinsic apoptosis, and autophagy initiation was largely mediated by increasing the levels of the intracellular accumulation of reactive oxygen species (ROS) in CRC cells. Taken together, these data suggest that ROS accumulation after treatment with compound 275# leads to mitochondria-mediated apoptosis and autophagy activation, highlighting the potential of compound 275# as a novel therapeutic agent for the treatment of CRC.

Keywords: compound 275#; CRC; apoptosis; ROS; autophagy

Citation: Yang, D.-L.; Li, Y.; Ma, S.-Q.; Zhang, Y.-J.; Huang, J.-H.; He, L.-J. Compound 275# Induces Mitochondria-Mediated Apoptosis and Autophagy Initiation in Colorectal Cancer Cells through an Accumulation of Intracellular ROS. Molecules 2023, 28, 3211. https://doi.org/10.3390/molecules28073211

Academic Editor: Andrea Ragusa

Received: 2 March 2023
Revised: 28 March 2023
Accepted: 30 March 2023
Published: 4 April 2023

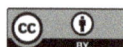

Copyright: © 2023 by the authors. Licensee MDPI, Basel, Switzerland. This article is an open access article distributed under the terms and conditions of the Creative Commons Attribution (CC BY) license (https://creativecommons.org/licenses/by/4.0/).

1. Introduction

Colorectal cancer (CRC), an aggressive primary gastrointestinal malignancy, has the third-highest incidence and second-highest mortality in all types of cancers worldwide. The number of CRC cases increases annually, and CRC poses a serious threat to human life and health [1]. Due to unknown etiology, lack of obvious symptoms in the early stage, and high level of metastasis, most CRC patients are diagnosed at advanced stages and have high mortality [2]. Despite the recent progress that has been made in treatment, the clinical outcomes and prognoses of patients with advanced-stage CRC remain extremely poor [3]. Thus, novel treatment regimens, such as the development of novel drugs that target proliferating tumor cells, may help to prolong the survival of CRC patients.

Reactive oxygen species (ROS) are a group of short-lived and highly reactive byproducts generated by aerobic metabolisms, which consist of hydroxyl radicals (OH$^\bullet$), superoxide ($^\bullet$O$_2^-$), hydroperoxy1 (HO$_2^\bullet$) radicals, and other nonradical members, such as hydrogen peroxide (H$_2$O$_2$) and singlet oxygen [4,5]. Cellular ROS are mainly originated from subcellular compartments or organelles, such as mitochondria, endoplasmic reticulum, lysosomes, and peroxisomes, by enzymatic reactions involving cyclooxygenases, oxidoreductases, NADPH oxidases, xanthine oxidases, and lipoxygenases and through the iron-catalyzed Fenton reaction [6]. As excellent significant intracellular signaling molecules, ROS play an important role in several physiological and pathological processes [7]. It is generally believed that low and moderate levels of ROS are required to promote tumor proliferation, survival, and metastasis [8,9]. In contrast, excessive ROS can lead to cellular oxidative stress and cell malfunction, which cause damage to DNA, proteins, or lipids, finally resulting in apoptotic or necrotic cell death [7,10]. Therefore, the identification of novel anticancer agents, which induce apoptotic cell death through the ROS generation mechanism, may be a necessary and effective treatment strategy for CRC.

In fact, many cancer therapeutic drugs often eliminate cancer cells and drug resistance through elevating ROS generation [11–13]. The aim of the present study was to synthesize a novel, small-molecule compound for potential future medical use, which is capable to induce excessive intracellular ROS. We investigated the anticancer activity of the novel, synthesized compound 275# against CRC in vitro and illustrated the underlying mechanism. Our data demonstrate that compound 275# suppresses the proliferation of CRC and acts as an inducer of ROS generation. Interestingly, ROS accumulation induced by compound 275# further triggered mitochondria-mediated intrinsic apoptosis and initiated autophagy, implying that compound 275# is a promising candidate as an anticancer agent.

2. Results

2.1. Synthesis of Compound 275#

The synthesis of compound 275# is indicated in Figure 1. Compound 1 (1 equivalents (equiv)) and compound 2 (1 equiv) were placed in PPA at 60 °C. The mixture was then heated at 100 °C for 1 h and followed at 125 °C for an additional 1.5 h. After cooling the mixture to room temperature, water was added, and the mixture was carefully neutralized with solid NaOH to pH~7.5–8.5. The formed precipitate was filtered off, suspended in 15% aqueous NaOH, filtered, washed with water, and dried. Crystallization from ethanol gave compound 3 in a 52% yield.

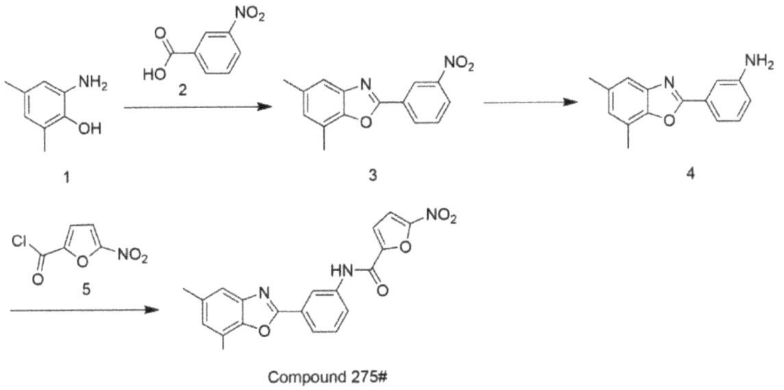

Figure 1. Strategy for the synthesis of compound 275#.

Compound 3 (1 equiv) was dissolved in hot CH_3OH. Then, ammonium formate (10 equiv) was added into the mixture followed by the portion-wise addition of a suspension of Pd/C (10%) (0.1 equiv) in water. The mixture was refluxed for 1 h, cooled to room temperature, filtered through celite, and concentrated in vacuo. The residue was suspended in water and extracted with ether. The combined ethereal extracts were dried over anhydrous Na_2SO_4 and concentrated to provide compound 4 in a yield of 90%.

The mixture of compound 4 (1 equiv) and acid chloride 5 (1.1 equiv) in dry DMF triethylamine (1.2 equiv) was added and stirred at 70 °C for 8 h. After quenching the reaction mixture with 3% Na_2CO_3, the precipitated product was filtered, washed with water, and dried. The product was recrystallized from the EtOH–EtOAc mixture to provide the target compound 275# in a 60% yield (Figure S1, Supplementary Materials).

2.2. Compound 275# Exhibits Cytotoxic Effects against CRC Cells

To explore the cytotoxicity of the novel, small-molecular compound 275# in CRC cells, an MTT assay was performed after exposure to this compound. As shown in Figure 2A,B, compound 275# dramatically reduced the cell viability in HCT116 and HCT8 cell lines in a dose- and time-dependent manner. In comparison, treatment with compound 275# was associated with a lower cytotoxicity in normal adult colonic epithelial cell line FHC (Figure 2C). Corresponding half-maximal inhibitory concentration (IC_{50}) values of compound 275 for the cell lines are shown in Figure 2D. To further examine its inhibitory effects, CRC cells were treated with different concentrations of compound 275# for 14 days, and the relationship between cell growth and concentration was evaluated. The colony formation assay showed that cells exposed to compound 275# exhibited markedly decreased cell growth in a dose-dependent manner, as convinced by the smaller colonies and reduced colony numbers compared with the control group (Figure 2E). Taken together, these results show that compound 275# could suppress cell proliferation and growth, suggesting that it has the potential as an inhibitor for the treatment of human CRC.

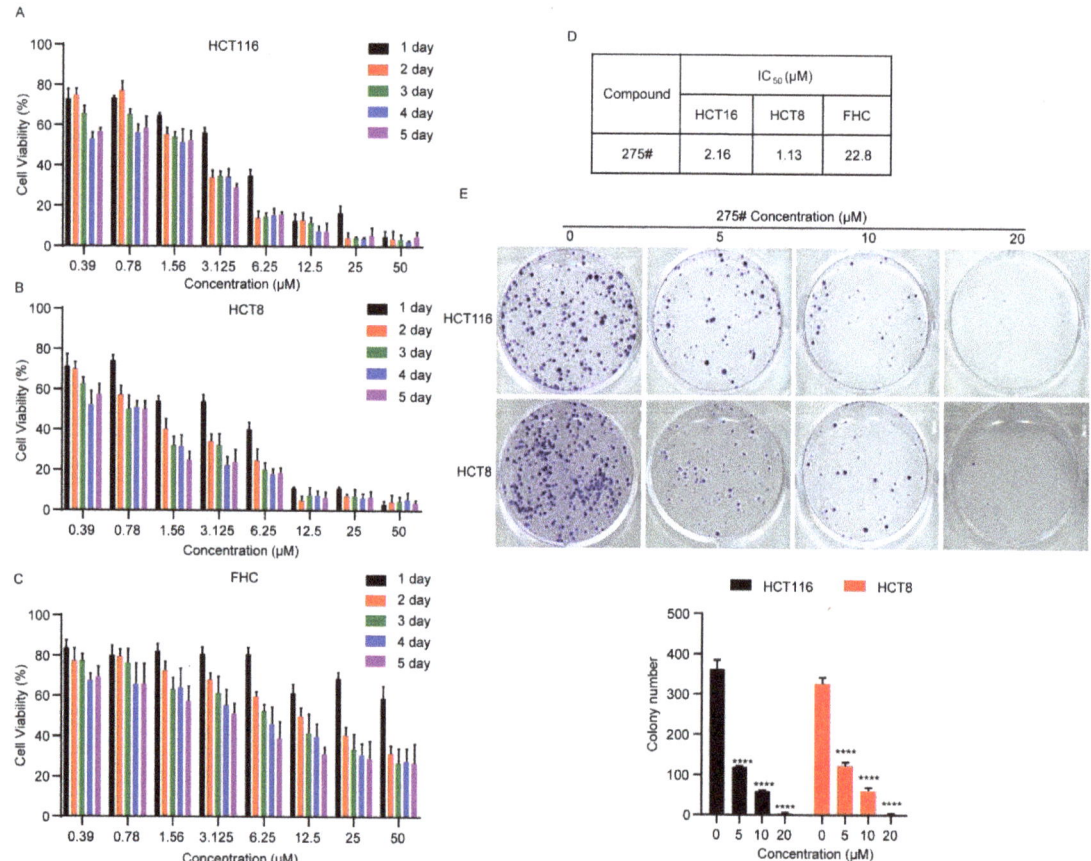

Figure 2. Compound 275# suppresses the proliferation and viability of CRC cells. (**A**,**B**) HCT116 and HCT8 cells were treated with the indicated concentrations of compound 275# for 1, 2, 3, 4, and 5 days. Relative cell viability was measured with MTT assay. (**C**) The cytotoxicity and specific effect of compound 275# on normal human rectal mucosal cells (FHC). (**D**) Calculated IC_{50} values of compound 275# for HCT116, HCT8, and FHC cell lines. (**E**) Colony formation assay was performed to evaluate growth in vitro after treatment with DMSO, 5, 10, and 20 µM compound 275# for 14 days. The colonies were visualized with the images. All data are presented as the mean ± SD of three independent experiments. **** $p < 0.001$ versus vehicle.

2.3. Compound 275# Promotes ROS Accumulation and ER Stress in CRC Cells

To gain insight into the action mode exhibited by compound 275# in CRC proliferative inhibition, we examined the intracellular ROS generation by flow cytometry after incubation with the specific ROS-detecting fluorescent dye (DCFH-DA) in HCT116 and HCT8 cells. As indicated in Figure 3A, ROS levels were considerably elevated in cells exposed to different concentrations of compound 275# when compared with control groups. In response to compound 275#, we found a time-dependent increase in intracellular ROS levels, and the earliest generation was detected at 0.5 h post treatment in CRC cells (Figure 3B). Next, flow cytometry indicated that pretreating the cells with NAC, a potent antioxidant and ROS scavenger, was capable to significantly reduce the number of DCFH-DA-positive HCT116 and HCT8 cells (Figure 3C). To further detect whether ROS specifically originate from mitochondria, MITOSOX, a novel fluorescent probe that specifically targets mitochondria in living cells, was used and found that most of ROS induced by compound 275# mainly originate from mitochondria (Figure S2, Supplementary Materials).

In light of previous studies showing that ROS accumulation is closely associated with the development of endoplasmic reticulum (ER) stress [14,15], we detected ER stress-related proteins in both HCT116 and HCT8 cells. As expected, compound 275# significantly increased the phosphorylation of eIF2α at Ser51 and the expression levels of several unfolded protein response (UPR)-associated proteins, such as BIP, CHOP, and ATF4, in a dose-dependent manner (Figure 3D), whereas NAC reduced its ability to upregulate ATF4 and CHOP (Figure 3E), suggesting that ER stress induced by compound 275# is dependent on excessive intracellular ROS.

2.4. Compound 275# Induces Mitochondria-Mediated Intrinsic Apoptosis in CRC Cells

A disproportional increase in ROS can induce the intrinsic apoptotic pathways mediated by mitochondria signaling [16–18]. Moreover, during ER stress, the level of CHOP expression is elevated, and CHOP functions to trigger mitochondria-mediated apoptosis by downregulating the prosurvival protein Bcl-2 [19]. Given the effects of compound 275# on the induction of ROS, apoptosis activation in response to compound 275# was evaluated. Of note, an Annexin V-FITC/PI assay was conducted using flow cytometry after HCT116 and HCT8 cells were exposed to compound 275# for 24 h. As indicated in Figure 4A, at a low dose of 5 µM, compound 275# induced 3.83% and 4.76% late-phase apoptosis (Annexin-V/PI double-positive cells) in HCT116 and HCT8 cell lines, respectively. At a dose of 20 µM, the percentage of both Annexin-V/PI-positive cells rose to 99.6% and 99.9%, respectively. Consistently, procaspase 3 and PARP were cleaved and activated in both HCT116 and HCT8 cells after treatment (Figure 4B), implying that compound 275# is capable to promote apoptosis.

Next, to evaluate whether the treatment with compound 275# affects depolarization of the mitochondrial membrane, the mitochondrial membrane potential (MMP, $\Delta\Psi m$) was measured with a fluorescent probe JC-1 in CRC cells treated with or without compound 275#. As hypothesized, 20 µM of compound 275# caused more than a 40% decrease in $\Delta\Psi m$ in CRC cells in comparison with the control group (Figure 4C), suggesting that the apoptosis triggered by compound 275# might be related to the mitochondrial pathway. Subsequently, the expression of mitochondrial signaling-associated proteins was detected to determine whether mitochondria was involved in apoptosis in response to compound 275#. As indicated in Figure 4D, we found that antiapoptotic proteins, such as Bcl-2 and Bcl-XL, were significantly reduced in a dose-dependent manner after exposure to compound 275#, while the proapoptotic protein Puma (p53 upregulated modulator of apoptosis) was dramatically elevated. Furthermore, compound 275# remarkably increased cytochrome c levels in a dose-dependent manner in CRC cells (Figure 4D), indicating that compound 275# may induce the release of cytochrome c from mitochondria to cytosol. In addition, the protein level of p53 was not influenced by compound 275#, and we inferred that the proapoptotic effect of compound 275# may be not mediated by p53 (Figure S3, Supplementary Materials). These results show that compound 275# might inhibit cell proliferation by inducing a mitochondrial-dependent apoptotic pathway in CRC cells.

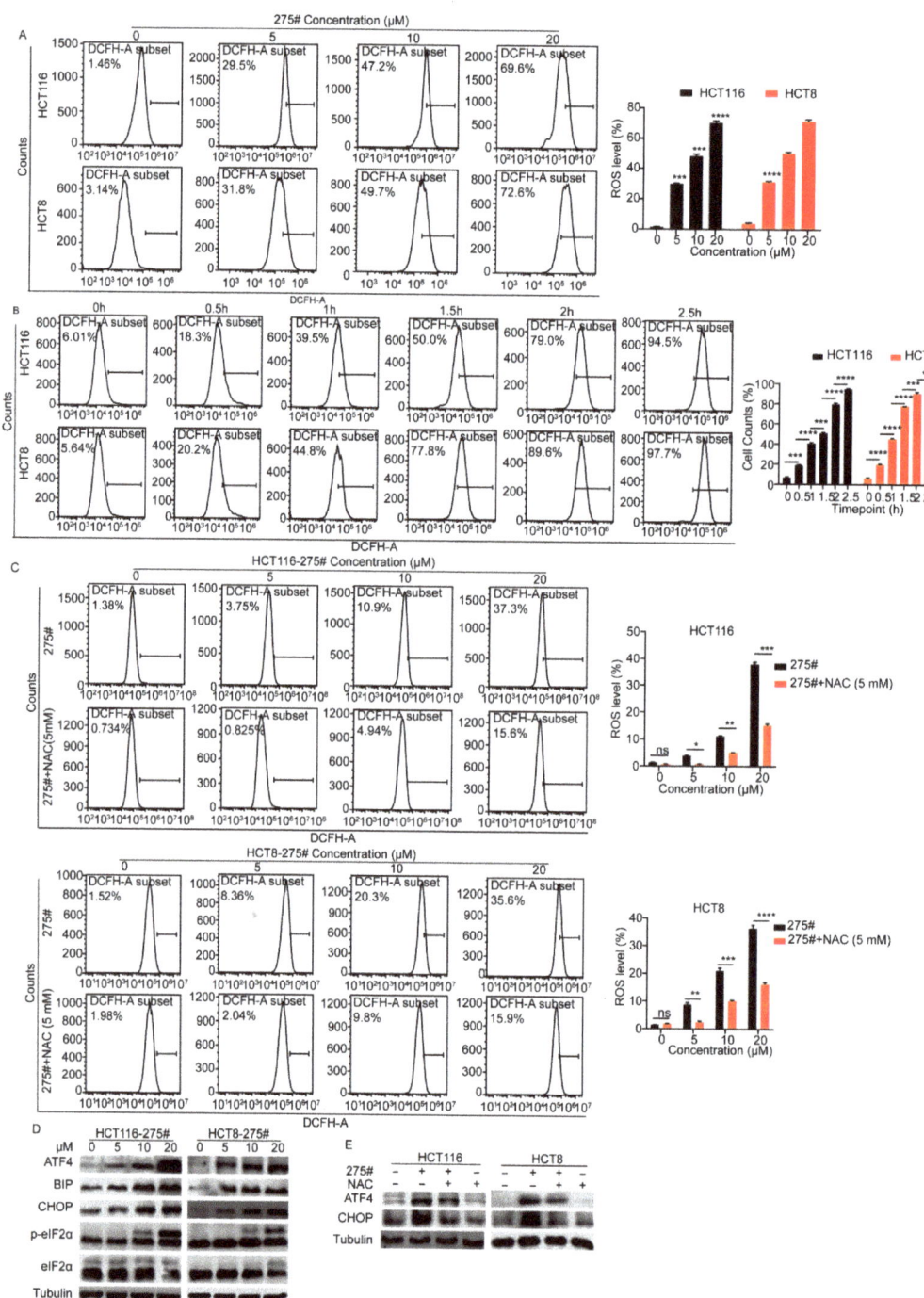

Figure 3. Compound 275# induces the accumulation of ROS and promotes ROS-dependent ER stress. (**A**) Compound 275# triggers ROS generation in a dose-dependent manner. HCT116 and HCT8 cells

were treated with the indicated concentrations of compound 275# for 2 h and then were exposed to DCFH-DA for another 20 min. Flow cytometry analysis was conducted to assess ROS generation. (**B**) Compound 275# triggers ROS generation in a time-dependent manner. (**C**) NAC, a potent antioxidant and ROS scavenger, was capable to reduce compound 275#-induced ROS accumulation in CRC cells. HCT116 and HCT8 cells were pretreated with or without NAC (5 mM) for 1 h and subsequently treated with compound 275# for 24 h before staining with DCFH-DA (10 μM) for 20 min. (**D**) Following treatment with different concentrations of compound 275#, cells were lysed, and expression of ER stress-related proteins was examined by Western blotting. (**E**) NAC can reverse compound 275#-triggered ER stress. β-tubulin was used as the loading control. Data are presented as the mean ± standard deviation of three independent experiments. * $p < 0.05$, ** $p < 0.01$, *** $p < 0.001$, and **** $p < 0.0001$ vs. control.

2.5. Induction of Intrinsic Apoptosis by Compound 275# Is Mediated through Excessive ROS

To further demonstrate whether the capability to induce mitochondria-mediated apoptosis by compound 275# in CRC cells was actually initiated by accumulating excessive cellular ROS, the proapoptotic effect of compound 275# on HCT116 and HCT8 cells after treatment with NAC was determined. As expected, flow cytometry showed that pretreating the cells with NAC significantly reduced the number of apoptotic cells induced by compound 275# (Figure 5A). Additionally, the effect of NAC on ΔΨm, which is reduced in response to compound 275#, was evaluated. We found that NAC pretreatment can obviously reverse the compound 275#-mediated decrease in ΔΨm in both HCT116 and HCT8 cells (Figure 5B). Subsequently, a caspase 3 inhibitor, Z-VAD-FMK, was used to detect the restorative effect on apoptosis caused by compound 275#. As shown in Figure 5C and Figure S4, Z-VAD-FMK can significantly rescue cell apoptosis induced by compound 275# and reduce the inhibitory effect of compound 275# on CRC cells. Consistently, immunoblotting results indicate that pretreating the cells with NAC dramatically downregulated the expression levels of Bax and cytochrome c and upregulated the antiapoptotic protein Bcl-2. Moreover, treatment with compound 275# alone considerably enhanced the cleavage of procaspase-3 and the downstream PARP, while combined treatment with compound 275# and NAC caused minimal proteolytic processing of procaspase-3 and cleavage of PARP (Figure 5D). Collectively, these results indicate that compound 275# induced mitochondria-mediated apoptosis in CRC cells by leading to the production of excessive ROS, which acts as a trigger of downstream caspase 3-dependent apoptosis.

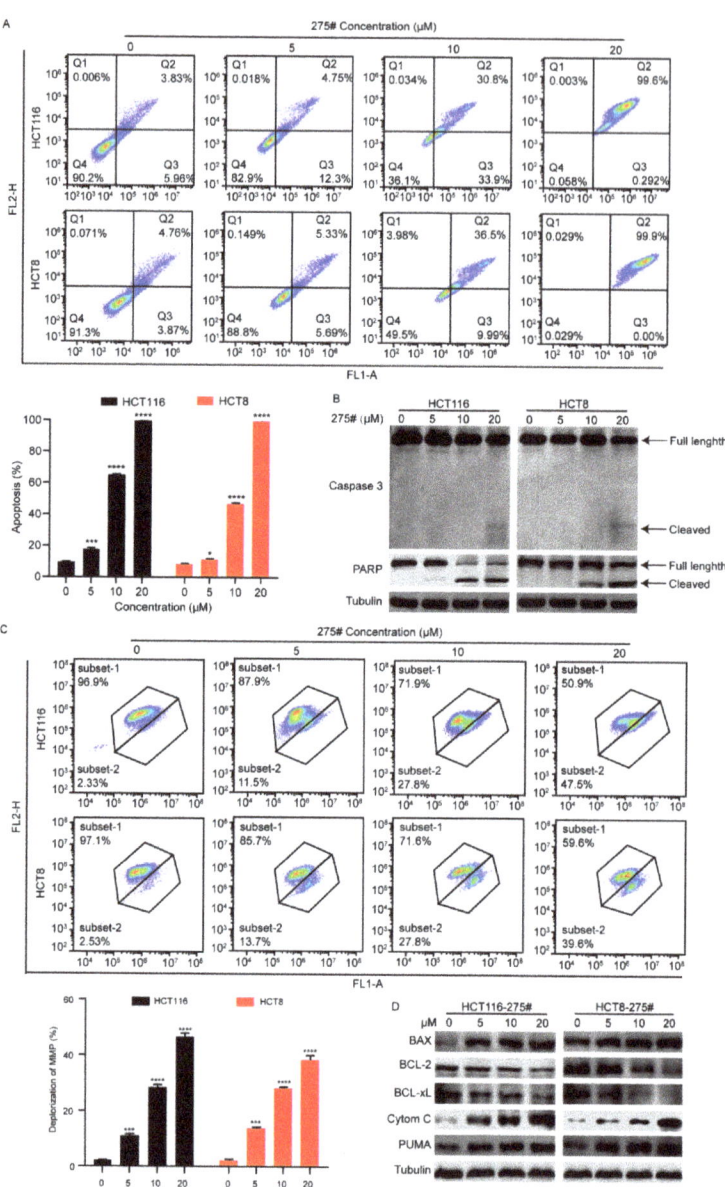

Figure 4. Compound 275# promotes mitochondria-mediated intrinsic apoptosis in both HCT116 and HCT8 cells. (**A**) Compound 275# triggers apoptosis in a dose-dependent manner in CRC cells. HCT116 and HCT8 cells were treated with the indicated concentrations of compound 275# for 24 h. Subsequently, cells were harvested and stained with annexin-V/PI. The color indicates the cell density and it changes from blue to red as the density increases. (**B**) Compound 275# can facilitate cleavage of caspase 3 and PARP. Cleaved forms of caspase 3 and PARP were detected using Western blotting after treatment with indicated doses of compound 275#. (**C**) Mitochondrial membrane potential (ΔΨm) is reduced after exposure to compound 275#. The ΔΨm was measured by flow cytometry after staining with fluorescent probe JC-1. Results indicating the intensity of green fluorescence show as folds of control

from three independent experiments. The color indicates the cell density and it changes from blue to red as the density increases. (**D**) Expression of mitochondria-mediated apoptosis-related proteins was examined using Western blotting after treatment with indicated concentrations of compound 275#. β-tubulin was used as the loading control. * $p < 0.05$, *** $p < 0.001$, and **** $p < 0.0001$ vs. control.

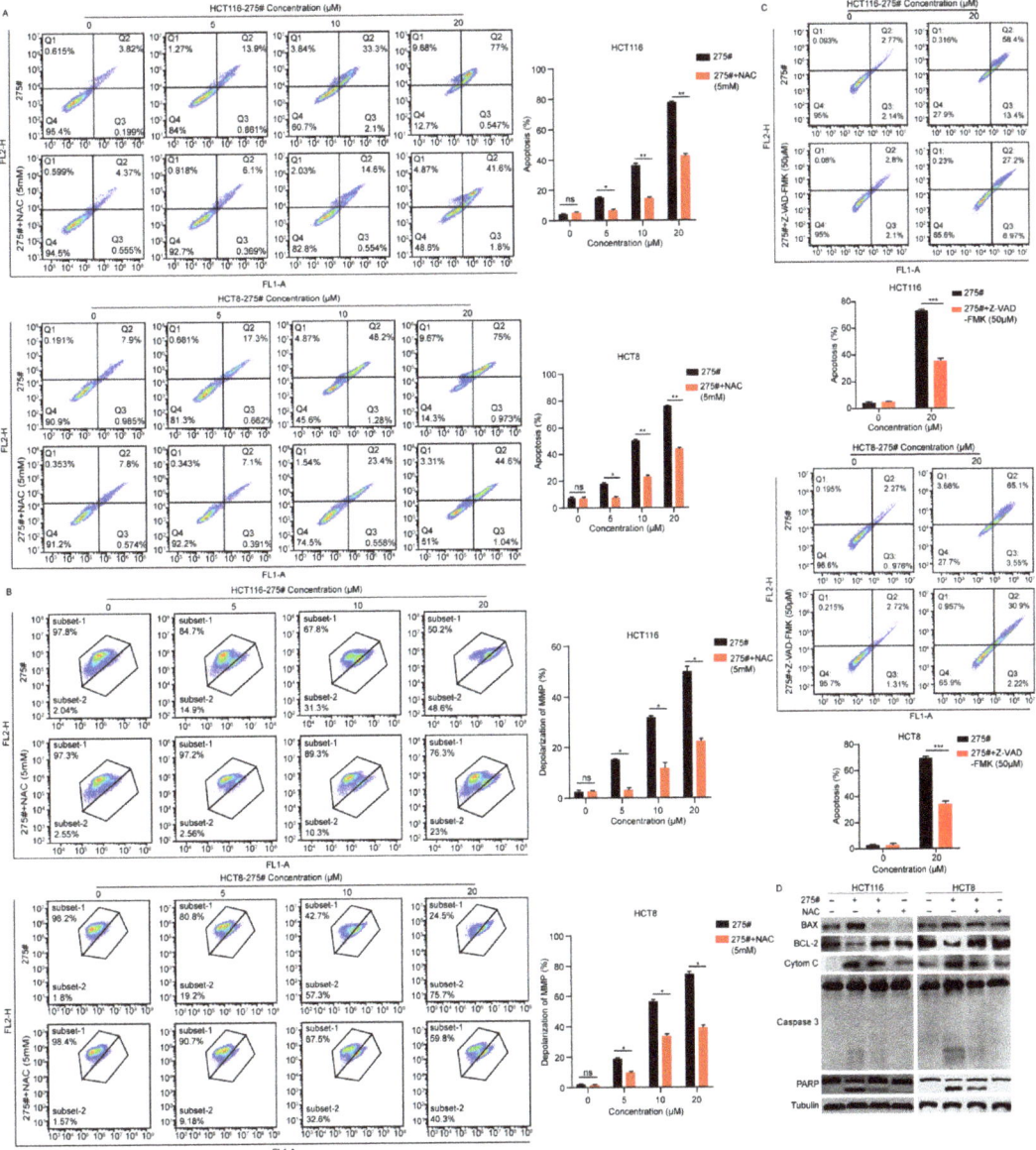

Figure 5. Induction of caspase-dependent intrinsic apoptosis by compound 275# is mediated through the accumulation of excessive ROS. (**A**) Blocking of ROS generation significantly decreased compound 275#-mediated apoptosis. HCT116 and HCT8 cells were pretreated with or without 5 mM NAC for 1 h and then treated with different concentrations of compound 275# for 24 h. Cell apoptosis was subsequently measured using flow cytometry. The color indicates the cell density and it changes

from blue to red as the density increases. (**B**) NAC significantly reversed ΔΨm decrease induced by compound 275#. The color indicates the cell density and it changes from blue to red as the density increases. (**C**) A specific caspase 3 inhibitor, Z-VAD-FMK, significantly decreased the rate of apoptosis triggered by compound 275# in HCT116 and HCT8 cells. Both HCT116 and HCT8 cells were treated with 20 µM compound 275#, with or without the inclusion of 50 µM caspase 3 inhibitor Z-VAD-FMK before staining with PI and Annexin V. The color indicates the cell density and it changes from blue to red as the density increases. (**D**) NAC could abrogate the effects of compound 275# on the expression levels of BCL-2 family proteins, cytochrome c, and apoptotic executor caspase 3. β-tubulin was used as the loading control. Data are presented as the mean ± standard deviation of three independent experiments. * $p < 0.05$, ** $p < 0.01$, and *** $p < 0.001$ vs. control.

2.6. Autophagy Initiation Triggered by Compound 275# Is Tightly Linked with Its Ability to Promote ROS Accumulation

Because the accumulation of ROS has been reported to exhibit a positive effect on autophagy activation [20,21], we investigated whether compound 275# can play a role in autophagy by generating excessive intracellular ROS. As indicated in Figure 6A, after exposure to compound 275#, the number of green puncta, which represent the formation of phagophores and autophagosomes, was remarkably increased in HCT116 cells transfected with the green fluorescent protein (GFP)-fused LC3B (GFP-LC3B) compared with the control group. Consistently, the autophagosome-associated form, LC3B-II, was obviously increased in CRC cells upon compound 275# treatment, whereas the level of p62, a specific marker of autophagic flux, was strongly downregulated in a dose-dependent manner (Figure 6B), indicating that autophagy was activated and autophagosomes were formed after treatment. To confirm whether or not compound 275# could regulate autophagic flux changes in CRC cells, we blocked autophagic flux by using chloroquine (CQ), a classical autophagic flux inhibitor. We found that the combined administration of both compound 275# and CQ exerted a cooperative enhancement of the LC3B-II expression level compared with either drug treatment alone. However, single-compound 275# treatment-induced p62 downregulation could be reversed by CQ (Figure 6C). Because autophagosomes can be formed by the activation of autophagy as well as by blocking autophagic flux, we next determined whether compound 275# activates or inhibits autophagy. Alternatively, 3-methyladenine (3-MA), an inhibitor of class III PI3K that inhibits autophagy initiation, was used to demonstrate compound 275#-induced autophagy. As shown in Figure 6D, 3-MA could mostly attenuate the GFP-LC3B-II puncta accumulation in CRC cells induced by compound 275#. To further confirm that compound 275# mainly plays a role in autophagy induction but not in the fusion process between autophagosome and lysosome, a tandem RFP-GFP-tagged LC3B autophagy reporter system was utilized as a dual-fluorescence pH sensor. Autophagosomes appear as yellow (both RFP and GFP signals) puncta, whereas autolysosomes appear as red (RFP-only signals) puncta. Of note, when the cells were treated with compound 275#, the number of red puncta was increased markedly without any significant increase in the number of yellow puncta (Figure 6E), whereas the autophagy promotion effect induced by compound 275# was dramatically attenuated by the cotreatment with 3-MA (Figure 6F). These results imply that compound 275# promotes fusion between autophagosome and autolysosome.

Next, cells were treated with 20 µM of compound 275# combined with 5 mM of NAC to determine the effect of NAC on autophagy. Notably, compound 275#-induced GFP-LC3B-II puncta accumulation was strongly abrogated by the cotreatment with NAC (Figure 6G). Consistently, we found that treatment with NAC was able to almost completely prevent the compound 275#-induced LC3-II accumulation (Figure 6H), implying that ROS accumulation mediated autophagy initiation in compound 275#-treated HCT116 cells. Furthermore, NAC could also greatly attenuate the enhanced autophagic flux progression caused by compound 275# treatment (Figure 6I). Collectively, these results demonstrate that excessive ROS induced by compound 275# participate in autophagy initiation.

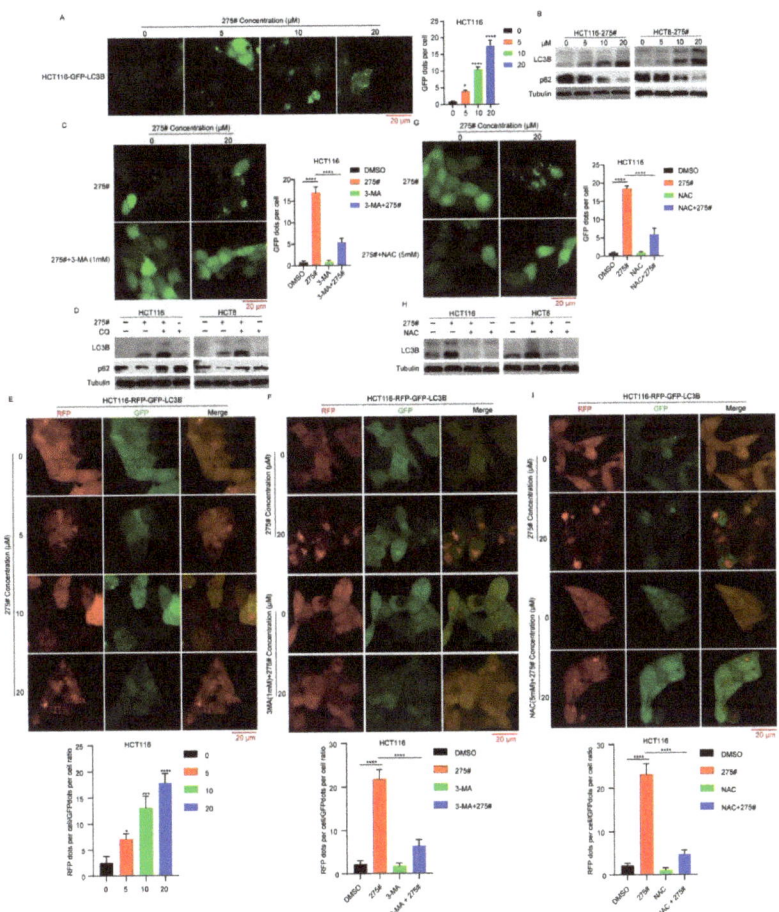

Figure 6. Compound 275# could promote the initiation of selective autophagy by inducing ROS accumulation. (**A**) Compound 275# markedly increased GFP-LC3B puncta. Fluorescence analysis was performed to evaluate the exogenous LC3 dot signals in HCT16 cells transfected with GFP-LC3 after treatment with or without compound 275#. Scale bar: 10 μm. (**B**) Western blotting analysis of LC3B and p62 in HCT116 cells treated with indicated concentrations of compound 275# for 12 h. β-tubulin level was used as internal load control. (**C**) 3-MA could strongly attenuate the GFP-LC3B puncta accumulation in HCT116 cells induced by compound 275#. (**D**) Compound 275# promoted LC3-II accumulation through autophagy initiation but not the inhibition of autophagic flux progression in CRC cells. HCT116 and HCT8 cells were treated with compound 202#, CQ, or a combination of them before detecting with Western blotting. (**E**) Compound 275# promoted the autophagic flux in HCT116 cells overexpressing RFP-EGFP-LC3. Scale bar, 10 μm. Yellow fluorescent dots represent the autophagosomes. Red fluorescent dots indicating autophagolysosomes were counted in three independent experiments. (**F**) Autophagy initiation effect induced by compound 275# was dramatically attenuated by cotreatment with 3-MA. (**G**) Compound 275#-induced accumulation of GFP-LC3B puncta was markedly abrogated by cotreatment with NAC. (**H**) Treatment with NAC was able to almost completely prevent the compound 275#-induced LC3-II accumulation. (**I**) NAC could greatly attenuate the enhanced autophagic flux progression caused by compound 275# treatment. Data are presented as the mean ± standard deviation of three independent experiments. * $p < 0.05$, *** $p < 0.001$, and **** $p < 0.0001$ vs. control.

3. Discussion

Chemotherapy resistance remains a major problem in limiting the efficacy of conventional and molecular-targeted cancer therapies. This problem is evident in colorectal cancer, in which, despite the advances in therapeutic options, such as EGFR inhibitors and drug combinations using EGFR inhibitor plus VEGF inhibitor/MEK inhibitor/BRAF inhibitor, the mortality rate remains high for cancer-related deaths [22,23]. Hence, there is an urgent need for therapeutic strategies to overcome drug resistance in CRC, such as the development of novel anticancer agents. In the present study, compound 275# was synthesized and exhibited some antiproliferative activity against CRC cells, facilitating further exploration of its antiproliferative effects and the underlying molecular mechanisms. Compound 275# had a structure that was similar to those previously reported benzoxazole derivatives. These derivatives possessed different inhibitory activities against cancer cells, *Trypan osoma brucei* [24] and *Visceral Leishmaniasis* [25], and selectively targeted tyrosine kinase [26], proteasome [25], and transthyretin amyloidogenesis [27]. The results from our analysis show that compound 275# can significantly inhibit CRC cell proliferation and growth, which is consistent with the above-mentioned data. However, in our current study, we failed to find the target of compound 275#. This compound may be a potential inhibitor of tyrosine kinase and proteasome, and we will demonstrate it in our future research.

It is well known that apoptosis is a fundamental regulatory process in multicellular organisms that plays a crucial role in the maintenance and development of homeostasis [28]. Moreover, apoptosis is involved in tumor formation and cancer therapy and is regarded as a main defense mechanism against tumorigenesis [29]. Numerous anticancer agents exert their inhibitory effects by triggering apoptosis [30–32]. It has been shown that two major apoptotic pathways are capable of initiating apoptosis: the mitochondrial-mediated intrinsic pathway and the death receptor-mediated extrinsic pathway [33]. Mitochondria-mediated apoptosis is fundamentally orchestrated by proapoptotic proteins and antiapoptotic proteins [34,35]. The production of cytochrome c from the mitochondrial intermembrane space into the cytoplasm induced by the intrinsic pathway can eventually activate the critical caspase cascade and the generation of the apoptosome, leading to the progression of apoptosis [36,37]. Accumulating evidence has indicated that certain pharmaceutical compounds cause apoptosis through the production of excessive intracellular ROS [38–41]. In agreement with these previous studies, the results of the present study show that compound 275# significantly downregulated antiapoptotic proteins, Bcl-2 and Bcl-XL, while it upregulated the proapoptotic proteins, Puma and Bax, and promoted the release of cytochrome c from mitochondria to cytosol, resulting in the decrease in $\Delta\Psi m$. Moreover, these effects exerted by compound 275# can be remarkably rescued in response to NAC treatment. Based on these data, it was hypothesized that compound 275# exerted its anticancer effects on CRC cells by inducing intrinsic apoptosis following treatment, and this was due to the intracellular accumulation of ROS.

Autophagy is a self-degradative process that is associated with cell proliferation, survival, tumorigenesis, development, and stress responses [42]. Interestingly, intracellular ROS accumulation has previously been reported to initiate autophagy [43]. In this study, we found that enhanced LC-3 II was induced by compound 275# treatment in vitro, while the autophagic flux marker, p62, was markedly reduced. Moreover, the fusion between autophagosome and lysosome was facilitated after treatment with compound 275#, supported by a tandem RFP-GFP-tagged LC3B autophagy reporter system. Surprisingly, the autophagy inhibitor 3-MA blocked the compound 275#-induced accumulation of LC-3-II. However, the antioxidants NAC markedly abolished compound 275#-induced ROS generation and autophagy. The present data clearly support our hypothesis that compound 275# primarily initiates autophagy rather than the late stage of autophagy, such as the fusion between autophagosome and lysosome, and autophagy activation is triggered by ROS accumulation. Considerable evidence has indicated that apoptosis and autophagy were thought to be two mutually cross-regulated cellular events because they share several critical molecular regulators, such as JNK1, Bcl-2, and Beclin 1 [44–47]. Hence, future experiments will be undertaken to clarify the complex mutual regulatory mechanism between autophagy and apoptosis induced by compound 275#.

4. Materials and Methods

4.1. Reagents and Antibodies

Methylthiazolyldiphenyl-tetrazolium bromide (MTT, ST316), N-Acetylcysteine (NAC, S0077), Z-VAD-FMK (C1202), and crystal violet staining solution (C0121) were obtained from Beyotime Biotechnology (Shanghai, China). 3-Methyladenine (3-MA, S2767) was purchased from Selleckchem (Houston, TX, USA). Anti-ATF4 (11815S), anti-BIP (3177S), anti-CHOP (2895S), anti-eIF2α (5324S), anti-Phospho-eIF2α (Ser51) (3398S), anti-Bax (41162S), anti-BCL2 (15071S), anti-Bcl-xL (2764S), anti-Puma (98672S), anti-LC3B (3868S), anti-SQSTM1/p62 (88588S), anti-Cytochrome c (4272S), anti-Caspase-3 (9662S), anti-PARP (9532S), and anti-β-Tubulin (2128S) antibodies were purchased from Cell Signaling Technology (Danvers, MA, USA).

4.2. Cell Lines and Culture

Human colorectal cancer cell lines HCT116 and HCT8 were obtained from the American Type Culture Collection (ATCC, Manassas, VA, USA). HCT116 and HCT8 cells were cultured in McCoy's 5a (FBS, 10100147, thermofisher Scientific, Waltham, MA, USA) and RPMI 1640 (Cytiva, SH30022.01, Xcellerex, MA, USA) medium supplemented with 10% fetal bovine serum (FBS, 10100147, thermofisher Scientific, Waltham, MA, USA), respectively. All cells were cultured in an incubator with a humidified atmosphere of 5% CO_2 at 37 °C.

4.3. Cell Viability Assay

The inhibitory effect of compound 275# on HCT116, HCT8, and normal adult colonic epithelial cell line FHC was determined by MTT assay. Cells were harvested at a density of 90% and counted and seeded into a 96-well plate (1×10^3 cells per well) containing 200 µL complete medium. After incubation for 24 h, cells were treated with compound 275# at various concentrations (0, 0.39, 0.78, 1.56, 3.125, 6.25, 12.5, 25, and 50 µM) and incubated for 1, 2, 3, 4, and 5 days, respectively. Subsequently, 20 µL MTT solution (5 mg/mL) was added to each well and incubated with the cells for 4 h. The medium was discarded, and 150 µL dimethylsulfoxide (DMSO) was added to each well to dissolve the formazan. The absorbance was measured at 570 nm using a microplate reader (Bio-Tek, Winooski, VT, USA). All experiments were performed in triplicate. The cell viability of the HCT116, HCT8, and FHC cell lines was calculated using GraphPad® Prism 9.0 software (Dotmatics, Boston, MA, USA).

4.4. Colony Formation Assay

For the colony formation assay, HCT116 and HCT8 cells were seeded into a 6-well plate at a density of 1000 cells per well supplemented with 2 mL complete medium, and the cells were subsequently incubated for 24 h. After exposure to compound 275# at concentrations of 0, 5, 10, or 20 µM for 14 days, the colonies formed were washed with cold phosphate-buffered saline (PBS), fixed with 4% paraformaldehyde for 25 min and then stained with 0.5% crystal violet for 30 min at room temperature. The plates were scanned and visualized using a Perfection V800 Photo scanning apparatus (Seiko Epson Corporation, Tokyo, Japan). All statistical measurements were performed in triplicate.

4.5. Immunoblotting

Both HCT116 and HCT8 cells were treated with compound 275# alone at concentrations of 0, 5, 10, and 20 µM for 12 h or in combination with 5 mM NAC for 4 h. Subsequently, the harvested cells were lysed in radioimmunoprecipitation assay (RIPA) buffer (150 mM NaCl, 1% Nonidet P-40 (NP-40), 1% sodium deoxycholate, 0.1% sodium dodecyl sulfate (SDS), 25 mM Tris-HCl (pH 7.4), and 1 mM EDTA (pH 8.0)) supplemented with Halt™ Protease and Phosphatase Inhibitor Cocktail (Thermo Fisher Scientific, Waltham, MA, USA) on ice for 30 min. The lysates were centrifuged at 15,000× g for 20 min, and the supernatants were collected. Total protein concentrations of supernatants were quantified using BCA (Bicinchoninic acid) Kit (Beyotime, P0010, Shanghai, China). An equal amount of total proteins for each sample (30 µg) was loaded, separated by 10% and 15% SDS-polyacrylamide gel electrophoresis, and transferred to polyvinylidene difluoride (PVDF) membranes (MilliporeSigma, St. Louis, MO, USA). After that, the membranes were blocked with 5% fat-free milk in TBST for 2 h at room temperature, incubated with the indicated primary antibodies overnight at 4 °C, and then incubated with the IRDye® 800CW goat anti-mouse IgG (H+L) or IRDye® 680LT donkey anti-rabbit IgG (H+L) (LI-COR Biosciences) secondary antibody at room temperature in a dark environment for 1 h. Finally, antibody-bound membranes were washed 3 times in TBST each for 5 min, and immunoreactivity was visualized using an Odyssey Two-Color Infrared fluorescence Imaging System (LI-COR Biosciences, Lincoln, NH, USA).

4.6. Cell Apoptosis Analysis

The apoptosis of HCT116 and HCT8 was assayed by the Annexin V-FITC Apoptosis Detection Kit (C1062S, Beyotime, Shanghai, China) according to the manufacturer's protocol. Briefly, cells were seeded into a 60 mm dish with a density of 2×10^6 cells per dish and cultured overnight. After pretreatment with NAC (5 mM) or Z-VAD-FMK (50 µM) for 1 h, cells were exposed to different concentrations of compound 275# for 24 h. All treated samples were collected and washed with PBS and then incubated with annexin V-FITC and PI for 30 min at room temperature in the dark. Finally, cells were measured with flow cytometry, and the apoptosis ratio was analyzed using FlowJo 7.6.1 analysis software (Becton Dickinson, San Jose, CA, USA).

4.7. Mitochondrial Membrane Potential (MMP, $\Delta\Psi m$) Assay

The $\Delta\Psi m$ of HCT116 and HCT8 was measured using an enhanced mitochondrial membrane potential assay kit with JC-1 (C2003S, Beyotime, Shanghai, China). Briefly, cells were seeded into a 60 mm dish with a density of 2×10^6 cells per dish and cultured overnight. Cells were pretreated with 5 mM NAC for 1 h and then treated with compound 275# for additional 24 h until harvested for further incubation with the mitochondria-specific fluorescent dye JC-1 for 20 min at 37 °C. Then, JC-1 dye was removed and washed twice with JC-1 buffer. Finally, the $\Delta\Psi m$ of cells was measured by flow cytometry and analyzed by FlowJo 7.6.1 analysis software.

4.8. Determination of ROS Formation

The amount of cellular ROS was measured by Reactive Oxygen Species Assay Kit (S0033S, Beyotime, Shanghai, China). Briefly, cells were seeded into a 60 mm dish with a density of 2×10^6 cells per dish and cultured for 24 h. Cells were pretreated with 5 mM NAC for 1 h or with DMSO alone (control) before adding compound 275# (up to 20 µM) for 2 h. After rinsing with PBS, the cells were incubated with 10 µM Dichloro-dihydro-fluorescein diacetate (DCFH-DA) for another 20 min in the dark at 37 °C, followed by flow cytometry detection to determine the level of cellular ROS. The analysis of cytometry data was achieved using FlowJo 7.6.1 software.

4.9. Fluorescence Observation of RFP-GFP-LC3B

For autophagy analysis, HCT116 cells stably expressed RFP-GFP-LC3B were constructed by lentivirus infection. Lentivirus packaging vectors (Pspax2, pMD2G) and RFP-GFP-LC3B were cotransfected into HEK293T cells using Lipo8000 Transfection Reagent (C0533, Beyotime, Shanghai, China) according to the manufacturer's protocols. Viral particles were harvested after 48 h transfection and then added directly into HCT116 cells with the assistance of Polybrene (10 µg/mL). Subsequently, cells were selected by 5 µg/mL puromycin to obtain the cell-stable expression clones. The stable RFP-GFP-LC3B-expressing cells were pretreated with 3-MA (1 mM) or NAC (5 mM) for 1 h and further incubated with or without compound 275# for 12 h. The fluorescent LC3B dots were captured and analyzed by the high-content analysis system-operetta CLSTM (Perkinelmer, Waltham, MA, USA).

4.10. Statistical Analysis

All experiments were performed in triplicate. GraphPad Prism version 9.0 (GraphPad Software, San Diego, CA, USA) was used for statistical analysis. Data were presented as mean ±standard deviation, and the ANOVA method was used to compare differences between groups. $p < 0.05$ was considered to be significant.

5. Conclusions

In summary, a novel compound, termed compound 275#, was synthesized using pharmaceutical methods, and we found that it exhibits inhibitory effects on CRC cells. Interestingly, compound 275# promoted a mitochondria-mediated intrinsic apoptosis pathway and autophagy initiation due to the intracellular accumulation of ROS. Therefore, our findings favorably imply the antitumor mechanism of compound 275# and offer evidence of its potential as a promising new lead compound in the discovery of chemotherapeutic agents for CRC.

Supplementary Materials: The following supporting information can be downloaded at: https://www.mdpi.com/article/10.3390/molecules28073211/s1, Figure S1: ^{1}H NMR and ^{13}C NMR spectra of compound 275#. Figure S2: Most of the ROS induced by compound 275# mainly originate from mitochondria. Figure S3: The protein level of p53 was not influenced by compound 275# and inferred that proapoptotic effect of compound 275# may be not mediated by p53. Figure S4: Pretreatment with Z-VAD-FMK can significantly improve cell viability and reduce the inhibitory effect of compound 275# on CRC cells.

Author Contributions: D.-L.Y., J.-H.H. and L.-J.H. designed and conceived the work. L.-J.H., Y.L., S.-Q.M. and Y.-J.Z. performed the experiments. D.-L.Y., L.-J.H., J.-H.H. and Y.L. analyzed and interpreted the data; D.-L.Y. and L.-J.H. prepared all figures and wrote the manuscript. All authors read and provided input on the manuscript. All authors have read and agreed to the published version of the manuscript.

Funding: This research was supported by the Basic Research and Frontier Program of Chongqing Science and Technology Bureau (CSTB2022NSCQ-MSX1293, cstc2020jcyj-msxmX0733 and cstc2020jcyj-msxmX0595), Science and Technology Research Program of Chongqing Municipal Education Commission (KJQN202201329, KJQN202201330, KJZD-K202001302, and KJQN201901331), The Science and Technology Program of Yongchuan Science and Technology Bureau (2022yc-jckx20014 and 2021yc-jckx20044), and Scientific Research Foundation of Chongqing University of Arts and Sciences (Y2020XY14).

Institutional Review Board Statement: Not applicable.

Informed Consent Statement: Not applicable.

Data Availability Statement: The datasets used and/or analyzed during the current study are available from the corresponding author on reasonable request.

Conflicts of Interest: The authors declare no conflict of interest.

Sample Availability: Compounds synthesized in this present study are available from the authors.

References

1. Sung, H.; Ferlay, J.; Siegel, R.L.; Laversanne, M.; Soerjomataram, I.; Jemal, A.; Bray, F. Global cancer statistics 2020: GLOBOCAN estimates of incidence and mortality worldwide for 36 cancers in 185 countries. *CA* **2021**, *71*, 209–249. [CrossRef]
2. Siegel, R.L.; Miller, K.D.; Goding Sauer, A.; Fedewa, S.A.; Butterly, L.F.; Anderson, J.C.; Cercek, A.; Smith, R.A.; Jemal, A. Colorectal cancer statistics, 2020. *CA* **2020**, *70*, 145–164. [CrossRef]
3. Yu, I.S.; Cheung, W.Y. Metastatic colorectal cancer in the era of personalized medicine: A more tailored approach to systemic therapy. *Can. J. Gastroenterol. Hepatol.* **2018**, *2018*, 9450754. [CrossRef]
4. Sies, H.; Jones, D.P. Reactive oxygen species (ROS) as pleiotropic physiological signalling agents. *Nat. Rev. Mol. Cell Biol.* **2020**, *21*, 363–383. [CrossRef]

5. D'Autréaux, B.; Toledano, M.B. ROS as signalling molecules: Mechanisms that generate specificity in ROS homeostasis. *Nat. Rev. Mol. Cell Biol.* **2007**, *8*, 813–824. [CrossRef]
6. Hayes, J.D.; Dinkova-Kostova, A.T.; Tew, K.D. Oxidative stress in cancer. *Cancer Cell* **2020**, *38*, 167–197. [CrossRef]
7. Schieber, M.; Chandel, N.S. ROS function in redox signaling and oxidative stress. *Curr. Biol.* **2014**, *24*, R453–R462. [CrossRef]
8. DeNicola, G.M.; Karreth, F.A.; Humpton, T.J.; Gopinathan, A.; Wei, C.; Frese, K.; Mangal, D.; Yu, K.H.; Yeo, C.J.; Calhoun, E.S. Oncogene-induced Nrf2 transcription promotes ROS detoxification and tumorigenesis. *Nature* **2011**, *475*, 106–109. [CrossRef]
9. Trachootham, D.; Alexandre, J.; Huang, P. Targeting cancer cells by ROS-mediated mechanisms: A radical therapeutic approach? *Nat. Rev. Drug Discov.* **2009**, *8*, 579–591. [CrossRef]
10. Dixon, S.J.; Stockwell, B.R. The role of iron and reactive oxygen species in cell death. *Nat. Chem. Biol.* **2014**, *10*, 9–17. [CrossRef]
11. Kirtonia, A.; Sethi, G.; Garg, M. The multifaceted role of reactive oxygen species in tumorigenesis. *Cell. Mol. Life Sci.* **2020**, *77*, 4459–4483. [CrossRef]
12. Shen, H.-M.; Liu, Z.-G. JNK signaling pathway is a key modulator in cell death mediated by reactive oxygen and nitrogen species. *Free. Radic. Biol. Med.* **2006**, *40*, 928–939. [CrossRef]
13. Donadelli, M.; Dando, I.; Zaniboni, T.; Costanzo, C.; Dalla Pozza, E.; Scupoli, M.; Scarpa, A.; Zappavigna, S.; Marra, M.; Abbruzzese, A. Gemcitabine/cannabinoid combination triggers autophagy in pancreatic cancer cells through a ROS-mediated mechanism. *Cell Death Dis.* **2011**, *2*, e152. [CrossRef]
14. Shen, M.; Wang, L.; Wang, B.; Wang, T.; Yang, G.; Shen, L.; Guo, X.; Liu, Y.; Xia, Y.; Jia, L. Activation of volume-sensitive outwardly rectifying chloride channel by ROS contributes to ER stress and cardiac contractile dysfunction: Involvement of CHOP through Wnt. *Cell Death Dis.* **2014**, *5*, e1528. [CrossRef]
15. Hasanain, M.; Bhattacharjee, A.; Pandey, P.; Ashraf, R.; Singh, N.; Sharma, S.; Vishwakarma, A.; Datta, D.; Mitra, K.; Sarkar, J. α-Solanine induces ROS-mediated autophagy through activation of endoplasmic reticulum stress and inhibition of Akt/mTOR pathway. *Cell Death Dis.* **2015**, *6*, e1860. [CrossRef]
16. Gorrini, C.; Harris, I.S.; Mak, T.W. Modulation of oxidative stress as an anticancer strategy. *Nat. Rev. Drug Discov.* **2013**, *12*, 931–947. [CrossRef]
17. Pelicano, H.; Feng, L.; Zhou, Y.; Carew, J.S.; Hileman, E.O.; Plunkett, W.; Keating, M.J.; Huang, P. Inhibition of mitochondrial respiration: A novel strategy to enhance drug-induced apoptosis in human leukemia cells by a reactive oxygen species-mediated mechanism. *J. Biol. Chem.* **2003**, *278*, 37832–37839. [CrossRef]
18. Moon, D.-O.; Kim, M.-O.; Choi, Y.H.; Hyun, J.W.; Chang, W.Y.; Kim, G.-Y. Butein induces G2/M phase arrest and apoptosis in human hepatoma cancer cells through ROS generation. *Cancer Lett.* **2010**, *288*, 204–213. [CrossRef]
19. Tabas, I.; Ron, D. Integrating the mechanisms of apoptosis induced by endoplasmic reticulum stress. *Nat. Cell Biol.* **2011**, *13*, 184–190. [CrossRef]
20. Salcher, S.; Hermann, M.; Kiechl-Kohlendorfer, U.; Ausserlechner, M.; Obexer, P. C10ORF10/DEPP-mediated ROS accumulation is a critical modulator of FOXO3-induced autophagy. *Mol. Cancer* **2017**, *16*, 95. [CrossRef]
21. Villar, V.H.; Merhi, F.; Djavaheri-Mergny, M.; Durán, R.V. Glutaminolysis and autophagy in cancer. *Autophagy* **2015**, *11*, 1198–1208. [CrossRef] [PubMed]
22. Kobayashi, S.; Boggon, T.J.; Dayaram, T.; Jänne, P.A.; Kocher, O.; Meyerson, M.; Johnson, B.E.; Eck, M.J.; Tenen, D.G.; Halmos, B. EGFR mutation and resistance of non–small-cell lung cancer to gefitinib. *N. Engl. J. Med.* **2005**, *352*, 786–792. [CrossRef] [PubMed]
23. Ali, A.; Levantini, E.; Teo, J.T.; Goggi, J.; Clohessy, J.G.; Wu, C.S.; Chen, L.; Yang, H.; Krishnan, I.; Kocher, O. Fatty acid synthase mediates EGFR palmitoylation in EGFR mutated non-small cell lung cancer. *EMBO Mol. Med.* **2018**, *10*, e8313. [CrossRef] [PubMed]
24. Ferrins, L.; Rahmani, R.; Sykes, M.L.; Jones, A.J.; Avery, V.M.; Teston, E.; Almohaywi, B.; Yin, J.; Smith, J.; Hyland, C. 3-(Oxazolo[4,5-b] pyridin-2-yl) anilides as a novel class of potent inhibitors for the kinetoplastid Trypanosoma brucei, the causative agent for human African trypanosomiasis. *Eur. J. Med. Chem.* **2013**, *66*, 450–465. [CrossRef] [PubMed]
25. Thomas, M.; Brand, S.; De Rycker, M.; Zuccotto, F.; Lukac, I.; Dodd, P.G.; Ko, E.-J.; Manthri, S.; McGonagle, K.; Osuna-Cabello, M. Scaffold-hopping strategy on a series of proteasome inhibitors led to a preclinical candidate for the treatment of visceral leishmaniasis. *J. Med. Chem.* **2021**, *64*, 5905–5930. [CrossRef]
26. Desai, S.; Desai, V.; Shingade, S. In-vitro Anti-cancer assay and apoptotic cell pathway of newly synthesized benzoxazole-N-heterocyclic hybrids as potent tyrosine kinase inhibitors. *Bioorg. Chem.* **2020**, *94*, 103382. [CrossRef]
27. Johnson, S.M.; Connelly, S.; Wilson, I.A.; Kelly, J.W. Biochemical and structural evaluation of highly selective 2-arylbenzoxazole-based transthyretin amyloidogenesis inhibitors. *J. Med. Chem.* **2008**, *51*, 260–270. [CrossRef]
28. Wu, D.; Si, W.; Wang, M.; Lv, S.; Ji, A.; Li, Y. Hydrogen sulfide in cancer: Friend or foe? *Nitric Oxide* **2015**, *50*, 38–45. [CrossRef]
29. Ashida, H.; Mimuro, H.; Ogawa, M.; Kobayashi, T.; Sanada, T.; Kim, M.; Sasakawa, C. Cell death and infection: A double-edged sword for host and pathogen survival. *J. Cell Biol.* **2011**, *195*, 931–942. [CrossRef]
30. Liu, Y.-L.; Tang, L.-H.; Liang, Z.-Q.; You, B.-G.; Yang, S.-L. Growth inhibitory and apoptosis inducing by effects of total flavonoids from Lysimachia clethroides Duby in human chronic myeloid leukemia K562 cells. *J. Ethnopharmacol.* **2010**, *131*, 1–9. [CrossRef]
31. Khanam, R.; Ahmad, K.; Hejazi, I.I.; Siddique, I.A.; Kumar, V.; Bhat, A.R.; Azam, A.; Athar, F. Inhibitory growth evaluation and apoptosis induction in MCF-7 cancer cells by new 5-aryl-2-butylthio-1, 3, 4-oxadiazole derivatives. *Cancer Chemother. Pharmacol.* **2017**, *80*, 1027–1042. [CrossRef]

32. Altıntop, M.D.; Özdemir, A.; Temel, H.E.; Cevizlidere, B.D.; Sever, B.; Kaplancıklı, Z.A.; Çiftçi, G.A. Design, synthesis and biological evaluation of a new series of arylidene indanones as small molecules for targeted therapy of non-small cell lung carcinoma and prostate cancer. *Eur. J. Med. Chem.* **2022**, *244*, 114851. [CrossRef]
33. El-Sayed, I.; Bassiouny, K.; Nokaly, A.; Abdelghani, A.S.; Roshdy, W. Influenza A virus and influenza B virus can induce apoptosis via intrinsic or extrinsic pathways and also via NF-κB in a time and dose dependent manner. *Biochem. Res. Int.* **2016**, *2016*, 1738237. [CrossRef]
34. Yang, J.; Liu, X.; Bhalla, K.; Kim, C.N.; Ibrado, A.M.; Cai, J.; Peng, T.-I.; Jones, D.P.; Wang, X. Prevention of apoptosis by Bcl-2: Release of cytochrome c from mitochondria blocked. *Science* **1997**, *275*, 1129–1132. [CrossRef]
35. O'Neill, K.L.; Huang, K.; Zhang, J.; Chen, Y.; Luo, X. Inactivation of prosurvival Bcl-2 proteins activates Bax/Bak through the outer mitochondrial membrane. *Genes Dev.* **2016**, *30*, 973–988. [CrossRef]
36. Liu, X.; Kim, C.N.; Yang, J.; Jemmerson, R.; Wang, X. Induction of apoptotic program in cell-free extracts: Requirement for dATP and cytochrome c. *Cell* **1996**, *86*, 147–157. [CrossRef]
37. Li, P.; Nijhawan, D.; Budihardjo, I.; Srinivasula, S.M.; Ahmad, M.; Alnemri, E.S.; Wang, X. Cytochrome c and dATP-dependent formation of Apaf-1/caspase-9 complex initiates an apoptotic protease cascade. *Cell* **1997**, *91*, 479–489. [CrossRef]
38. Hang, W.; Yin, Z.-X.; Liu, G.; Zeng, Q.; Shen, X.-F.; Sun, Q.-H.; Li, D.-D.; Jian, Y.-P.; Zhang, Y.-H.; Wang, Y.-S. Piperlongumine and p53-reactivator APR-246 selectively induce cell death in HNSCC by targeting GSTP1. *Oncogene* **2018**, *37*, 3384–3398. [CrossRef]
39. Zhao, Y.; Zhou, Y.; Wang, M. Brosimone I, an isoprenoid-substituted flavonoid, induces cell cycle G1 phase arrest and apoptosis through ROS-dependent endoplasmic reticulum stress in HCT116 human colon cancer cells. *Food Funct.* **2019**, *10*, 2729–2738. [CrossRef]
40. Yang, Y.; Zhang, Y.; Wang, L.; Lee, S. Levistolide A induces apoptosis via ROS-mediated ER stress pathway in colon cancer cells. *Cell. Physiol. Biochem.* **2017**, *42*, 929–938. [CrossRef]
41. Colin, D.; Limagne, E.; Ragot, K.; Lizard, G.; Ghiringhelli, F.; Solary, E.; Chauffert, B.; Latruffe, N.; Delmas, D. The role of reactive oxygen species and subsequent DNA-damage response in the emergence of resistance towards resveratrol in colon cancer models. *Cell Death Dis.* **2014**, *5*, e1533. [CrossRef] [PubMed]
42. Xie, C.-M.; Liu, X.-Y.; Sham, K.W.; Lai, J.M.; Cheng, C.H. Silencing of EEF2K (eukaryotic elongation factor-2 kinase) reveals AMPK-ULK1-dependent autophagy in colon cancer cells. *Autophagy* **2014**, *10*, 1495–1508. [CrossRef] [PubMed]
43. Scherz-Shouval, R.; Elazar, Z. Regulation of autophagy by ROS: Physiology and pathology. *Trends Biochem. Sci.* **2011**, *36*, 30–38. [CrossRef] [PubMed]
44. Wei, Y.; Sinha, S.C.; Levine, B. Dual role of JNK1-mediated phosphorylation of Bcl-2 in autophagy and apoptosis regulation. *Autophagy* **2008**, *4*, 949–951. [CrossRef]
45. Levine, B.; Sinha, S.C.; Kroemer, G. Bcl-2 family members: Dual regulators of apoptosis and autophagy. *Autophagy* **2008**, *4*, 600–606. [CrossRef]
46. Eisenberg-Lerner, A.; Bialik, S.; Simon, H.-U.; Kimchi, A. Life and death partners: Apoptosis, autophagy and the cross-talk between them. *Cell Death Differ.* **2009**, *16*, 966–975. [CrossRef]
47. Nikoletopoulou, V.; Markaki, M.; Palikaras, K.; Tavernarakis, N. Crosstalk between apoptosis, necrosis and autophagy. *Biochim. Biophys. Acta (BBA)—Mol. Cell Res.* **2013**, *1833*, 3448–3459. [CrossRef]

Disclaimer/Publisher's Note: The statements, opinions and data contained in all publications are solely those of the individual author(s) and contributor(s) and not of MDPI and/or the editor(s). MDPI and/or the editor(s) disclaim responsibility for any injury to people or property resulting from any ideas, methods, instructions or products referred to in the content.

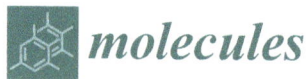

Article

Oxidative Stress and Multi-Organel Damage Induced by Two Novel Phytocannabinoids, CBDB and CBDP, in Breast Cancer Cells

Maria Salbini [1], Alessandra Quarta [1], Fabiana Russo [2], Anna Maria Giudetti [3], Cinzia Citti [1], Giuseppe Cannazza [1,4], Giuseppe Gigli [1,5], Daniele Vergara [3] and Antonio Gaballo [1,*]

[1] CNR Nanotec, Institute of Nanotechnology, Via Monteroni, 73100 Lecce, Italy; maria.salbini@nanotec.cnr.it (M.S.); alessandra.quarta@nanotec.cnr.it (A.Q.); cinzia.citti@nanotec.cnr.it (C.C.); giuseppe.cannazza@unimore.it (G.C.); giuseppe.gigli@unisalento.it (G.G.)
[2] Clinical and Experimental Medicine PhD Program, University of Modena and Reggio Emilia, 41125 Modena, Italy; fabiana.russo@unimore.it
[3] Department of Biological and Environmental Sciences and Technologies, University of Salento, Via Monteroni, 73100 Lecce, Italy; anna.giudetti@unisalento.it (A.M.G.); daniele.vergara@unisalento.it (D.V.)
[4] Department of Life Sciences, University of Modena and Reggio Emilia, Via G. Campi 103, 41125 Modena, Italy
[5] Dipartimento di Matematica e Fisica E. de Giorgi, Università Del Salento, 73100 Lecce, Italy
* Correspondence: antonio.gaballo@nanotec.cnr.it

Abstract: Over the last few years, much attention has been paid to phytocannabinoids derived from Cannabis for their therapeutic potential. Δ^9-tetrahydrocannabinol (Δ^9-THC) and cannabidiol (CBD) are the most abundant compounds of the *Cannabis sativa L.* plant. Recently, novel phytocannabinoids, such as cannabidibutol (CBDB) and cannabidiphorol (CBDP), have been discovered. These new molecules exhibit the same terpenophenolic core of CBD and differ only for the length of the alkyl side chain. Roles of CBD homologs in physiological and pathological processes are emerging but the exact molecular mechanisms remain to be fully elucidated. Here, we investigated the biological effects of the newly discovered CBDB or CBDP, compared to the well-known natural and synthetic CBD (nat CBD and syn CBD) in human breast carcinoma cells that express CB receptors. In detail, our data demonstrated that the treatment of cells with the novel phytocannabinoids affects cell viability, increases the production of reactive oxygen species (ROS) and activates cellular pathways related to ROS signaling, as already demonstrated for natural CBD. Moreover, we observed that the biological activity is significantly increased upon combining CBD homologs with drugs that inhibit the activity of enzymes involved in the metabolism of endocannabinoids, such as the monoacylglycerol lipase (MAGL) inhibitor, or with drugs that induces the activation of cellular stress pathways, such as the phorbol ester 12-myristate 13-acetate (PMA).

Keywords: MCF-7; cannabidiol; ROS; oxidative stress; autophagy; altered mitochondria; cytoplasmic vacuole; MAGL; MJN110

1. Introduction

Cannabinoids include a wide group of organic molecules, including those that are physiologically produced in the human body, called endocannabinoids, those extracted primarily from the *Cannabis sativa L.* plant, named phytocannabinoids, and synthetic cannabinoids [1]. Recently, phytocannabinoids, in particular cannabidiol (CBD) and Δ^9-tetrahydrocannabinol (THC), have been widely exploited in several research and clinical fields [2]. In the last few years, the homologous series of CBD has been expanded by the isolation in a medicinal cannabis variety of novel phytocannabinoids such as cannabigerol (CBG), cannabichromene (CBC), cannabinol (CBN) and cannabidivarin (CBDV) [3–8]. Although these compounds have similar chemical structures, they can elicit different biological actions. Phytocannabinoids demonstrated a selective anti-cancer activity in many cancer cell lines, by affecting cell proliferation, differentiation, and death [9]. In light of this, a possible role as an adjuvant in many cancer therapies has been proposed. Recently, it was found that the co-administration of cannabinoids with chemotherapeutic drugs enhanced their efficiency, especially in chemotherapy-refractory tumors [10,11]. Phytocannabinoids may act via dependent and/or independent cannabinoid receptor mechanisms [12,13]. CB1 and CB2 are the first cannabinoids receptors described. These are G-protein coupled receptors (GPCR) that can be activated by endogenous and exogenous cannabinoids. More recently, studies have shown that cannabinoids can activate other receptors, i.e., GPR55, TRPM8 as well as other ion channels of the transient receptor potential superfamily as vanilloid type 1–4 (TRPV1, TRPV2, TRPV3 and TRPV4) [12,14–17]. In the context of breast cancer, the biological role of CBD in the regulation of epithelial tumor pathophysiology has clearly emerged [18,19]. Tumor cells express CBD receptors and respond to these molecules by activating specific signaling pathways. For instance, Shrivastava A. et al., [20] described that in breast cancer cells, cannabidiol induces the generation of reactive oxygen species (ROS), endoplasmic reticulum (ER)-stress and subsequently the activation of autophagic processes. Here, we investigated in vitro the biological effects of CBD homologs, the newly discovered CBDB or CBDP, in breast cancer models. We observed that CBD homologs induced changes in ROS levels and cellular processes related to ROS signaling. Furthermore, CBD homologs affected the morphology and functionality of several cell structures, such as mitochondria and ER, as already demonstrated for natural CBD [21]. The combination of CBD homologs with drugs that inhibit the activity of enzymes involved in the metabolism of endocannabinoids, such as the monoacylglycerol lipase (MAGL), or with drugs that induce the activation of cellular stress pathways, such as the phorbol ester 12-myristate 13-acetate (PMA), is associated with an extensive vacuolization, hyper-increased ROS levels, and multiple alterations in organelles structure. In summary, we investigated the biological effects of two novel CBD homologs in breast cancer cells and reported, for the first time, the activation of catastrophic processes after the combination of CBDB or CBDP with drugs that modulate the metabolism of endocannabinoids or regulate the activation of specific protein kinases.

2. Results

2.1. Synthesis and Characterization of Phytocannabinoids

CBD of both synthetic and natural origin, syn CBD and nat CBD respectively, are commercially available, while cannabidibutol (CBDB) and cannabidiphorol (CBDP) have been recently discovered and isolated from the Italian medicinal variety FM2 of *Cannabis sativa* L. [4,6,7]. In these works, the stereoselective synthesis of the same compounds allowed absolute stereochemistry by comparison of their spectroscopic and optical properties [4,6,7]. Nat CBD and syn CBD are identical molecules, therefore we expect to see no difference in their biological behavior. However, high-performance liquid chromatography coupled to high-resolution mass spectrometry (HPLC-HRMS) analyses has recently shown that nat CBD contains small amounts (0.1–0.5%, w/w) of two impurities corresponding to CBD propyl and butyl homologs, cannabidivarin (CBDV) and CBDB respectively [4]. The CBD homologs under investigation in the present work differ only by the length of the alkyl side chain on the resorcinyl moiety. In particular, CBDB has a linear C4 (butyl) side chain, both nat CBD and syn CBD have a C5 (pentyl) chain, and CBDP has a C7 (heptyl) chain (Figure 1). The four cannabinoids present similar physicochemical and spectroscopic properties: UV and FT-IR spectra are perfectly superimposable, while Nuclear Magnetic Resonance (NMR) spectroscopy shows a difference only in the signal corresponding to the alkyl chain; HRMS data highlight a perfect match of all m/z of the fragments with the difference only in the number of methylene units [4,6,7]. The length of the alkyl side chain could dramatically affect the affinity for the biological targets as it has been demonstrated for THC, a CBD isomer [22].

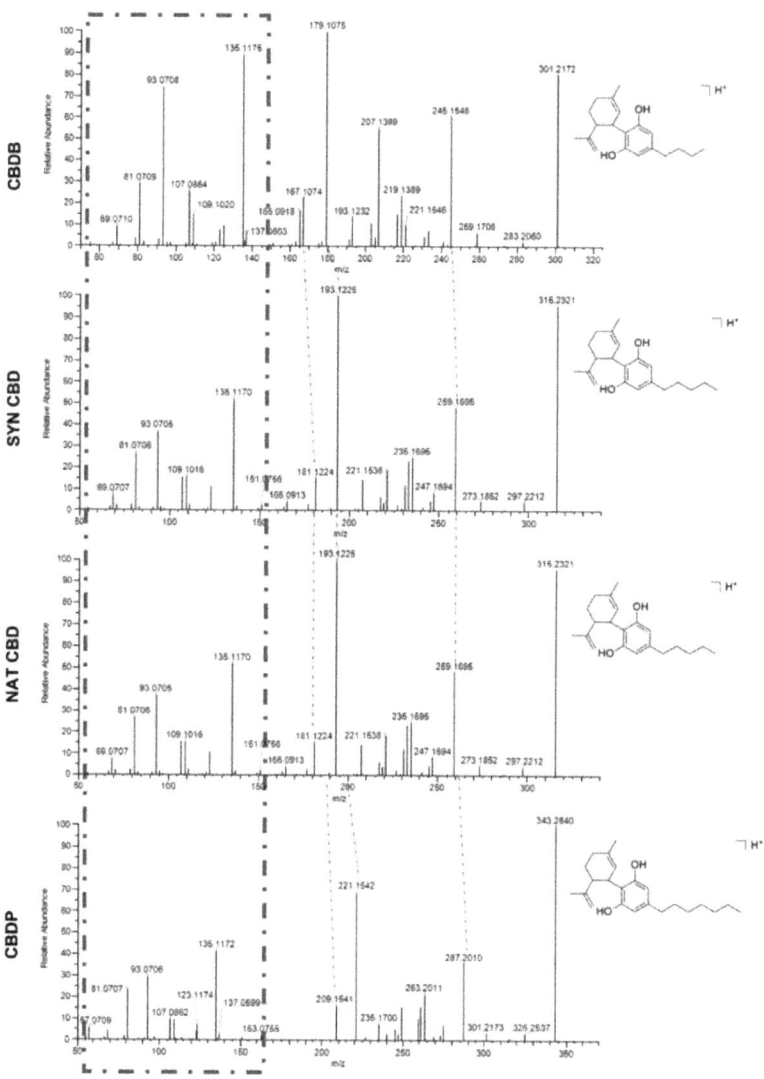

Figure 1. HPLC-HRMS analysis in positive ionization mode of the four CBD homologs under investigation. Blue dotted lines highlight the common pattern, while red dotted lines show the difference in the fragments due to the number of methylene units on the alkyl side chain.

2.2. CBD Homologs Treatment Significantly Decreased Cancer Cell Viability

The biological effects of phytocannabinoids are thought to be due to their affinity to CB1 and CB2 receptors. The expression of these proteins was investigated in vitro using a panel of breast cancer cell models (estrogen and progesterone receptor positive: MCF-7, MDA-MB-361; and estrogen and progesterone receptor negative: MDA-MB-231). Qualitative analysis of cannabinoid targets in vitro showed that the three breast cancer cells express both CB1 and CB2 receptors (Figure 2A).

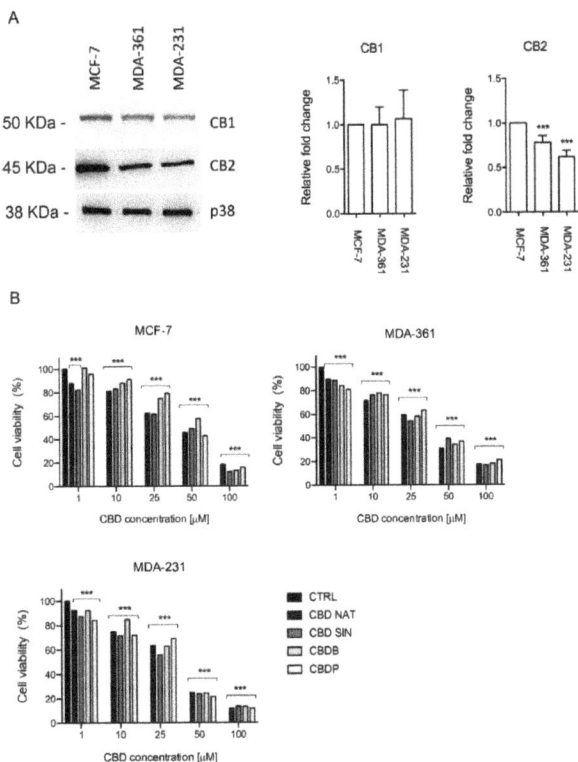

Figure 2. (A) Immunoblot analysis of CB1 and CB2 receptors in MCF-7, MDA-MB-361 and MDA-MB-231 breast cancer cell lines, p38 was used as a loading control. Densitometric quantification of the band intensity was normalized to p38 levels using ImageJ. p-value *** < 0.001 by t-test. Effect of cannabinoid treatment on cell viability: (B) MCF-7, MDA-MB-361 and MDA-MB-231 cells. All the cell lines were treated with different concentrations of nat CBD, syn CBD, CBDB and CBDP for 24 h; the cell viability was measured using the MTT assay. Values are the mean ± SD. *** $p < 0.0001$ compared with controls.

Subsequently, before investigating the specific activity of the CBD homologs on cancer cell lines, we screened their cytotoxicity on two different epithelial and one mesenchymal breast cancer cell lines namely MCF-7, MDA-MB-361 and MDA-MB-231, using the metabolism-dependent MTT viability assay. Cells were treated with various concentrations (from 1 to 100 μM) of nat CBD, syn CBD, CBDB and CBDP, for 24 h. All CBD homologs inhibited the viability of breast cell lines with lower activity in MCF-7 and MDA-MB-361 cells, while the higher effect was observed in MDA-MB-231 (Figure 2B). Table 1 summarizes the IC_{50} values for all the tested molecules. The striking behavior of CBD homologs treatments was the occurrence of massive cytoplasmic vacuolation in the epithelial MCF-7 cells (Figure S1). Vacuoles already appeared after 2 h of treatment and their number and size increased after 24 h. The same changes were less pronounced in mesenchymal MDA-MB-231 cells, while in the epithelial MDA-MB-361 cells no vacuolation occurred (Figure S1). This preliminary analysis evidenced that MCF-7 cells while preserving their viability, displayed macroscopic morphological alterations upon CBD homologs administration. To shed light on the possible intracellular effects, we focused on the comparative analyis of the four CBD homologs on this cellular model. Indeed, while nat CBD and syn CBD are identical and quite known molecules, the cellular effects of the newly isolated CBDB and CBDP are not investigated yet. The nat and syn CBD are used as reference molecules.

All the experimental data presented in the following sections have been performed using the four CBD homologs, although particular attention will be dedicated to the two new ones, at a concentration of 10 µM. In line with the literature [18,23,24], this is a working concentration that induces biological responses without dramatic effects on cell viability.

Table 1. IC_{50} values (µM) are reported as mean ± S.D. of three independent experiments ($n = 3$). MCF-7, MDA-MB-361 and MDA-MB-231 cells were treated with nat CBD, syn CBD, CBDB and CBDP (from 0 to 100 µM) for 24 h.

Compounds	MCF-7	MDA-MB-361	MDA-MB-231
NAT CBD	58.6 ± 0.1	49.8 ± 1.5	46.6 ± 1.0
SYN CBD	59.0 ± 1.2	53.2 ± 0.8	45.3 ± 0.9
CBDB	57.4 ± 1.2	56.4 ± 1.2	48.4 ± 0.6
CBDP	56.7 ± 0.4	60.9 ± 0.4	49.3 ± 1.4

2.3. CBD Homologs Treatment Significantly Increased ROS Production in MCF-7 Cells

An increase in the oxidative stress has been detected in cancer cells after CBD treatment due to a massive increase of ROS production that leads to the activation of apoptosis and autophagy [14,16,17]. Starting from these data, we analyzed ROS levels in MCF-7 cells treated with 10 µM nat CBD, syn CBD, CBDB and CBDP for 24 h using the 2′,7′-dichlorodihydrofluorescein diacetate (DCFH-DA) staining. The DCFH-DA probe is nonfluorescent in its initial form, but it can be easily oxidized by intracellular ROS, leading to the formation of the fluorescent product dichlorofluorescein (DCF). The antioxidant N-acetyl cysteine (NAC) was used to counteract ROS production. As shown in Figure 3A,C, a significant increase in intracellular ROS levels was observed in MCF-7 cells treated with CBD homologs. On the contrary, NAC treatment in association with CBD homologs reverted the relative fluorescence intensity to a value lower than control, due to a remarkable ROS scavenging effect (Figure 3B,C).

2.4. CBD Homologs Treatment Altered Mitochondria and ER in MCF-7 Cells

To establish if there is a correlation between ROS production and impaired mitochondrial functions, we used two mitochondria stains, Mitotracker Red and MitoTracker Green. The first is an indicator of mitochondrial membrane potential that selectively stains active mitochondria, while MitoTracker Green allows the detection of the mitochondrial morphology and mass. When MCF-7 cells were exposed to 10 µM CBDB or CBDP for 24 h, the Mitotracker red fluorescence intensity dramatically dropped as compared to the control (Figure 4A). Similar results were obtained with nat CBD and syn CBD (data not shown). On the other hand, the MitoTracker Green fluorescence signal remained similar in control and treated cells (Figure 4B). These observations suggest that the treatment with CBD homologs leads to an alteration of the mitochondrial functionality without an appreciable decrease of the mitochondrial mass. The loss of the mitochondrial function was also accompanied by a substantial decrease of ATP, whose levels dropped by approximately 35–40% compared to controls in MCF-7 cells treated with all CBD homologs (Figure 4C).

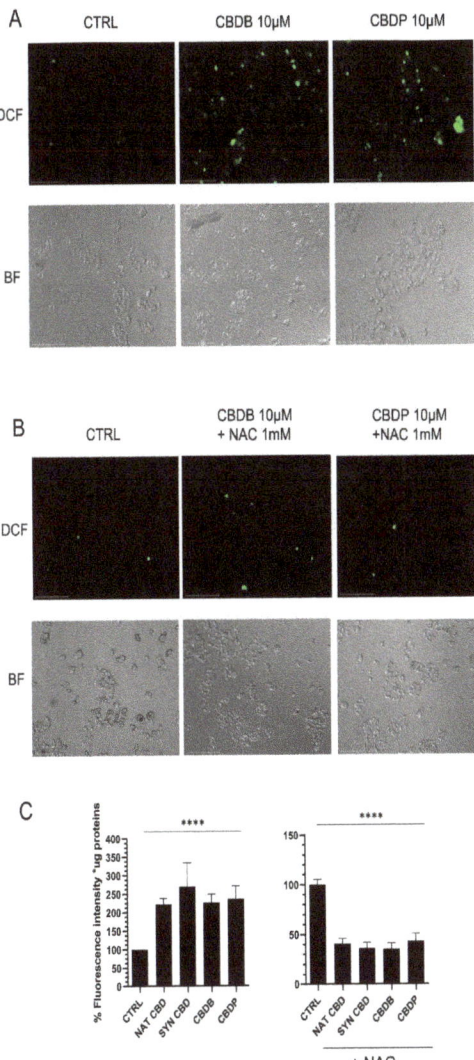

Figure 3. Representative fluorescent images of 2′,7′-dichlorodihydrofluorescein diacetate (DCFH-DA) staining in MCF-7 cells and its corresponding image in bright field (BF). (**A**) MCF-7 cells treated for 24 h with vehicle (CTRL), CBDB or CBDP (10 µM). (**B**) MCF-7 cells treated with CBDB or CBDP (10 µM) and 1 mM N-acetylcysteine (NAC), for 24 h. All images were taken by Evos m7000 fluorescence microscope objective 10x, scale bar 275 µm. (**C**) Fluorescence intensity quantification by a fluorescence microplate reader for DCF staining in MCF-7 cells control and after CBD, and NAC+ CBD homologs, after 24 h. Values are the mean ± SD. **** $p < 0.0001$ compared with controls.

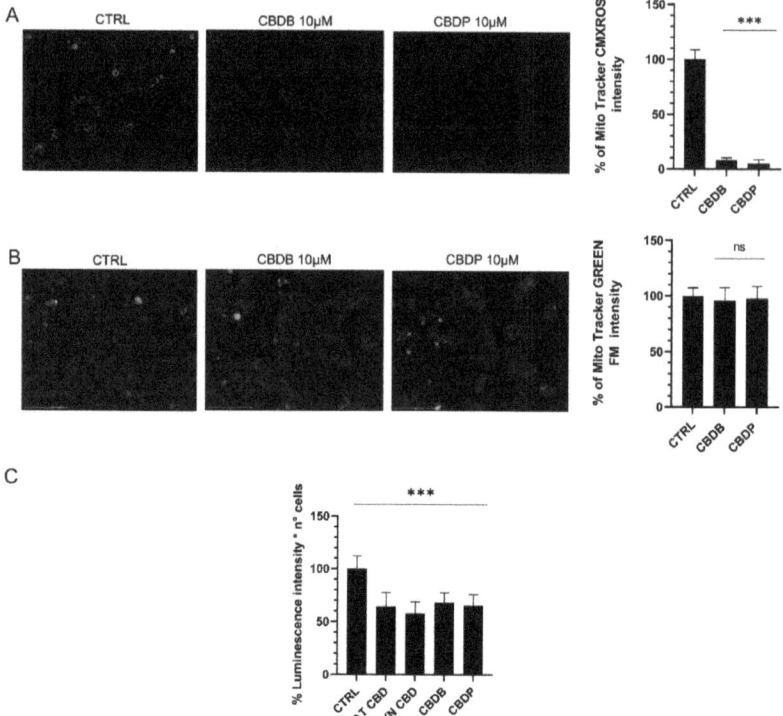

Figure 4. Representative fluorescent images of the mitochondrial function. MCF-7 cells were treated with vehicle (CTRL), CBDB and CBDP (10 μM) for 24 h. (**A**) Cells were stained with the membrane potential-dependent dye MitoTracker CMXRos. (**B**) Cells were stained with the MitoTracker Green FM. Both fluorescent markers were imaged with an Evos m7000 fluorescence microscope. Scale bar 150 μm, objective 20x. (**C**) After treatments, the cellular ATP level was measured with the CellTiter-Glo 2.0 cell viability luminescence assay. Values are the mean ± SD. *** $p < 0.001$ compared to controls; ns not significant.

To further elucidate the effects of CBDB and CBDP treatment in MCF-7 cells, ultrastructural analysis employing transmission electron microscopy (TEM) was performed. TEM imaging revealed multiple damages to cellular organelles. Interestingly, as already observed by optical imaging, cytoplasmic vacuolations were detected. In addition, mitochondria with altered morphology, such as rounded and rod-like mitochondria and dilated cristae were distinguished (Figure 5B, panel a, red arrow). Figure 5B (panel a–e, black arrows) displays swollen mitochondria, with broken cristae and decreased electron density of the lumen.

TEM imaging also revealed multiple dramatic changes in other cellular compartments after CBDB or CBDP (10 μM) exposure. Figure 6B shows the accumulation of double-membrane (Figure 6B, red asterisk) autophagic vacuoles containing cellular organelles and electron-dense material (Figure 6B, black arrows). Figure 6C shows that the ER also appears enlarged and disassembled (red arrows). These data were confirmed by ER staining with ER tracker which exhibited an increased fluorescence signal surrounding the vacuole membrane, suggesting that some cytoplasmic vacuolations can also arise from the ER membranes, due to a massive ER stress (Figure 7A).

The presence of late autophagic vesicles in cells treated with CBD homologs was also indirectly confirmed through staining with LysoTracker Red, as it is selective for acidic organelles. Cell nuclei were stained with Hoechst 33342. MCF-7 cells treated with CBD homologs displayed a higher number of lysosomes, compared to the control (Figure 7B). This observation suggests a massive presence/accumulation of autophagolysosomes.

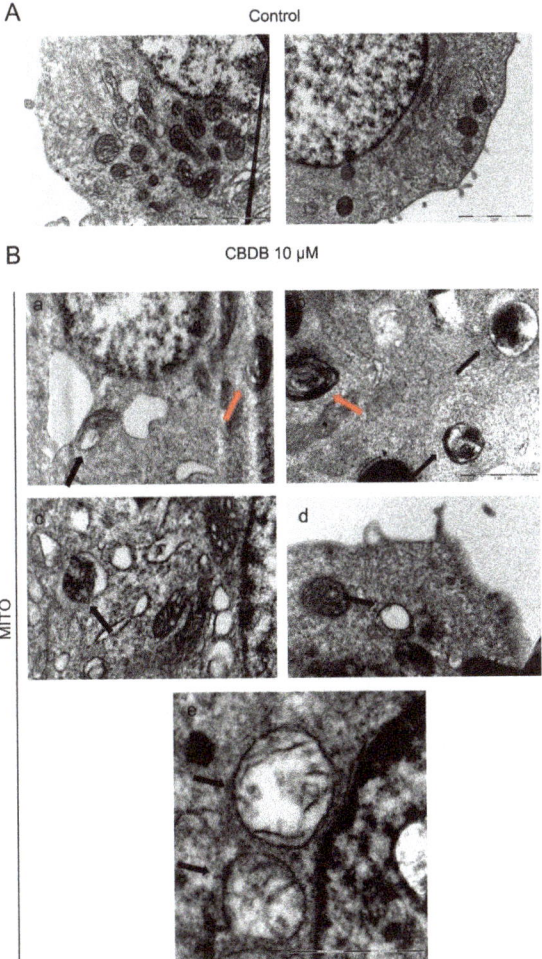

Figure 5. Representative TEM images of cell morphology. (**A**) MCF-7 control cells (treated with DMSO as a vehicle). Scale bar 2 µm. (**B**) MCF-7 cells exposed to CBDB or CBDP (10 µM) for 24 h. Mitochondria with dilated cristae(panel **a,b**, red arrows); swollen mitochondria with crests in the process of breaking (panel **a–e**; black arrows). Scale bar 1 µm.

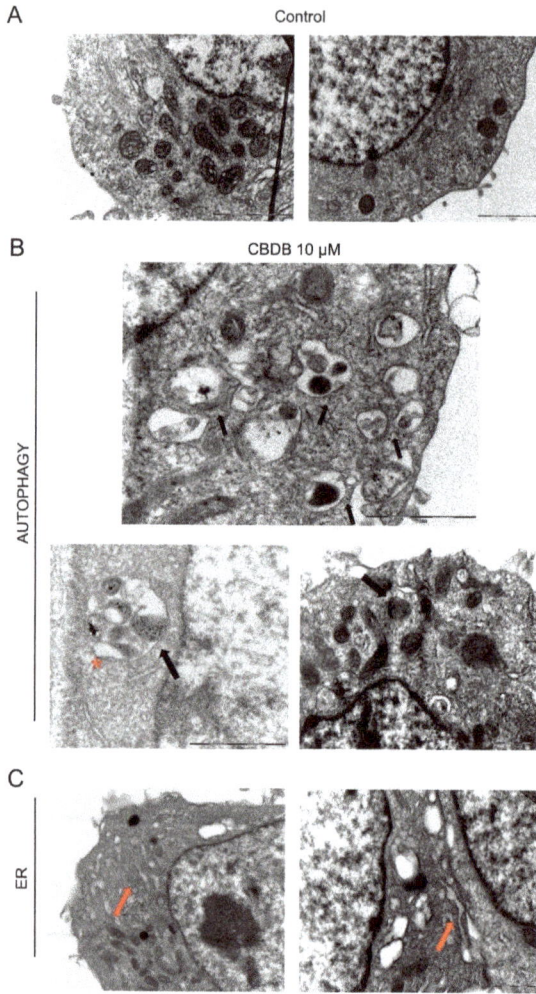

Figure 6. Representative TEM images of cell morphology. (**A**) MCF-7 control cells (treated with DMSO, as vehicle). Scale bar 2 μm. (**B,C**) MCF-7 cells fixed exposed to CBDB or CBDP (10 μM) for 24 h; (**B**) double-membrane autophagic vacuoles red asterisk, autophagosomes black arrows, (**C**) outstretched ER red arrows.

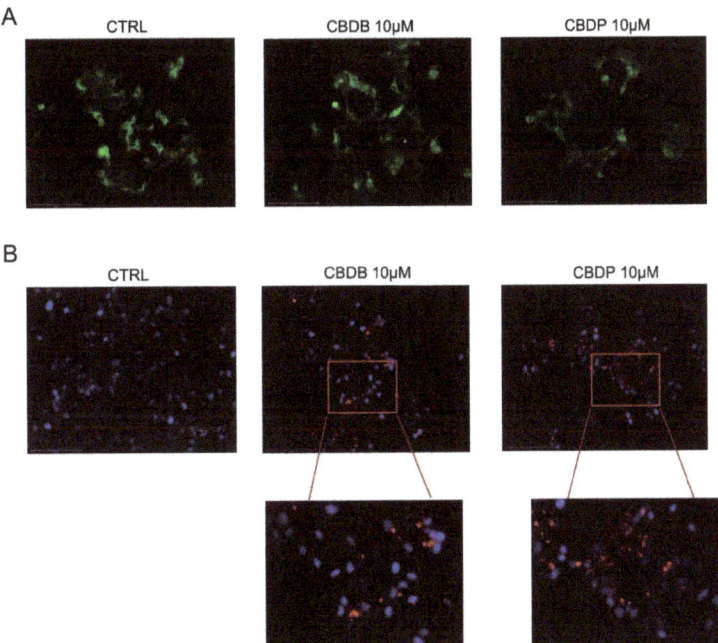

Figure 7. Representative fluorescent images of organelle structures. MCF-7 cells were treated with vehicle (CTRL) or CBDB and CBDP (10 µM) for 24 h. (**A**) Cells were stained with ER TrackerTM to visualize endoplasmic reticulum membranes. (**B**) Cells were stained with Hoechst (0.5 mg/mL) and Lysotracker Red DND-99 (100 nM) according to the manufacturer's recommendations and imaged with an Evos m7000 fluorescence microscope. Scale bar 150 µm, objective 20×.

2.5. Biological Effects of CBD Homologs in Combination with Either an MAGL Inhibitor 2,5-Dioxopyrrolidin-1-yl 4-(bis(4-chlorophenyl)methyl)piperazine-1-carboxylate (MJN110) and Phorbol Ester 12-Myristate 13-Acetate (PMA)

We analyzed the effect of CBD homologs on MCF-7 cells in combination with MJN110 (2,5-dioxopyrrolidin-1-yl 4-(bis(4-chlorophenyl) methyl)piperazine-1-carboxylate), a MAGL inhibitor. MAGL is an enzyme that, in addition to its ability to hydrolyse monoglycerides, has been shown to have a role in endocannabinoid catabolism. Indeed it can hydrolyse 2-arachidonoyl glycerol into arachidonic acid [25]. In particular, the treatment with MJN110 (1 µM) in combination with CBDB or CBDP induced severe cellular morphological changes, with an increase of about 30% in the number of cytoplasmic vacuolations, as compared to the treatments with the individual molecules (i.e., CBD homologs or MJN110) (Figure S2A,B). A similar effect, with a more prominent increase in cytoplasmic vacuolations (about 60%) was observed by treating the cells with CBDB or CBDP in combination with PMA (100 nM), a drug that has been shown to induce the activation of different cellular stress pathways [26,27] (Figure S2A,C). Furthermore, we observed a rise in ROS levels in MCF-7 cells treated with both MJN110 and PMA (Figure 8). Dramatic changes in cell morphology, as well as in organelle structures, were confirmed by TEM imaging of MCF-7 cells treated with CBDB or CBDP in the presence of MJN110 (Figure S3). In addition, double-membrane vacuoles, containing degrading materials, were much more increased in MJN110-CBD homologs treated cells, as compared to their control. Treatment with PMA, in the same way, highlighted the presence of cytoplasmic vacuolations related to disassembled ER and mitochondria (Figure 9). The dramatic changes in cell morphology, as well as in organelle structures, appeared more catastrophic than those previously observed after the treatments with CBDB or CBDP alone or with MJN110 or PMA alone. As we mentioned before, the treatment of MCF-7 cells with CBDB or CBDP also induced ER and/or mitochondria dilation. Notably, after the combined exposure to CBD homologs and the two drugs, the morphological changes at the ER level and the quantitative increase of the lysosomes were even more remarkable (Figures S4 and S5).

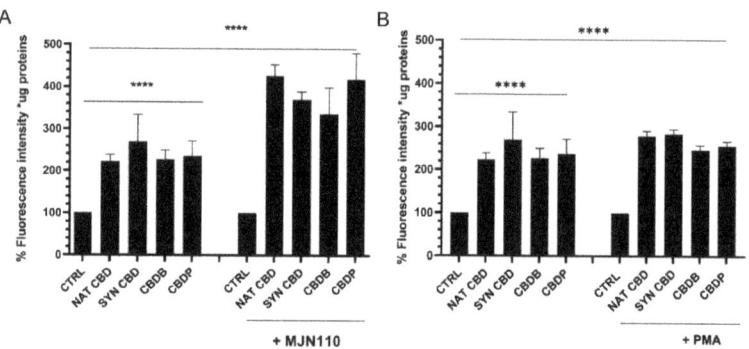

Figure 8. (**A**) Intensity quantification by a fluorescence microplate reader for DCFH-DA staining in MCF-7 cells after 24 h treatment with CBD (10 µM), and MJN110 (1 µM) + CBD homologs. Values are the mean ± SD. **** $p < 0.0001$ compared with controls. (**B**) Intensity quantification by a fluorescence microplate reader for DCFH-DA staining in MCF-7 cells, including control samples (DMSO) and cells treated for 24 h with CBD (10 µM), and PMA (100 nM) + CBD homologs. Values are the mean ± SD. **** $p < 0.0001$ compared with controls.

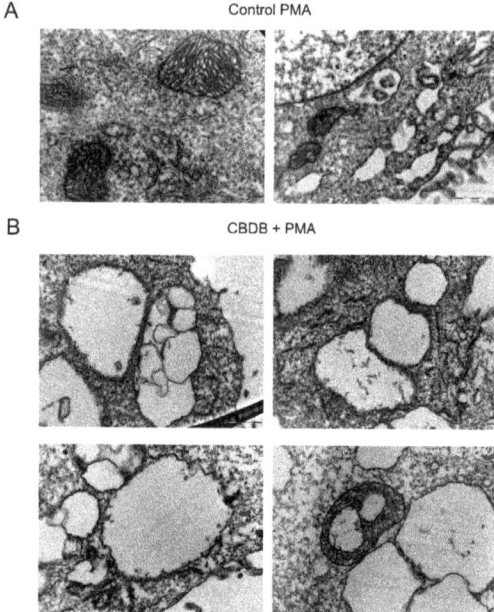

Figure 9. Representative TEM images of cell morphology. (**A**) MCF-7 cells were treated with vehicle (DMSO) and PMA (100 nM), showing normal cell organelles. Scale bar 2 µm. (**B**) MCF-7 cells were incubated with CBDB + PMA (100 nM), highlighting the presence of cytoplasmic vacuolations related to disassembled ER and mitochondria. Scale bar 1 µm.

3. Discussion

Here we conducted an in vitro study to investigate the biological effects of the newly discovered CBDB or CBDP, compared to the well-known nat CBD and syn CBD. As already mentioned, the CBD homologs under investigation differ only by the length of the alkyl side chain on the resorcinyl moiety. CBDB has a linear C4 (butyl) side chain, both nat CBD and syn CBD have a C5 (pentyl) chain, and CBDP has a C7 (heptyl) chain. The length of the alkyl side chain may affect the affinity for some biological targets as it has been demonstrated for THC, which is a CBD isomer [22]. Furthermore, due to their implication in the control of cell growth and death, cannabinoids have been proposed as a new adjuvant in cancer therapy of various malignancies, such as prostate and breast cancer [17,28]. As already described, phytocannabinoids may act via dependent and/or independent cannabinoid receptor mechanisms [13,15]. In the context of breast cancer, the biological effect of CBD in the regulation of epithelial tumor pathophysiology has clearly emerged [18,19] and is thought to be due to multiple molecular targets including the CB1 and CB2 receptors. The expression of these proteins was investigated in vitro using a panel of breast cancer cell models (estrogen and progesterone receptor positive: MCF-7, MDA-MB-361; and estrogen and progesterone receptor negative: MDA-MB-231). Qualitative analysis of cannabinoid targets in vitro showed that CB1 and CB2 were expressed in all breast cancer cells confirming already published data [29] (Figure 2A).

Within this frame, the cellular effects of the newly isolated CBDB or CBDP are not investigated yet. First we tested the antiproliferative effects of the four CBD homologs, using the metabolism-dependent MTT viability assay. For this aim, we treated MCF-7, MDA-MB-361 and MDA-MB-231 (Figure 2B) with different concentrations (1–100 µM) of nat CBD, syn CBD, CBDB and CBDP, for 24 h.

All tested molecules showed an anti-proliferative effect in triple negative, estrogen receptor positive (ER+) and progesteron receptor positive (PR+) breast tumor cell lines. More in detail, MCF-7 and MDA-MB-361 showed a lower sensitivity to CBDB or CBDP treatment in comparison to MDA-MB-231, as described in Table 1. Additional investigations are needed to gain further insights into the cellular mechanisms and the role of ER/PR signalling in CBD homologs sensitivity. Taken together, these preliminary data show that the three cellular models were sensitive to CBD homologs treatment *in vitro*, despite their different regulation of intracellular signaling pathways.

This is consistent with previous work which cannabinoids affect breast cancer growth with both ER-dependent and -independent mechanisms [20,30].

The microscopic examination of the cells treated with 10 µM CBD homologs revealed massive cytoplasmic vacuolation, especially in MCF-7 cells, a clear signal of cellular stress (Figure S1). A similar effect was observed in mesenchymal MDA-MB-231 cells but in a milder way, while in the epithelial MDA-MB-361 cells no vacuolation occurred (Figure S1). The latter interesting observation needs further investigations that are not included in the present study. In a recent paper similar vacuolar structures were observed in MCF-7 cells treated with a cannabinoid combination: the authors did not determine the origin of these structures but excluded a possible origin from the plasma membrane [31]. They proposed that the cytoplasmic vacuoles could be derived from the ER; they also detected an increased number of lysosomes and the dilation of both ER and mitochondria, resulting in the activation of autophagy and paraptosis pathways. Similarly, Fang W. et al., [32] found that CBD could activate the mitochondrial apoptosis pathway and cause cell damage due to the continuous increase of intracellular ROS. This increase led to the reduction of the mitochondrial transmembrane potential, the opening of the mitochondrial permeability transition pore (mPTP) with subsequent release of cytochrome C into the cytoplasm [33,34], finally resulting in the activation of the mitochondrial-dependent apoptosis pathway. The apoptotic event is preceded by the cell cycle arrest in various cancer models [1,17,35]. Another recent study confirmed that the CBD treatment triggered multiple intracellular effects in MCF-7 cells, such as increased Ca^{2+} levels, ROS accumulation and ER stress, finally leading to the induction of apoptosis [14].

The present study shows that under the tested conditions, all the four CBD homologs exhibited similar behavior, though only the results obtained with the two novel phytocannabinoids have been presented herein. The CBD homologs induced a significant boost of ROS production (Figure 3A), lowering of the mitochondrial functionality (Figure 4), alteration of cell organelles (Figures 5 and 6), ER modification (Figure 7A) and increase in the number of lysosomes (Figure 7B). By the DCFH-DA test the intracellular increase of ROS levels upon CBDB or CBDP treatment was detected (Figure 3C). In addition, the combined treatment of cells with the CBD homologs and NAC evidenced a significant decrease in the relative fluorescence intensity, thanks to the ROS scavengering effect of NAC (Figure 3C). Furthermore, the CBD-driven ROS production is related to the activation of apoptosis, due to impaired mitochondrial function [36], but it is also associated with autophagy [37]. To investigate whether the new CBDB and CBDP led to an impaired mitochondrial function we used two mitochondria stains, Mitotracker Red and MitoTracker Green. In particular, MitoTracker Red is a membrane potential-sensitive dye and is non-fluorescent until entering an actively respiring cell, while MitoTracker Green covalently binds to mitochondrial matrix proteins and allows to monitor the mitochondrial morphology. Figure 4A,B shows that the treatment with both CBDB or CBDB leads to an alteration of the mitochondrial functionality without an appreciable decrease of the mitochondrial mass. The functional loss was also accompanied by a substantial decrease of ATP whose levels dropped by approximately 35–40% in MCF-7 cells treated with all CBD homologs, compared to controls (Figure 4C). A recent study have documented that CBD directly targets mitochondria, revealing multiple dramatic changes in their function and morphology such as swelling and lacking cristae in Jurkat cells [34]. Moreover, the presence of double-membrane vacuoles, containing degrading material (autophagosomes), and the disassembly of Golgi and ER was described. Through the ultrastructural analysis of the CBD homolog-treated cells, we detected multiple damages to cell organelles. First of all, mitochondria with altered morphology were distinguished: in particular the presence of dilated cristae, rounded, rod-like and swollen mitochondria with broken cristae and decreased electron density of the lumen was recognized (Figure 5). TEM imaging also revealed multiple dramatic changes in other cellular compartments. Figure 6B shows the accumulation of double-membrane autophagic vacuoles containing cellular organelles and electron-dense material, while Figure 6C reveals that the ER appears enlarged and disassembled. This data was confirmed by ER staining with an ER tracker. Indeed, in treated cells, an intense fluorescence signal, likely due to massive ER stress, was detected (Figure 7A). These findings are in accordance with the literature [31]. In addition, the presence of autophagic vesicles in cells exposed to CBD homologs was confirmed through staining with LysoTracker Red, as it is selective for acidic organelles. This optical analysis denotes the accumulation of autophagolysosomes that could be due to an impairment of the autophagic process. Indeed, Shrivastava et al. [20] have shown that CBD may affect the complex cross-talk between autophagy and apoptosis. More recently, Huang et al. reported that CBD, acting via TRPV4, caused mitochondrial dysfunction and lethal mitophagy arrest leading to autophagic cell death in glioma cells [38].

In human cancer cells, the enzyme MAGL plays a major role in the regulation of several processes including cell growth, survival, migration, and invasion [39]. The combination of CBD homologs with drugs that inhibit the activity of enzymes involved in the metabolism of endocannabinoids, such as MAGL inhibitor (MJN110), or with drugs that induce the activation of cellular stress pathways [26,27], such as PMA, is associated with an extensive vacuolization, increased ROS levels, and multiple alterations in cellular organelles, whose effects look more dramatic than those observed when cells were exposed to the CBD homologs alone. Indeed, the combined treatment with CBD homologs and with the drugs (either MJN110 (1 µM) or PMA (100 nM)) induced severe cellular morphological changes, with an increase of about respectively 30% and 60% in the number of cytoplasmic vacuolations (Figure S2). Furthermore, a remarkable rise of ROS levels (Figure 8) and dramatic changes of the organelles structure (Figure S3) were detected in the combined treatment. In the case of PMA treatments, the effects on the cell structures appeared even more catastrophic. In particular, Figure 9 displays a huge number of double-membrane vacuoles containing degrading materials, and the presence of cytoplasmic vacuolations, likely associated with disassembled ER and mitochondria. Further morphological changes at the ER level and an increased number of lysosomes are shown in Figures S4 and S5, respectively. It has been reported that phytocannabinoids exert their action via CB receptor-dependent and independent ways [13,15]. In this regard, it has been also described that mitochondria are the primary CBD target in Jurkat cells [34] and our results are in line with these results.

Hence, CBDB and CBDP are two phytocannabinoids discovered only recently [4,6,7], thus their pharmacological activity is still to be investigated. It is conceivable that both CBDB and CBDP have on the one hand biological properties similar to those of CBD but a different affinity for the target receptors. As for their pharmacokinetics, since CBDB and CBDP are respectively less and more lipophilic than CBD, it is believable that they may have have different absorption rate, metabolism, binding to plasma proteins and elimination rate. However, so far there is no scientific evidence in this sense, and this manuscript represents the first study on the biological activity of these new CBD counterparts

4. Materials and Methods

- Cell Culture and Chemicals

The human breast cancer cell lines MCF-7, MDA-MB-361 and MDA-MB-231 were purchased from the American Type Culture Collection (ATCC). These cell lines were maintained in high-glucose Dulbecco's Modified Eagle's Medium (DMEM), supplemented with 10% (v/v) fetal bovine serum, 2% (v/v) L-glutamine 200 mM and 1% (v/v) penicillin-streptomycin (5000 U/mL). Cells were maintained in a humidified incubator with 5% CO_2 at 37 °C. The monoacylglycerol lipase (MAGL) inhibitor, MJN110, was purchased from SIGMA and used at the concentration of 1 µM. N-acetyl cysteine (NAC) was purchased from SIGMA and used at 1 mM and 1–0.1 mM, respectively. Nat CBD and syn CBD were kindly provided by CBDepot (Teplice, Czech Republic). Reagents and solvents used in the synthesis were of reagent grade and used without further purification.

- Synthesis and Characterization of CBD Homologs: CBDB and CBDP

CBDB and CBDP were synthesized as reported in previous works [4,7]. Briefly, the synthetic procedure to obtain CBD involved a dropwise addition of a solution of (1S,4R)-1-methyl-4-(prop-1-en-2-yl) cycloex-2-enol and 5-butylbenzene-1,3-diol (76 mg, 0.50 mmol, 1 eq.) in 5 mL of dry drydichloromethane (DCM) to a solution of 5-butylbenzene-1,3-diol (83 mg, 0.50 mmol, 1eq.) and p-toluenesulfonic acid (9 mg, 0.05 mmol, 0.1 eq.) in DCM (5 mL) at −10 °C, under argon atmosphere. The mixture was stirred for 1 h and then quenched with saturated $NaHCO_3$ (10 mL). Extraction of the mixture with diethylether (2 × 10 mL) was followed by purification over silica gel (crude:silica gel ratio 1/200, eluent: cyclohexane:DCM 8/2). The chromatographic fractions were analyzed by HPLC-UV and HPLC-HRMS and those containing exclusively CBDB without impurities were collected to give 48 mg of a reddish oil (32% yield, purity > 99%). The same procedure was carried out for the synthesis of CBDP, but 5-heptylbenzene-1,3-diol was used in place of 5-butylbenzene-1,3-diol to obtain a linear heptyl side chain. CBDP was obtained with a 23% yield (76 mg) as a colorless oil (purity > 99%).

The purity of CBDB and CBDP was checked by HPLC-HRMS analysis using an Ultimate 3000 liquid chromatograph (Thermo Fisher Scientific, Grand Island, NY, USA), equipped with a vacuum degasser, a binary pump, a thermostated autosampler, and a thermostated column compartment. The chromatographic system was interfaced to a heated electrospray ionization source and a Q-Exactive Orbitrap mass spectrometer (HPLC-HRMS). The chromatographic separation was carried out on a Poroshell 120 SB-C18 (3.0 × 100 mm, 2.7 µm, Agilent, Milan, Italy). The same instrumental parameters used in previous works were applied to confirm the identity of the synthesized compounds [4,7].

In detail, an isocratic elution of 30% water with 0.1% formic acid (A) and 70% acetonitrile (ACN) with 0.1% of formic acid (B) was set for 10 min, then 95% B was pumped for 5 min and lastly, the column was re-equilibrated for 2 min with the initial conditions for a total run time of 17 min. The flow rate was maintained constant at 0.5 mL/min. 5 µL of 0.1 µg/mL solutions of CBDB and CBDP were separately injected into the analytical system. The parameters of the heated electrospray ionization source were set as follows: capillary temperature, 320 °C; vaporizer temperature, 280 °C; electrospray voltage, 4.2 kV for positive mode and 3.8 kV for negative mode; sheath gas, 55 arbitrary units; auxiliary gas, 30 arbitrary units; S lens RF level, 45. Analyses were acquired using the Xcalibur 3.0 software (Thermo Fisher Scientific, San Jose, CA, USA) in full scan data-dependent acquisition (FS-dd-MS^2) in positive and negative mode at a resolving power of 70,000 FWHM at m/z 200. The parameters of the Orbitrap mass analyzer were as follows: scan range of m/z 250–400, AGC of 3e6, injection time 100 ms, and isolation window for the filtration of the precursor ions of m/z 0.7. Normalized collision energy (NCE) of 20 was used to fragment the precursor ions. Extracted ion chromatograms (EIC) of the [M + H]+ and [M − H]− molecular ions were derived from the total ion chromatogram with a 5-ppm mass tolerance.

- Western Immunoblot Analysis

Cells were lysed in a RIPA buffer (Cell Signaling) supplemented with protease inhibitors Cocktail (1×) and sodium fluoride (NaF, 16 µL/mL). Protein concentration was determined by the Bradford protein assay (BIO-RAD, Hercules, CA, USA). Samples were mixed 1:1 with Laemmli buffer (SIGMA, St. Louis, MO, USA), boiled for 5 min, 90 °C and 25 µg of proteins were separated onto Mini-PROTEAN® TGX™ Precast Gels (BIO-RAD, Hercules, CA, USA). Electrophoresis was run at 200 V for 60 min (IEF Cell Protean System, BIO-RAD, Hercules, CA, USA) and consequently total protein bands were visualized by 2.5 min of UV exposure, for gel activation. The bands were then transferred to the Midi Nitrocellulose membrane Trans-Blot Turbo (BIO-RAD, Hercules, CA, USA). The membranes were blocked for 1 h in Blotto A (Santa Cruz, CA, USA) at room temperature and subsequently probed for 1 h by the appropriately diluted primary antibodies. After three washes with a solution containing 10 mM Tris, pH 8.0, 150 mM NaCl, 0.5% Tween 20 (TBST solution), blots were incubated with secondary antibody HRP-conjugated for 1 h at room temperature (1:2000 dilution). Blots were then developed using the Clarity Enhanced chemiluminescence (ECL) (BIO-RAD, Hercules, CA, USA). Primary antibodies (1:1000 dilution) were: from Santa Cruz CB1 (2F9) sc-293419, CB2 (3C7) sc-293188 and from cell signaling p38 MAPK (#8690). Secondary antibodies (HRP-conjugated) were from Bethyl Laboratories (1:5000 dilution) (mouse IgG-heavy and light chain antibody, A90-116P). Images shown in the paper are representative of three independent replicates. Densitometric quantification of the band intensity was normalized to p38 levels using ImageJ.

- Cell Viability Assay

Changes in viability after the various treatments were measured using the Thiazolyl blue tetrazolium bromide (MTT) assay. Cells were seeded in 96-well plates at a density of 1×10^4/well and incubated at 37 °C in 5% CO_2. After overnight incubation, the medium was replaced with vehicle control or drug at different concentrations in DMEM and supplemented with 10% (v/v) fetal bovine serum, 2% (v/v) L-glutamine 200 mM and 1% (v/v) penicillin-streptomycin (5,000 U/mL). The cell lines were maintained in a humidified incubator with 5% CO_2 at 37 °C. After 24 h, upon completion of the drug treatments, the medium was removed and replaced with a serum-free medium containing 2 mg/mL MTT and incubated for 2 h at 37 °C. The MTT reagent was then removed and the formazan crystals were solubilized using dimethyl sulfoxide. The absorbance was read using the CLARIO star Plus microplate reader (570 nm). The absorbance of the vehicle control was subtracted and the percentage control was calculated as the absorbance of the treated cells/control cells × 100.

- Measurement of Reactive Oxygen Species (ROS)

To detect the changes in intracellular ROS levels, 2′,7′-dichlorofluorescein diacetate (DCFH-DA, Sigma-Aldrich) staining was used (Hyeoncheol Kim et al.). DCFH-DA is a stable, fluorogenic and non-polar compound that can readily diffuse into the cells and get deacetylated by intracellular esterases to a non-fluorescent 2′,7′-dichlorodihydrofluorescein (DCFH) which is later oxidized by intracellular ROS into highly fluorescent 2′,7′-dichlorofluorescein (DCF). The intensity of fluorescence is proportional to intracellular ROS levels. MCF-7 cells were seeded at a density of 2×10^5 cells per well in 24 well plates and were allowed to attach overnight. On the first day of treatment, the medium was replaced with the fresh ones containing the vehicle control, CBD homologs (10 µM), NAC (1 mM), PMA (1 µM) and MJN110 (1 µM) respectively. After 24 h, upon completion of the drug treatment, the spent medium was removed. The cells were washed once with fresh DMEM, and twice with 1X PBS and incubated with DCFH-DA in a final concentration of 10 µM for 30 min. Cells were rinsed with PBS and representative fluorescent images for each well using the green fluorescent protein (GFP) channel on an Evos m7000 fluorescence microscope were taken. After taking images, PBS was removed and a radioimmunoprecipitation assay (RIPA) buffer was added to each well. The collected cells were incubated at −80 °C for 20 min and then centrifuged at $21{,}130\times g$ for 10 min at 4 °C. The collected supernatant was transferred to a black 96 well plate and the fluorescence intensity measured using the CLARIO star Plus microplate reader at an excitation wavelength of 485 nm and an emission wavelength of 530 nm. After fluorescence recording, 5 µL of supernatant were transferred to a clear 96 well plate containing 195 µL of 1× protein assay solution to measure the protein concentration using the BCA assay. The fluorescence intensity was normalized to the protein concentration.

- MitoTracker Staining

The determination of the mitochondrial membrane potential was performed with the Mitotracker assay. MCF-7 cells were seeded at a density of 2×10^5 cells per well in a 24-well plate and were allowed to attach overnight, 37 °C. On the first day of treatment, the medium was replaced with vehicle control or CBD homologs (10 µM) in DMEM. After 24 h, upon completion of drug treatments, the spent medium was removed. The cells were then washed with fresh DMEM prior to incubating them with 75 nM of either MitoTracker™ Green FM or MitoTracker™ Red CMXRos in pre-warmed medium, without FBS, for 30 min, at 37 °C. Then the medium was removed, the cells were rinsed with PBS and representative fluorescent images for each well using respectively the GFP and the RFP channel on an Evos m7000 fluorescence microscope were taken.

- CellTiter-Glo 2.0 Cell Viability Assay

The quantification of the cellular ATP was performed using the CellTiter-Glo 2.0 cell viability assay. Cells were seeded in 96-well plates at a density of 1×10^4 /well and incubated at 37 °C in 5% CO_2. After overnight incubation, the medium was replaced with either vehicle control or drug at different concentrations in DMEM and supplemented with 10% (v/v) fetal bovine serum, 2% (v/v) L-glutamine 200 mM and 1% (v/v) penicillin-streptomycin (5000 U/mL). The cell lines were maintained in a humidified incubator with 5% CO_2, at 37 °C. After 24 h, upon completion of the drug treatments, the CellTiter-Glo 2.0 reagent was added into each well at the equivalent volume of cell culture medium in the well. Then, the contents were mixed vigorously for 5 min to induce cell lysis, and the plate was incubated at room temperature for an additional 25 min to stabilize the luminescent signal. Afterward, the supernatants were transferred in technical replicates into the 96-well opaque white-walled plate and the luminescence was measured using the CLARIO star Plus microplate reader.

- Ultrastructural Analysis of the Cellular Samples

MCF-7 cells were seeded at a density of 5×10^5 cells in Primo TC flasks 25 cm^2 and were allowed to attach overnight. Control and CBD homologs treated cells were grown to 80% confluency and fixed with 2.5% glutaraldehyde in 0.1 M cacodylate buffer, pH 7.4, for 2 h at 4 °C. The cells were washed three times, 5–10 min each, in ice-cold PBS buffer and then post-fixed in ice-cold 1% osmium tetroxide. After 1 h, the samples were washed three times in PBS and dehydrated in an acetone series for 15 min each with 25, 50, 75, 90 and 100% acetone. Three steps of infiltration in a mixture of resin/acetone (1/2, 1/1 and 2/1 ratios) were performed and finally, the specimens were embedded in 100% resin at 60 °C for 48 h. Ultrathin sections (70 nm thick) were cut with an Ultramicrotome. TEM images were recorded on a JEOL Jem1011 microscope operating at an accelerating voltage of 100 kV (Tokyo, Japan).

- Lysotracker Assay

The mitochondrial-lysosomal axis theory of aging postulates that oxidized material accumulates in lysosomes as cells age, which results in a decreased degradative capacity of lysosomes. This behavior was studied using Lysotracker staining. MCF-7 cells are seeded at a density of 2×10^5 cells per well in a 24-well plate and are allowed to attach overnight, at 37 °C. On the first day of treatment, the medium was replaced with vehicle control, CBD homologs (10 µM), NAC (1 mM), PMA (1 µM) and MJN110 (1 µM) in DMEM. After 24 h, upon completion of the drug treatments, spent media was removed. The cells were washed once with fresh DMEM. Cells were incubated with HOECHST (0.5 mg/mL in PBS), for 5 min, at 37 °C. The Hoechst was removed and replaced with a pre-warmed medium, without FBS, containing 100 nM LysoTracker Red DND-99 (Cat. No. L-7528). Cells are incubated at 33 °C for 30 min with LysoTracker. Then the medium was removed, the cells were rinsed with PBS and representative fluorescent images for each well using the RFP channel on an Evos m7000 fluorescence microscope were taken.

- Endoplasmic Reticulum Staining

MCF-7 cells are seeded at a density of 2×10^5 cells per well in a 24-well plate and are allowed to attach overnight, at 37 °C. On the first day of treatment, the medium was replaced with vehicle control, CBD homologs (10 µM), NAC (1 mM), PMA (1 µM) and MJN110 (1 µM) in DMEM. After 24 h, upon completion of the drug treatments, spent media was removed. The cells were washed once with fresh DMEM. Cells were stained with ER-Tracker™ Green (glibenclamide BODIPY® FL), 1 µM in pre-warmed medium, without FBS for 15 min at 37 °C. Then the medium was removed, the cells were rinsed with PBS and representative fluorescent images for each well using the GFP channel on an Evos m7000 fluorescence microscope were taken.

5. Conclusions

Data collected in this study suggest that the treatment of MCF-7 cells with CBDB and CBDP activates catastrophic intracellular processes. Though the newly discovered CBDB and CBDP differ from the well-known nat CBD and syn CBD only for the length of the alkyl side chain on the resorcinic portion, their biological effects look comparable to those observed in cancer cells exposed to nat and syn CBD. Additionally, our results provide evidence that CBD homologs alter the morphology and the structure of multiple organelles, affecting cell homeostasis. These preliminary results represent the first step of further in-depth studies required to confirm the potential use of these homologs as an adjuvant in anticancer chemotherapy.

Supplementary Materials: The following are available online. Figure S1: Representative images of MCF-7, MDA-MB-361 and MDA-MB-231 cells treated with cannabinoid homologs, Figure S2: Quantification of vacuolated cells and representative images of MCF-7 cells treated with either MJN110 or PMA, Figure S3: Representative TEM images of cell morphology, Figure S4: Representative fluorescent images of organelles structures from MCF-7 cells treated with MJN110, Figure S5: Representative fluorescent images of organelles structures from MCF-7 cells treated with PMA.

Author Contributions: Conceptualization, A.Q., D.V. and A.G.; methodology, M.S., A.Q., A.G., A.M.G., D.V., C.C. and F.R.; validation: A.G., A.Q. and D.V.; formal analysis, A.G., A.Q.; investigation, A.Q., D.V. and A.G.; resources, A.G.; data curation, A.G., A.Q. and D.V. writing—original draft preparation, M.S., A.Q., and A.G.; writing—review and editing, A.Q., D.V. and A.G.; visualization, A.Q. and A.G.; supervision, A.Q., A.G. and D.V.; project administration A.G.; funding acquisition, A.G., G.G. and G.C. All authors have read and agreed to the published version of the manuscript.

Funding: This research was funded by the UNIHEMP research project "Use of iNdustrIal Hemp biomass for Energy and new biocheMicals Production" (ARS01_00668) funded by Fondo Europeo di Sviluppo Regionale (FESR) (within the PON R&I 2017–202 –Axis 2–Action II–OS 1. b). Grant decree UNIHEMP prot. n. 2016 of 27 July 2018; CUP B76C18000520005.

Institutional Review Board Statement: Not applicable.

Informed Consent Statement: Not applicable.

Acknowledgments: The authors would like to acknowledge the support of the following Italian projects: "Tecnopolo per la medicina di precisione" (TecnoMed Puglia)—Regione Puglia: DGR n.2117 del 21/11/2018 (CUP: B84I18000540002), and "Tecnopolo di Nanotecnologia e Fotonica per la medicina di precisione" (TECNOMED)—FISR/MIUR-CNR: delibera CIPE n. 3449 del 7-08-2017(CUP: B83B17000010001).

Conflicts of Interest: The authors declare no conflict of interest.

Sample Availability: Not applicable.

References

1. Kisková, T.; Mungenast, F.; Suváková, M.; Jäger, W.; Thalhammer, T. Future aspects for cannabinoids in breast cancer therapy. *Int. J. Mol. Sci.* **2019**, *20*, 1673. [CrossRef] [PubMed]
2. Freeman, T.P.; Hindocha, C.; Green, S.F.; Bloomfield, M.A.P. Medicinal use of cannabis based products and cannabinoids. *BMJ* **2019**, *365*, l1141. [CrossRef] [PubMed]
3. Pisanti, S.; Malfitano, A.M.; Ciaglia, E.; Lamberti, A.; Ranieri, R.; Cuomo, G.; Abate, M.; Faggiana, G.; Proto, M.C.; Fiore, D.; et al. Cannabidiol: State of the art and new challenges for therapeutic applications. *Pharmacol. Ther.* **2017**, *175*, 133–150. [CrossRef] [PubMed]
4. Citti, C.; Russo, F.; Linciano, P.; Strallhofer, S.S.; Tolomeo, F.; Forni, F.; Vandelli, M.A.; Gigli, G.; Cannazza, G. Origin of Δ9-Tetrahydrocannabinol Impurity in Synthetic Cannabidiol. *Cannabis Cannabinoid Res.* **2021**, *6*, 28–39. [CrossRef] [PubMed]
5. Citti, C.; Linciano, P.; Russo, F.; Luongo, L.; Iannotta, M.; Maione, S.; Laganà, A.; Capriotti, A.L.; Forni, F.; Vandelli, M.A.; et al. A novel phytocannabinoid isolated from Cannabis sativa L. with an in vivo cannabimimetic activity higher than Δ9-tetrahydrocannabinol: Δ9-Tetrahydrocannabiphorol. *Sci. Rep.* **2019**, *9*, 1–13. [CrossRef]
6. Linciano, P.; Citti, C.; Luongo, L.; Belardo, C.; Maione, S.; Vandelli, M.A.; Forni, F.; Gigli, G.; Laganà, A.; Montone, C.M.; et al. Isolation of a High-Affinity Cannabinoid for the Human CB1 Receptor from a Medicinal Cannabis sativa Variety: Δ9-Tetrahydrocannabutol, the Butyl Homologue of Δ9-Tetrahydrocannabinol. *J. Nat. Prod.* **2019**, *83*, 88–98. [CrossRef]
7. Citti, C.; Linciano, P.; Forni, F.; Vandelli, M.A.; Gigli, G.; Laganà, A.; Cannazza, G. Chemical and spectroscopic characterization data of 'cannabidibutol', a novel cannabidiol butyl analog. *Data Brief* **2019**, *26*, 104463. [CrossRef]
8. Citti, C.; Linciano, P.; Forni, F.; Vandelli, M.A.; Gigli, G.; Laganà, A.; Cannazza, G. Analysis of impurities of cannabidiol from hemp. Isolation, characterization and synthesis of cannabidibutol, the novel cannabidiol butyl analog. *J. Pharm. Biomed. Anal.* **2019**, *175*, 112752. [CrossRef] [PubMed]
9. Nigro, E.; Formato, M.; Crescente, G.; Daniele, A. Cancer Initiation, Progression and Resistance: Are Phytocannabinoids from Cannabis sativa L. Promising Compounds? *Molecules* **2021**, *26*, 2668. [CrossRef] [PubMed]
10. Fraguas-Sánchez, A.I.; Martín-Sabroso, C.; Fernández-Carballido, A.; Torres-Suárez, A.I. Current status of nanomedicine in the chemotherapy of breast cancer. *Cancer Chemother. Pharmacol.* **2019**, *84*, 689–706. [CrossRef]
11. Donadelli, M.; Dando, I.; Zaniboni, T.; Costanzo, C.; Pozza, E.D.; Scupoli, M.T.; Scarpa, A.; Zappavigna, S.; Marra, M.; Abbruzzese, A.; et al. Gemcitabine/cannabinoid combination triggers autophagy in pancreatic cancer cells through a ROS-mediated mechanism. *Cell Death Dis.* **2011**, *2*, e152. [CrossRef]
12. Luongo, M.; Marinelli, O.; Zeppa, L.; Aguzzi, C.; Morelli, M.B.; Amantini, C.; Frassineti, A.; Costanzo, M.; Fanelli, A.; Santoni, G.; et al. Cannabidiol and Oxygen-Ozone Combination Induce Cytotoxicity in Human Pancreatic Ductal Adenocarcinoma Cell Lines. *Cancers* **2020**, *12*, 2774. [CrossRef]
13. Nabissi, M.; Morelli, M.B.; Santoni, M.; Santoni, G. Triggering of the TRPV2 channel by cannabidiol sensitizes glioblastoma cells to cytotoxic chemotherapeutic agents. *Carcinogenesis* **2013**, *34*, 48–57. [CrossRef]
14. Harpe, A.d.l.; Beukes, N.; Frost, C.L. CBD activation of TRPV1 induces oxidative signaling and subsequent ER stress in breast cancer cell lines. *Biotechnol. Appl. Biochem.* **2021**. [CrossRef]

15. Marinelli, O.; Morelli, M.B.; Annibali, D.; Aguzzi, C.; Zeppa, L.; Tuyaerts, S.; Amantini, C.; Amant, F.; Ferretti, B.; Maggi, F.; et al. The effects of cannabidiol and prognostic role of TRPV2 in human endometrial cancer. *Int. J. Mol. Sci.* **2020**, *21*, 5409. [CrossRef]
16. Calvaruso, G.; Pellerito, O.; Notaro, A.; Giuliano, M. Cannabinoid-associated cell death mechanisms in tumor models (Review). *Int. J. Oncol.* **2012**, *41*, 407–413. [CrossRef]
17. Mangal, N.; Erridge, S.; Habib, N.; Sadanandam, A.; Reebye, V.; Sodergren, M.H. Cannabinoids in the landscape of cancer. *J. Cancer Res. Clin. Oncol.* **2021**, *147*, 2507–2534. [CrossRef]
18. McAllister, S.D.; Murase, R.; Christian, R.T.; Lau, D.; Zielinski, A.J.; Allison, J.; Almanza, C.; Pakdel, A.; Lee, J.; Limbad, C.; et al. Pathways mediating the effects of cannabidiol on the reduction of breast cancer cell proliferation, invasion, and metastasis. *Breast Cancer Res. Treat.* **2011**, *129*, 37–47. [CrossRef] [PubMed]
19. Caffarel, M.M.; Andradas, C.; Mira, E.; Pérez-Gómez, E.; Cerutti, C.; Moreno-Bueno, G.; Flores, J.M.; García-Real, I.; Palacios, J.; Mañes, S.; et al. Cannabinoids reduce ErbB2-driven breast cancer progression through Akt inhibition. *Mol. Cancer* **2010**, *9*, 1–11. [CrossRef] [PubMed]
20. Shrivastava, A.; Kuzontkoski, P.M.; Groopman, J.E.; Prasad, A. Cannabidiol induces programmed cell death in breast cancer cells by coordinating the cross-talk between apoptosis and autophagy. *Mol. Cancer Ther.* **2011**, *10*, 1161–1172. [CrossRef] [PubMed]
21. Lee, X.C.; Werner, E.; Falasca, M. Molecular Mechanism of Autophagy and Its Regulation by Cannabinoids in Cancer. *Cancers* **2021**, *13*, 1211. [CrossRef]
22. Bow, E.W.; Rimoldi, J.M. The Structure-Function Relationships of Classical Cannabinoids: CB1/CB2 Modulation. *Perspect. Med. Chem.* **2016**, *8*, 17–39. [CrossRef]
23. Grimaldi, C.; Pisanti, S.; Laezza, C.; Malfitano, A.M.; Santoro, A.; Vitale, M.; Caruso, M.G.; Notarnicola, M.; Iacuzzo, I.; Portella, G.; et al. Anandamide inhibits adhesion and migration of breast cancer cells. *Exp. Cell Res.* **2006**, *312*, 363–373. [CrossRef]
24. Lin, Y.; Xu, J.; Lan, H. Tumor-associated macrophages in tumor metastasis: Biological roles and clinical therapeutic applications. *J. Hematol. Oncol.* **2019**, *12*, 1–16. [CrossRef]
25. Deng, H.; Li, W. Monoacylglycerol Lipase Inhibitors: Modulators for Lipid Metabolism in Cancer Malignancy, Neurological and Metabolic Disorders. *Acta Pharm. Sin. B* **2019**, *10*, 582–602. [CrossRef]
26. Pandur, S.; Ravuri, C.; Moens, U.; Huseby, N.-E. Combined incubation of colon carcinoma cells with phorbol ester and mitochondrial uncoupling agents results in synergic elevated reactive oxygen species levels and increased γ-glutamyltransferase expression. *Mol. Cell. Biochem.* **2014**, *388*, 149–156. [CrossRef]
27. Vergara, D.; Ravaioli, S.; Fonzi, E.; Adamo, L.; Damato, M.; Bravaccini, S.; Pirini, F.; Gaballo, A.; Barbano, R.; Pasculli, B.; et al. Carbonic Anhydrase XII Expression Is Modulated during Epithelial Mesenchymal Transition and Regulated through Protein Kinase C Signaling. *Int. J. Mol. Sci.* **2020**, *21*, 715. [CrossRef] [PubMed]
28. Fogli, S.; Breschi, M.C. The molecular bases of cannabinoid action in cancer. *Cancer Ther.* **2008**, *6*, 103–116.
29. Chakravarti, B.; Ravi, J.; Ganju, R.K. Cannabinoids as therapeutic agents in cancer: Current status and future implications. *Oncotarget* **2014**, *5*, 5852–5872. [CrossRef] [PubMed]
30. Dobovišek, L.; Krstanović, F.; Borštnar, S.; Debeljak, N. Cannabinoids and Hormone Receptor-Positive Breast Cancer Treatment. *Cancers* **2020**, *12*, 525. [CrossRef]
31. Schoeman, R.; Beukes, N.; Frost, C. Cannabinoid Combination Induces Cytoplasmic Vacuolation in MCF-7 Breast Cancer Cells. *Molecules* **2020**, *25*, 4682. [CrossRef] [PubMed]
32. Ma, Y.; Fang, W.; Wang, J.; Yang, X.; Gu, Y.; Li, Y. In vitro and in vivo antitumor activity of neochlorogenic acid in human gastric carcinoma cells are complemented with ROS generation, loss of mitochondrial membrane potential and apoptosis induction. *JBUON* **2019**, *24*, 221–226.
33. Chung, Y.M.; Bae, Y.S.; Lee, S.Y. Molecular ordering of ROS production, mitochondrial changes, and caspase activation during sodium salicylate-induced apoptosis. *Free. Radic. Biol. Med.* **2003**, *34*, 434–442. [CrossRef]
34. Olivas-Aguirre, M.; Torres-López, L.; Valle-Reyes, J.S.; Hernández-Cruz, A.; Pottosin, L.; Dobrovinskaya, O. Cannabidiol directly targets mitochondria and disturbs calcium homeostasis in acute lymphoblastic leukemia. *Cell Death Dis.* **2019**, *10*, 1–19. [CrossRef] [PubMed]
35. Zhang, X.; Qin, Y.; Pan, Z.; Li, M.; Liu, X.; Chen, X.; Qu, G.; Zhou, L.; Xu, M.; Zheng, Q.; et al. Cannabidiol Induces Cell Cycle Arrest and Cell Apoptosis in Human Gastric Cancer SGC-7901 Cells. *Biomolecules* **2019**, *9*, 302. [CrossRef]
36. Zorov, D.B.; Filburn, C.R.; Klotz, L.O.; Zweier, J.L.; Sollott, S.J. Reactive oxygen species (ROS)-induced ROS release: A new phenomenon accompanying induction of the mitochondrial permeability transition in cardiac myocytes. *J. Exp. Med.* **2000**, *192*, 1001–1014. [CrossRef] [PubMed]
37. Chen, Y.; Gibson, S.B. Is mitochondrial generation of reactive oxygen species a trigger for autophagy? *Autophagy* **2008**, *4*, 246–248. [CrossRef]
38. Huang, T.; Xu, T.; Wang, Y.; Zhou, Y.; Yu, D.; Wang, Z.; He, L.; Chen, Z.; Zhang, Y.; Davidson, D.; et al. Cannabidiol inhibits human glioma by induction of lethal mitophagy through activating TRPV4. *Autophagy* **2021**, 1–15. [CrossRef]
39. Nomura, D.K.; Long, J.Z.; Niessen, S.; Hoover, H.S.; Ng, S.-W.; Cravatt, B.F. Monoacylglycerol lipase regulates a fatty acid network that promotes cancer pathogenesis. *Cell* **2010**, *140*, 49–61. [CrossRef]

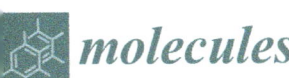

Review

Olive Tree in Circular Economy as a Source of Secondary Metabolites Active for Human and Animal Health Beyond Oxidative Stress and Inflammation

Rosanna Mallamaci [1], Roberta Budriesi [2], Maria Lisa Clodoveo [3], Giulia Biotti [2], Matteo Micucci [2], Andrea Ragusa [4], Francesca Curci [5], Marilena Muraglia [5], Filomena Corbo [5,*] and Carlo Franchini [5]

[1] Department of Bioscience, Biotechnology and Biopharmaceutics, University Aldo Moro Bari, 70125 Bari, Italy; rosanna.mallamaci@uniba.it
[2] Department of Pharmacy and Biotechnology, Food Chemistry & Nutraceutical Lab, Alma Mater Studiorum-University of Bologna, 40126 Bologna, Italy; roberta.budriesi@unibo.it (R.B.); giulia.biotti@studio.unibo.it (G.B.); matteo.micucci2@unibo.it (M.M.)
[3] Interdisciplinary Department of Medicine, University Aldo Moro Bari, 702125 Bari, Italy; marialisa.clodoveo@uniba.it
[4] Department of Biological and Environmental Sciences and Technologies, Campus Ecotekne, University of Salento, 73100 Lecce, Italy; andrea.ragusa@unisalento.it
[5] Department of Pharmacy-Drug Sciences, University Aldo Moro Bari, 70125 Bari, Italy; francesca.curci@uniba.it (F.C.); marilena.muraglia@uniba.it (M.M.); carlo.franchini@uniba.it (C.F.)
* Correspondence: filomena.corbo@uniba.it; Tel.: +39-0805442746

Abstract: Extra-virgin olive oil (EVOO) contains many bioactive compounds with multiple biological activities that make it one of the most important functional foods. Both the constituents of the lipid fraction and that of the unsaponifiable fraction show a clear action in reducing oxidative stress by acting on various body components, at concentrations established by the European Food Safety Authority's claims. In addition to the main product obtained by the mechanical pressing of the fruit, i.e., the EVOO, the residual by-products of the process also contain significant amounts of antioxidant molecules, thus potentially making the *Olea europea* L. an excellent example of the circular economy. In fact, the olive mill wastewaters, the leaves, the pomace, and the pits discharged from the EVOO production process are partially recycled in the nutraceutical and cosmeceutical fields also because of their antioxidant effect. This work presents an overview of the biological activities of these by-products, as shown by in vitro and in vivo assays, and also from clinical trials, as well as their main formulations currently available on the market.

Keywords: *Olea europea* L.; olive oil; olive mill wastewater (OMW); olive leaf extract (OLE); hydroxytyrosol; oleuropein; polyphenols; pit; by-products

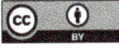

1. Introduction

Olive oil is the main product obtained from olives, fruits that come from the *Olea europaea* L. evergreen trees [1]. Olive oil is a characteristic element of the Mediterranean Diet (MD) because of the health-beneficial effects deriving from its chemical composition [2–4] as well as its appreciable taste and usefulness in flavoring a large variety of foods. In particular, the constituents of both lipidic and unsaponifiable fractions in extra-virgin olive oils (EVOOs) have been demonstrated to be able to reduce oxidative stress by acting on various biomolecules in the body, as also stated by the European Food Safety Authority (EFSA) [5].

During the production process of EVOOs, olive milling yields a mixture of olive paste and water. Subsequent malaxation of the olive paste allows for the separation of three phases: (i) the olive oil, (ii) a solid residue, and (iii) the olive mill wastewater (OMW). The last two components are produced in large quantities, and they are considered an agro-industrial waste whose disposal represents an important environmental problem as the plant material is usually subjected to microbial deterioration [6,7].

Currently, in the linear economy, agricultural by-products are mainly used as combustion feedstock for biofuels (Figure 1) [8,9].

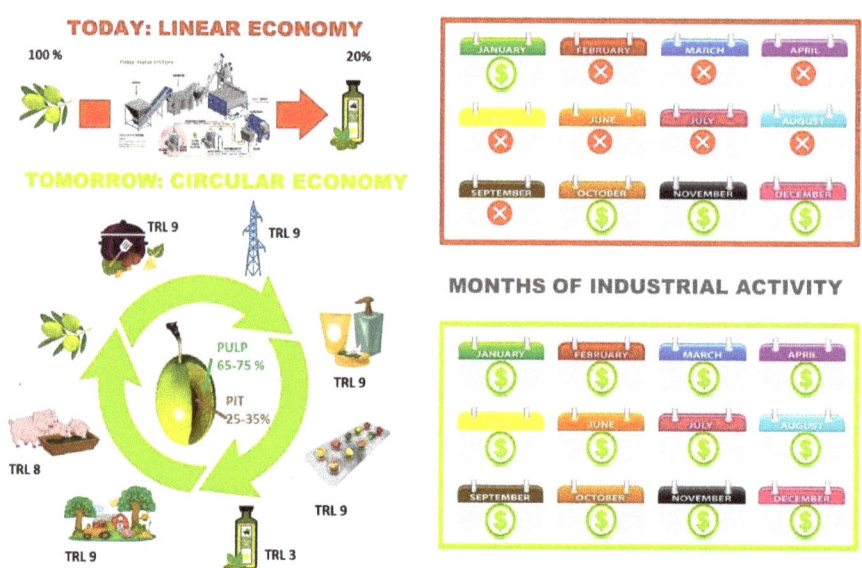

Figure 1. From linear to the circular economy in the olive oil sector.

The most important biomasses are residues from wood working (wood shavings and sawdust) or forestry activities, wastes from farms and agro-business, the organic fraction of municipal solid wastes, and plants deliberately grown for energetic purposes. Similarly, pruning wastes from olive trees are also used as biomass. However, in coherence with the "circular economy" principle, it is important to valorize these waste products containing high levels of secondary metabolites, thus accelerating the implementation of the "Transforming our world: the 2030 Agenda for Sustainable Development" [10,11].

Nevertheless, the transition from linear to the circular economy requires a cultural and structural change: a deep revision and innovation of production, distribution, and consumption models [12]. Furthermore, from a circular economy perspective, the added value of materials and energy must be maintained for as long as possible over multiple productions and use cycles, representing a new opportunity also for seasonal sectors, such as the EVOOs manufacturing industry.

Olive mill waste, olive pomace (exhausted pulp, kernel, and seeds), and vegetative water are significant by-products of the olive oil-producing countries in the Mediterranean basin, with a high environmental impact if not properly treated. In addition, these wastes are rich in high-value compounds, which can be either used directly after extraction or exploited as ingredients with different applications, e.g., as food supplements, nutraceuticals, cosmeceuticals, and animal feed.

The transition from linear to the circular economy, largely desired from stakeholders in the olive oil sector, requires a multidisciplinary approach that exploits know-how harmonically from different fields (Figure 2).

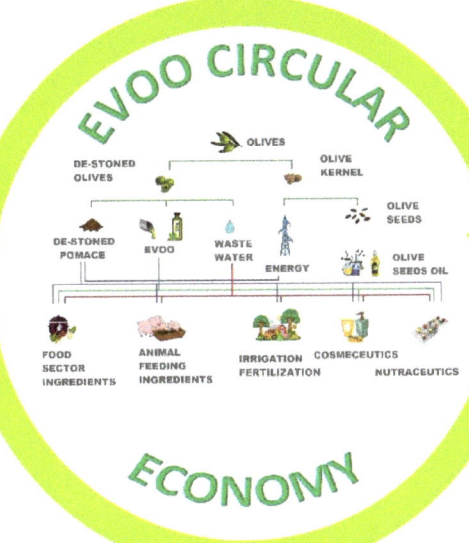

Figure 2. Extra virgin olive oil's (EVOO's) circular economy: overview of an integrated olive tree exploitation.

This transition would also bring an additional value, represented by the possibility that each oil mill can integrate new processes with the pre-existing ones, with the resulting economic advantages, guaranteeing both product diversification and fair income for all stakeholders, who are currently threatened by the increasing oil price trend and the emerging Xylella pandemic.

In this review, we focused our attention on the secondary metabolites contained in waste materials derived from the olive oil production process and their ability to reduce oxidative stress, both in vitro and in vivo. Particular attention has been paid to their potential exploitation in the circular economy by obtaining new high-value ingredients for health-related products (nutraceuticals, pharmaceuticals, and cosmeceuticals).

2. *Olea europea* L.: Overview on Its Chemical Compounds

The most represented chemical classes in *Olea europea* L. tree are mainly classified as nonpolar compounds (present in the lipophilic oil fraction, such as squalene, tocopherols, sterols, and triterpenic compounds) and polar phenolic compounds [13].

Among the polyphenolic compounds, the most abundant and studied in olives are tyrosol (TY), hydroxytyrosol (HT), oleuropein (OL), oleocanthal, and verbascoside (Figure 3).

The secondary metabolites from *Olea europea* L. have high biological value, and they are present in different concentrations in the various parts of the olive plant (Table 1); as such, many of them are present in the derived EVOOs, but they can also be found in the waste products from the production process.

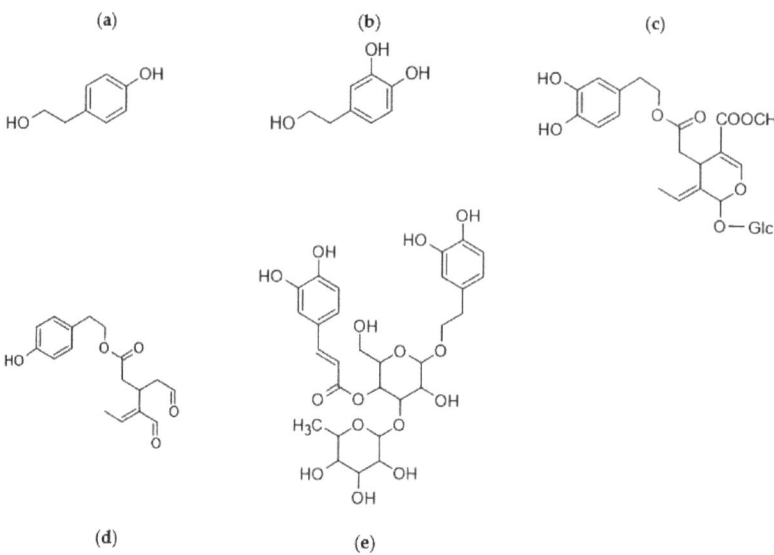

Figure 3. Most abundant polyphenols in olives: (**a**) tyrosol; (**b**) hydroxytyrosol; (**c**) oleuropein; (**d**) oleocanthal; (**e**) verbascoside.

Table 1. Distribution of the main classes of metabolites in the different parts of the plant *Olea europea* L. [13–21].

Seed Oil	Virgin Olive Oil	Skin	Pulp	Wood	Leaves
Phenolic acid/aldehydes	Phenolic acid/aldehydes	Phenolic acid/aldehydes	Phenolic acid/aldehydes Tocopherols	Phenolic acid/aldehydes	Phenolic acid/aldehydes
Tocopherols	Tocopherols	Organic acid and coumarins	Organic acid and coumarins	Organic acid and coumarins	Organic acid and coumarins
Sterols	Sterols	Flavonoids	Simple phenols and derivatives	Simple phenols and derivatives	Simple phenols and derivatives
		Lignans	Secoiridoids and derivatives	Secoiridoids and derivatives	Secoiridoids and derivatives
		Fatty acids and derivatives		Flavonoids	Flavonoids
		Pentacyclic triterpenes			Tocopherols

For this reason, all the materials involved in olive oil manufacturing represent a precious reservoir that could supply extracts reusable for health purposes. The most studied secondary metabolites are the polyphenols (or biophenols, as they are often referred to in EVOOs) that represent a group of molecules with one or more phenolic rings [14]. These compounds can be defined as nutraceuticals for their biological/pharmacological actions [15], mostly derived from their antioxidant properties, that play a protective role against oxidative stress [16] and extend the shelf-life of olive oil [17].

The antioxidant activity is mainly due to five classes of polyphenols identified as simple phenols, phenolic acids, secoiridoids, flavonoids, and lignans [18]. Among these, OL represents the principal biophenol in the olive leaf [19], followed by other constituents such as verbascoside, luteolin-7-O-glucoside, apigenin-7-O-glucoside, and TY [20]. Their antioxidant activity is even higher than that of antioxidants, such as vitamins E and C [21].

3. *Olea europea* L. By-Products for Human Health

The plant *Olea europea* L. is a genus that comprises more than 40 species. To this genus belong plants that are typical of temperate regions in the European continent, Asia, and

Africa. We focused on *Olea europaea* L. because it is the only species used for obtaining oil by pressing their fruit (i.e., the olive). On the other hand, other species, such as *O. capensis*, *O. dioica*, *O. brachiata*, and *O. obvata*, are not used for oil production. Currently, there are almost 400 cultivars of *Olea europaea* L. used all over the world, of which about 100 are planted in Italy.

Olive products, such as olive oil and table olives, are functional foods because of their beneficial effects, mostly due to mono- and poly-unsaturated fatty acids and, last but not least, the presence of polyphenols and other secondary metabolites. During the olive oil production process, some polyphenols remain in the oil-water emulsion, but most of them, being hydrophilic, end up in the OMW. Sometimes olive leaves are also added to the olives before milling in order to enrich the resulting oil in polyphenols. In addition, many production factors (e.g., cultivar, ripening time, and extraction method), as well as environmental factors (e.g., climate, precipitations, and age of the trees), are responsible for the different content and composition of polyphenols in oil [22].

The nutritional and health-promoting effects of olives and olive oils are well-established and recognized [23], such as their antioxidant [24,25], anti-inflammatory [26,27], cardioprotective [28,29], anticancer [30], antidiabetic, and neuroprotective effects [31,32]. Thanks to these properties, these compounds positively contribute to the beneficial effects of the MD [33]. To confirm the significant role of olive oil components as responsible for the benefits of the MD, Fernandes et al. examined the outcome from randomized controlled trials on the effect of regular dietary EVOO intake on inflammatory markers [34]. Recently, Storniolo and co-workers demonstrated that the role of oleic acid in the colon cancer cells growth is reverted in the presence of olive oil representative minor components, suggesting that the consumption of seed oils, high oleic acid seed oils, or olive oil will probably have different effects on colorectal cancer [35,36]. The presence of secondary metabolites also in the by-products of olive oil production makes OMW, leaves, pomace, and kernels raw materials exploitable in the nutraceutical, food, cosmetic, feed, and energy sectors. The scientific evidence related to the health-promoting effects of these by-products is detailed below.

3.1. Secondary Metabolites in Olive Mill Wastewater

OMW is a by-product of olive oil production, rich in water-soluble bioactive compounds that could be separated by industrial membrane technology [37]. This procedure, based on the different capabilities of the substances in a mixture to cross the polymeric or inorganic semipermeable membrane at different rates, allows a cost-effective purification of the OMW phenolic pool because of the low operative temperature needed [38].

Nanofiltration has also been successfully employed for concentrating phenolic compounds extracted from the same raw material. The extracts are fractionated across different membranes to get microfiltration, followed by ultrafiltration and nanofiltration [39]. The total phenolic content is then analyzed using high-performance liquid chromatography (HPLC) [40].

OMW has long been considered a waste whose disposal requires high economic costs. Recently, numerous studies have shown its content in polyphenols and other biologically important molecules, shifting its perspective from waste to an economical and natural source of antioxidants [41]. The typical composition of OMW is reported in Table 2. As can be observed, OL, abundant in leaves, is absent in OMW, while are present several low molecular weight phenolic compounds, such as TY and HT, which are formed by enzymatic hydrolysis during the milling process. Phenolic compounds with molecular weights in the range of 600–5000 Da and other molecules, such as verbascoside, its isomers, and oxidation products, as well as higher molecular weight phenols deriving from the oxidative polymerization of hydroxytyrosol and elenolic acid, are also present [42,43].

Table 2. Chemical composition of olive mill wastewater (OMW) extracts obtained by different techniques.

Composition	OMW [a]	UF [b]	AIR [c]	WSF [c]	WIF [c]	UF HSF			UF ETNA O1PP			NF 90	
						F [a]	P [a]	R [a]	F [a]	P [a]	R [a]	F [a]	R [a]
Total phenols	1409.0	1692.0	3.2	2.8	1.9	81.3	79.5	81.3	75.5	62.2	77.4	65.6	86.2
Hydroxytyrosol	3.8	n.d.	-	-	-	3.8	3.7	3.9	3.5	3.0	3.8	3.2	4.0
Protocatechuic acid	25.0	-	-	-	-	25.0	24.0	24.5	27.0	20.6	26.0	22.0	30.0
Catechol	7.5	-	-	-	-	7.5	7.1	7.2	6.0	5.0	6.2	5.5	7.5
Tyrosol	39.0	n.d.	-	-	-	39.0	38.7	39.6	34.2	30.0	36.0	31.0	40.0
Caffeic acid	5.0	-	-	-	-	5.0	4.9	5.2	4.0	3.0	4.4	3.2	3.7
p-Cumaric acid	1.0	-	-	-	-	1.0	0.9	0.9	0.8	0.6	1.0	0.7	1.0
Verbascoside	-	n.d.	-	-	-	-	-	-	-	-	-	-	-
Isoverbascoside	-	n.d.	-	-	-	-	-	-	-	-	-	-	-
Carbohydrates	-	-	25.0 [d]	60.0 [d]	5.1 [d]	-	-	-	-	-	-	-	-
Fucose	-	-	0.5	0.6	0.4	-	-	-	-	-	-	-	-
Rhamnose	-	-	14.3	13.7	16.4	-	-	-	-	-	-	-	-
Arabinose	-	-	14.1	10.7	17.6	-	-	-	-	-	-	-	-
Galactose	-	-	12.6	13.1	5.9	-	-	-	-	-	-	-	-
Glucose	-	-	42.2	45.1	47.7	-	-	-	-	-	-	-	-
Mannose	-	-	5.5	5.4	4.4	-	-	-	-	-	-	-	-
Xylose	-	-	5.0	4.9	5.3	-	-	-	-	-	-	-	-
Galacturonic acid	-	-	4.9	5.0	1.4	-	-	-	-	-	-	-	-
Glucuronic acid	-	-	1.0	1.1	0.7	-	-	-	-	-	-	-	-
Proteins	-	-	3.2	11.0	0.3	-	-	-	-	-	-	-	-

UF = ultrafiltration residue; AIR = alcohol insoluble OMW residue; WSF = water-soluble fraction; WIF = water-insoluble fraction; UF HSF = ultrafiltration performed with HSF membrane type; UF ETNA O1PP = ultrafiltration performed with ETNA 01PP membrane type; NF 90 = nanofiltration performed with NF90 membrane type; F = feed; P = permeate; R = retentate. [a] Expressed as mg/L; [b] expressed as ppm; [c] expressed as g/100 g of fraction; [d] expressed as mol%; n.d. = not determined.

OMW also contains significant amounts of monosaccharides, such as glucose, galactose, arabinose, rhamnose, and galacturonic acid, and polysaccharides, whose prebiotic and antioxidant activities have been evaluated [44–47]. Among simple sugars, arabinose, in particular, showed to be able to reduce the concentration of hydroxyl radicals by chelating Fe^{2+} ions [48] significantly. Many studies on various matrices also showed the antioxidant capacity of polysaccharides [49–51]. Therefore, the remarkable antioxidant activity of OMW can be attributed not only to its polyphenolic content but probably also to the polysaccharide and protein content. Furthermore, polysaccharides in OMW assimilated to dietary fibers owed additional biological and physiological functions, such as antimetastatic, immunostimulating, and anti-ulcer activity, as well as reduction of serum cholesterol, inhibition of hyaluronidase, and release of histamine [45,52].

3.2. Biological Activity of Olive Mill Wastewater Extracts

Recently, many research groups have tested OMW, in which both HT and its precursors are much more concentrated with respect to olive oil, on numerous biological targets. A study on two OMW mixtures with a polyphenol content of 100 and 36 g/kg (MOMAST® HY100 and MOMAST® HP30, respectively) found a significant antioxidant and anti-inflammatory effect in an ex vivo model of rat colon, liver, heart, and prefrontal cortex [53]. After treatment, the levels of the several inflammatory markers, i.e., prostaglandin (PGE_2), lactate dehydrogenase (LDH), nitric oxide synthase (iNOS), COX-2, and TNFα, decreased drastically.

Other studies on purified extracts of OMW have shown additional anti-angiogenic and chemopreventive effects, both in vitro and in vivo [54,55], as well as inhibition of the proliferation, migration, and invasion of endothelial cells [56]. Furthermore, the antiproliferative activity of OMW against MDA-MB-231 breast cancer cells has been also demonstrated [57]. Chemopreventive effects of OMW rich in HT have also been observed in HL60 human promyelocytic leukemia cells, HT-29, and DLD1 colon adenocarcinoma cells, reducing cell proliferation by inducing apoptosis [58].

Noteworthy, OMW extracts were shown to have neuroprotective effects both in vitro and in vivo on dissociated brain cells (DBC) of NMRI mice. Even though the mechanism of action is not yet fully understood, it is likely that the biological effect is due to its antioxidant and anti-inflammatory action by inhibiting lipid peroxidation and restoring glutathione concentrations. The secoiridoids in OMW are also responsible for the beneficial effects in delaying cellular aging in neurodegenerative disease. For example, they were able to interfere with aggregation of amylin [31], tau [59], and Aβ peptides in vitro [60], in C. elegans [61], and in the mouse model TgCRND8 of Aβ deposition [62], which appears to be dose-dependent [63]. Neuroprotection exerted by biophenols has also been demonstrated in neuroblastoma cells by reducing the oxidative stress induced by H_2O_2 and the toxicity induced by copper (Cu) [64]. The cytoprotective effects of formulations containing both HT and OMW were compared on the same cell line by inducing toxicity after 24 h of exposure to cadmium (Cd), mercury (Hg), and lead (Pb), showing that the polyphenols could slow down or even halt the progression of the disease aggravated by heavy metals [65].

OMW phenolic compounds were also able to reduce risk factors for coronary heart disease and stroke prevention [66]. Furthermore, Storniolo et al. highlighted that HT and other polyphenols play an important role in preventing the negative consequences of diets rich in fats and/or sugars [67]. They showed that treatment with HT or OMW could reduce significantly the level of nitric oxide (NO) and the increase of endothelin-1 (ET-1) by modulating the intracellular levels of Ca^{2+} and the endothelial phosphorylation of nitric oxide synthase, changes induced by high levels of glucose and free fatty acids (as in diabetic patients).

Due to its antioxidant properties, OMW could easily find applications in the food, pharmaceutical, and cosmetic industries. For example, it could be used to better preserve the quality and shelf life of food [68,69]. Production of functional foods from OMW extracts represents a crucial alternative to transform this agro-industrial waste into a useful and relevant ingredient [70,71]. An interesting approach for fortifying food products with phenolic substances involves their direct addition [72]. In this regard, OMW phenolic extracts were added to milk to study their effect in modulating the Maillard reaction when milk is heated at very high temperatures. The authors reported that the phenolic extracts were able to trap the reactive carbonyl species responsible for the unpleasant taste and to inhibit the formation of Amadori products [73]. The use of OMW phenolic compounds in milk-based beverages has also been reported to improve their nutritional properties; in fact, as the concentration of more complex phenolic compounds decreased during storage, the level of HT increased due to the hydrolysis of its precursors [74].

In light of all these pieces of evidence, it can be hypothesized that the phenolic compounds present in OMW, such as HT and OL, could soon be considered raw materials for nutraceutical supplements or formulations. Several HT-containing products, such as Mediteanox®, Hydrox®, and Hytolive®, are already on the market in pharmaceutical forms, such as capsules, elixirs, creams, and even in EVOOs with a very high HT content (over 500 mg/kg). Hydrox® and Hytolive® have been licensed as "generally recognized as safe (GRAS)" ingredients. Pure synthetic hydroxytyrosol, marketed by SEPROX BIOTECH, has also achieved this status and has recently been proposed in the EU for Novel Food. Some of these products have already been tested successfully [75,76].

Polyphenols are massively used as cosmetic ingredients. In fact, it is known that UV irradiation and oxidative stress are the main causes of extrinsic aging and of diseases such as skin cancer [77]. The protective action against UV damage, inhibition of the antimicrobial activity of dermal proteinases, and the anti-carcinogenic action have been demonstrated in vitro on skin cell lines. These findings could be exploited for preparing novel topical formulations. The protective effect exerted by polyphenols against lipid oxidation on cell membranes, an effect that mimics the protection from the oxidation of oil lipids by polyphenols, can also prevent oxidative phenomena in the formulation during storage [78,79]. The topical application of active antioxidant ingredients can support the skin's own antioxidant system against oxidative stress and may protect the skin from long-term photoaging.

High reactive oxygen species (ROS) production also results in the expression of collagenase (MMP-1) and elastase, leading to accelerated degradation of the corresponding proteins. Lee et al. showed that polyphenols effectively inhibit elastase and hyaluronidase, exerting an anti-aging effect [80]. Treatment of HaCaT keratinocytes with polyphenolic extracts resulted in a reduced formation of intracellular ROS after UV irradiation [81–83]. Finally, Potapovich et al. showed that post-treatment with polyphenols of normal human epidermal keratinocytes (NHEKs) after UV exposure was effective in abolishing the overproduction of peroxides and inflammatory mediators [84]. In this regard, considering the composition of OMW, it would be interesting to investigate more in detail this aspect as OMW could also present similar anti-aging effects.

3.3. Secondary Metabolites and Biological Activity of Olive Pomace Extracts

The main destiny of olive pomace in the linear economy is its transfer to an olive pomace factory, where it is dried and then used for extracting with organic solvents (usually hexane) the residual fat (crude pomace oil), which will be then rectified before marketing. In recent times, the price of pomace oil has significantly dropped, making, in some cases, its extraction uneconomical. In addition, the sector had already been experiencing great difficulties because of the increased water content in virgin pomace due to the increasingly widespread use of two-phase decanters. The opportunity to consider the pomace not only as a source of fats but also of a complex mixture of bio-compounds can be advantageous for both the environment and the miller's income. In fact, the possibility to implement a new production process into the mill could potentially provide an additional source of profit for both olive oil producers and olive millers, thus closing the supply chain at the production site.

In this regard, Nunes et al. investigated the chemical composition of the bioactive compounds in olive pomace (e.g., fatty acids, vitamin E, and phenolic compounds) and its nutritional profile and they also developed a sustainable process for extracting the antioxidants (the Multi-frequency Multimode Modulated Ultrasonic technique) [85]. Moreover, they discovered that the vitamin E profile of the olive pomace contained high amounts of α-tocopherol (2.63 mg/100 g), although β- and γ-tocopherol and α-tocotrienol were present in lower concentrations (less than 0.1 mg/100 g of pomace). Oleic acid was the most abundant lipid, followed by palmitic, linoleic, and stearic acid (10%, 9%, and 3%, respectively), while the polyphenols were mainly represented by HT and comsegoloside (making together about 79% of the total content). A year before, Goldsmith et al. had already tested an innovative ultrasound method with the aim to increase the aqueous extraction of phenolic compounds from olive pomace [86]. Application of a Design of Experiments allowed the authors to find the optimal extraction conditions, although the process was not very efficient (2 g of dried pomace/100 mL of water at 250 W for 75 min at 30 °C), thus limiting the technological transfer to an industrial level.

Recently, the interest in the water-soluble fraction from olive pomace is high because numerous authors are demonstrating the potential beneficial effects of the contained sugars, polyphenols, and minerals. Ribeiro et al. investigated the effect of the gastrointestinal tract on its bioactive composition, demonstrating that about 50% of the water-soluble compounds remained active, especially of HT and potassium [87]. In addition, the recovered antioxidant activity in the serum was about almost 58%, and more than 50% of the initial α-glucosidase inhibition activity was maintained, as well as its ACE inhibitory activity. The colon-available fraction presented a substantial concentration of polyphenols and minerals, evidencing that OMW liquid-enriched powder could be potentially useful to prevent both cardiovascular and gut diseases. The potential effects in terms of liquid-enriched powder marketing are interesting, although further studies are needed to confirm preliminary results.

Other authors investigated even simpler techniques to make the extraction process more convenient. Cea Pavez et al. exploited pressurized liquid extraction (PLE) for extracting phenolic compounds from olive pomace [88]. Despite the extraction protocol showed great compositional variability of the obtained mixtures depending on the experimental conditions used; after optimization, PLE allowed the obtaining of a higher polyphenolic content compared to the traditional extraction method (1659 mg/kg and 282 mg/kg, respectively), also yielding three- and four-times higher concentrations of secoiridoids and flavonoids, as well as a significant HT enrichment.

In the context of environment-friendly green technologies, the use of deep eutectic solvents (DESs) has been gaining prominence in recent years. DESs have several advantages, including very low toxicity, ease of preparation, low cost, high biodegradability, and stability in the presence of water. In 2018, Chanioti et al. employed natural deep eutectic solvents (NADES) constituted by choline chloride with citric acid, lactic acid, maltose and glycerol, and water combined with homogenization (HAE), microwave (MAE), ultrasound (UAE), or high hydrostatic pressure (HHPAE) [89]. Choline chloride with citric acid and lactic acid showed the best extraction efficiency in terms of total phenolic content and antioxidant activity of the extracts, while HAE proved to be the best extraction technique. Extracts with NADES were generally richer in polyphenols compared to conventional solvent extraction procedures, and HPLC analysis confirmed that proposed methods are effective and sustainable alternatives for their extraction from natural sources.

The exploitation of compounds with high biological and commercial value is certainly the direction in which to push the transition of the oil sector. Many studies agree on the beneficial properties of these substances. Vergani et al. carried out a study on the biological effects of polyphenols extracted from olive pomace and on the effects of single phenolic compounds present in the extract (i.e., TY, apigenin, and OL) in protecting hepatocytes against fat excess and oxidative stress [90]. The polyphenols were extracted in ethanol/water (50:50 v/v) at high pressure-temperature (25 bar, 180 °C for 90 min), obtaining a total concentration of 5.77 mg of caffeic acid equivalent/mL. In order to test the biological effects of the extract, FaO cells exposed for 3 h to a mixture of oleate/palmitate (2:1 molar ratio) were used as a model for hepatic steatosis. The cells were incubated with TY, apigenin, or OL (10, 13, and 50 µg/mL, respectively), and the content of intra- and extra-cellular triglycerides (TGs) and other oxidative stress markers measured after 24 h. The preliminary results showed that olive pomace extract ameliorated lipid accumulation and lipid-dependent oxidative unbalance, suggesting them as potential therapeutic agents. The direct correlation between an MD supplemented with EVOO and a reduced prevalence of hepatic steatosis in older individuals at high cardiovascular risk was recently investigated in a clinical trial comprising one hundred men and women (mean age: 64 ± 6 years old) at high cardiovascular risk (62% with type 2 diabetes) [91].

The biological activity of polyphenols recovered from olive oil by-products was also investigated by Romani et al., who studied the cardioprotective effects of hydroxytyrosol, oleuropein, oleocanthal, and lignans in the MD [92]. Moreover, recent European projects, such as EPIC (European Prospective Investigation into Cancer and Nutrition) and EPICOR (long-term follow-up of antithrombotic management patterns in acute coronary syndrome patients), focused on the functional and health-promoting properties of EVOOs, showing the relationship between cancer and nutrition and the existent link between the consumption of EVOO, fresh fruits, and vegetables, and the incidence of coronary heart diseases. Results evidenced that both the EVOO and the by-products of the olive oil extraction process are precious sources of bioactive compounds that can be recovered applying green technologies and used for food, agronomic, nutraceutical, and biomedical applications, in agreement with the circular economy strategy.

3.4. Secondary Metabolites in Olive Leaves

Leaves represent an important quote of the total harvest weight. Therefore, it is important to develop efficient extraction methods that can assure high yields of polyphenols, secoiridoids, and other bioactive molecules that can be exploited in nutraceutical products, cosmetics, and functional foods (see Table 1). *Olea europaea* L. leaves are a potentially inexpensive, renewable, and abundant source of biophenols [93]. The importance of this agricultural and industrial waste needs to be emphasized and better understood, considering the benefits that we can get from it in health terms and also regarding the environment. Due to its antioxidant, antimicrobial, and anti-inflammatory effects, olive leaf extract (OLE) is considered a natural supplement. Several studies already showed the pharmaceutical and nutraceutical potentials of the secondary metabolites extracted from olive leaves. Microfiltration, ultrafiltration, and nanofiltration are all techniques able to provide OLEs with high amounts of polyphenols that could be exploited by cosmetic, food, and pharmaceutical industries.

Because natural active compounds are safer to use than synthetic chemicals, there is a growing interest in extracting oleuropein from olive leaves. However, the high operational cost, as well as the toxicity and flammability of the organic solvents usually employed, limits their exploitation. Nevertheless, the utilization of novel techniques, e.g., NADES, might bring a change [94]. In order to use these extracts for nutraceutical and pharmacological purposes, another crucial point to address is their bioavailability. In fact, when assumed orally, secondary metabolites in olive leaf should resist the gastric acid in the stomach before reaching the bloodstream. However, it has been observed that the amount of OL and verbascoside at the end of the digestion processes are almost negligible, mainly due to their chemical instability [95]. On the other side, luteolin-7-O-glucoside (Figure 4) was fairly resistant to digestion and, therefore, it can be considered an interesting polyphenol for oral administration.

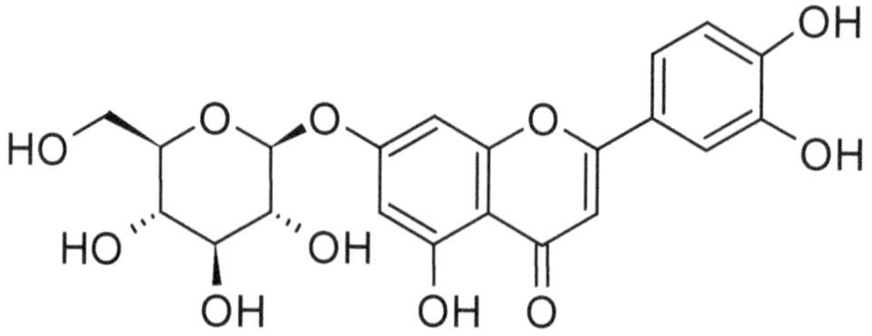

Figure 4. Chemical structure of luteolin 7-O-glucoside.

The same study also analyzed if different extraction methods could influence the total amount of obtained polyphenols, either processing the olive leaves by freeze-drying at −20 °C or by hot air drying (70–120 °C), although the final concentration was nearly the same.

In order to determine the total polyphenol content of the leaves, a wide research study was performed on seventeen cultivars planted in Iran, including some varieties that are also present in Italy [96]. The total phenolic content and antioxidant activity of the leaves' extracts were determined, showing that the Coratina cultivar has one of the highest content of polyphenols and the maximum radical scavenging activity. The OLE composition was mainly characterized by vanillin, rutin, luteolin 7-O-glucoside, oleuropein, and quercetin. High OL concentrations were also detected in other cultivars, such as the Mishen, Beleidi, Kalamon, and Roghani cultivars, while it was not detected in the Conservolea, Amigdalolia, Leccino, and Fishomi cultivars (Table 3).

Table 3. Total phenols contents and antioxidant activities of different cultivars of olive leaves extracts.

Cultivars	Total Phenol [1]	FRAP [2]	DPPH [3]
Manzanilla	134.50 ± 0.01	1107.71 ± 0.01	33.93
Conservolea	92.35 ± 0.01	1277.33 ± 0.01	62.94
Arbequina	42.35 ± 0.02	1760.57 ± 0.01	62.56
Mishen	71.93 ± 0.01	1971.37 ± 0.01	63.48
Coratina	155.91 ± 0.06	358.66 ± 0.01	22.95
Roghani	121.75 ± 0.02	1400.76 ± 0.01	29.58
Kalamon	190.65 ± 0.03	532.76 ± 0.01	26.74
Amphissis	50.70 ± 0.01	1110.38 ± 0.01	95.39
Yellow	73.85 ± 0.01	1400.95 ± 0.01	53.80
Amigdalolia	42.73 ± 0.01	1341.05 ± 0.01	74.30
Mary	62.24 ± 0.01	1203.81 ± 0.01	60.26
Leccino	59.23 ± 0.01	568.28 ± 0.01	69.30
Shenge	61.97 ± 0.01	614.19 ± 0.01	60.18
Gordal	184.72 ± 0.01	450.86 ± 0.01	20.66
Sevillenca	83.63 ± 0.01	432.19 ± 0.01	34.92
Fishomi	109.98 ± 0.06	1794.57 ± 0.01	32.82

[1] Expressed as mg GAE/g dry extract. [2] Expressed as µmol Fe II/g dried extract. [3] Concentration expressed in IC_{50}: µg/mL.

Itrana, Apollo, and Maurino cultivars were the ones with the highest content of polyphenols, mainly quinic acid, oleuropein, and luteolin 7-O-glucoside, and also the ones with the strongest antioxidant activity. Italian olive cultivars, namely Dritta, Leccino, Caroleo, Coratina, Castiglionese, Nebbio, and Grossa di Cassano were also studied to determine their OL concentration in the extracts. Leaves from Nebbio, Grossa di Cassano, and Castiglionese olive trees revealed the highest oleuropein content. On the other hand, Caroleo, Leccino, and Dritta leaf extracts showed the lowest OL amounts.

Concluding, polyphenols have a wide range of bioactivities, and the olive leaf extracts could be either used as such in cosmetics, or they could be mixed with olives that are too ripe to produce oils with great resistance to oxidation, thus using them directly as olive oil supplements [97]. Alternatively, their phenolic extracts could be employed to produce dietetic tablets and food supplements, pharmaceuticals, and also to improve the shelf-life of foods.

In general, green leaves seem to have a higher OL content compared to the yellow ones [98]. Since leaves represent a significant part of the total harvest weight, it is of paramount importance to exploit them in the best way possible, as already stated, according to a circular economy approach.

3.5. Biological Activity of Olive Leaf Extracts

Olive leaves have been widely used in popular medicine to treat diseases like fever and other inflammation-related situations. The ancient Greeks and Romans used OLE as a natural remedy for treating hypertension. Leaves were also used in the past to prepare infusions.

It has been shown that olive leaf extract can lower blood pressure in animal models, alleviate arrhythmia, and exert spasmolytic activity on intestinal muscle [99]. Several studies attest to the antihypertensive effect of olive leaf extract by reducing systolic and diastolic blood pressure and even improving plasma TGs and LDL levels. Moreover, the antihypertensive effect did not show side effects on liver or renal functions in subjects with stage-1 hypertension, attesting its potential use as a preventive nutraceutical for chronic diseases [100].

Among the *Olea europea* L. polyphenols, oleuropein is a secoiridoid present as glucosylated derivatives in the olive fruit, while its dihydroxytyrosol and non-glucosylated secoiridoids were found in the leaf. OLE is a natural supplement that can be used either alone or in combination with other extracts, mainly in formulations that do not require a medical prescription. To support the key nutraceutical role of EVOO in the MD, Storniolo et al.

recently analyzed whether it induced changes on endothelial physiology elements, such as NO, ET-1, and ET-1 receptors, which are involved in controlling blood pressure [101]. Some in vitro studies confirmed this action by analyzing a commercial extract on cardiomyocytes of rabbits' hearts. As a result, OLE caused a concentration-depended decrease in systolic left ventricular pressure and heart rate, as well as an increase in relative coronary flow, maybe because of the direct and reversible suppression of the L-type calcium channel [102].

The vasorelaxant activity of OLE has also been investigated on aorta sections in addition to the inotropic and chronotropic effects measured on atria [103]. The vasorelaxant activity was related to the mechanism involving voltage and receptor operated Ca^{2+} calcium channels. The calcium antagonist activity is always to be considered in addition to the antioxidant activity and to other mechanisms involved in the same pharmacological direction, such as the direct effect on endothelium cells. The leaf extract was also shown to act by reducing the spontaneous contractility of the vessels, thus indirectly acting positively on the pressure exerted by the blood flow on the vessels [104].

OLE and *Hybiscus sabdariffa* L. flower extracts also showed calcium antagonistic properties [103]. Before the idea of formulating a nutraceutical product that synergizes the two activities, several in vitro and *ex-vivo* studies were conducted to verify the antagonist action directed to calcium channels. These two extracts have already been developed in a nutraceutical product, registered as "Pres Phytum" and already commercialized in Italy. In particular, the biological activity of the nutraceutical formulation led to vasorelaxant effects on smooth muscles in different districts of the body (IC_{50} 2.38 mg/mL) and to a negative chronotropic effect (IC_{50} 1.04 mg/mL) that could be exploited in the treatment of preclinical hypertension, without leading to a negative inotropic effect.

As we know, natural molecules do not only have an antioxidant effect; but we have to study and analyze their multitarget profile in order to understand what their real potential is [105]. Olive leaves phenols also reduce blood pressure with NO bioavailability modulation that is increased after a 28 day long dietary assumption [106]. Oleuropein and hydroxytyrosol induced the NO synthase and also had effects on NADPH, which also augmented the quote of superoxide.

OLE has also been studied in humans, and results are significantly positive in terms of cardioprotection [107]. When assumed as a dietary supplement (chronic consumption), the phenolic compounds contained in the olive leaf extract led to a reduction in LDL and TGs concentration that could be attributed to the antioxidant and calcium antagonist properties, but, in diabetic people, they also led to a reduction of the glucose concentration, probably because of the α-amylases inhibition, and to a reduction of glycosylated hemoglobin (HbAlc) and plasma insulin [106,108].

The anti-inflammatory effect on monocytes, the reduction of adhesion molecules, such as ICAM-1 and VCAM-1, and the inhibition of platelet aggregation are aspects that contribute to the cardioprotective effects of olive tree leaves [109]. As reported above, OL has activity on calcium channels; this evidence opens up new perspectives for using this molecule in many pathologies and also neurodegenerative diseases, such as Alzheimer's disease (AD). In fact, neurodegenerative pathologies are often caused by calcium cytotoxicity, and in this case, the olive's polyphenols, such as oleuropein, could play an important role.

Several studies have already been performed in this direction, and the results are encouraging. Transgenic mice (APPswe/PS1dE9) received, from 7 to 23 weeks of age, 50 mg/kg of oleuropein contained in OLE compared to a control diet [110]. OLE-treated mice showed significantly reduced ($p < 0.001$) amyloid plaque deposition in cortex and hippocampus compared to control mice, providing a basis for considering natural and low cost biophenols from olive as a promising drug candidate against AD. Nevertheless, additional studies are needed to validate these results and determine the anti-amyloid mechanism, bioavailability as well as permeability of olive biophenols to the blood brain barrier (BBB) in AD.

Oxidative stress certainly contributes to the onset of neurodegenerative diseases. OLE, in combination with hibiscus flower extract, has been shown to prevent the degeneration of cerebral cells following insult in vitro studies, thus exerting a neuroprotective action [111]. The action of the pool of molecules that these extracts contain is related to the bioavailability often impaired by oral administration. With a "drug like" approach, the components of the phytocomplexes were tested for their ability to permeate the BBB using an in silico predictive model. Oleuropein, contained in the mix, was shown to be able to pass the BBB and, using adequate doses of leaf extract, it was possible to reach biologically active concentrations in the brain, demonstrating the neuroprotective efficacy in the brain and its permanence even after oral intake, as confirmed by in vivo studies [63].

The anti-inflammatory effect of OLE has been investigated by screening all diseases in which inflammatory mechanisms are involved. In order to demonstrate the anti-inflammatory properties of OLE on upper respiratory illness (URI), very common among teenagers and especially in young athletes, a study was performed on high school students by treating for nine weeks the groups either with 100 mg of oleuropein or with placebo [112]. The young athletes were monitored during training, and the illness incidence was the same in both groups, but the treatment with OL led to a reduction of the sick days, resulting in a quicker recovery.

OLE also plays an important role against osteoarthritis (OA) [113]. A study revealed as an olive oil supplemented diet could improve cartilage recovery after anterior cruciate ligament transection [114]. In particular, the polyphenols inhibited the development of proinflammatory cytokines, including IL-1β, TNF-α, IL-6, and prostaglandin E$_2$, and other synthetic pathways involved in the development and progression of OA [115,116].

Table 4 summarizes the principal biological activities of OLE reported in the literature.

Table 4. Biological effects of olive leaf extracts (OLEs).

Disease	Type of Experiment	Dose	Effects
Hypertension [100]	Human clinical trial	1000 mg OLE/die	Lowering systolic and diastolic blood pressures, significant reduction of triglyceride (TG) levels.
Atherosclerosis [107]	in vivo	100 mg OLE/kg body weight	Reduction of the levels of cholesterol, TGs, and LDL cholesterol, and block of the inflammatory response.
Thrombosis [109]	in vitro	1% v/v OLE	Significant dose-dependent reduction in platelet activity.
Hypocholesterolemia [111]	Human studies	1.2 g OLE/die	Reduction of total cholesterol, decreased LDL cholesterol.
Diabetes [106,108]	in vitro	IC$_{50}$ = 4.0–0.02 mg/mL OLE	Inhibition of the activities of α-amylases from human saliva and pancreas.
	Human clinical trial	500 mg OLE/die	Significant reduction in HbA1C values.
Alzheimer [110]	in vivo	50 mg OLE/kg	Reduction of amyloid plaque deposition in cortex and hippocampus.
Upper respiratory illness [112]	Randomized controlled trials	100 mg oleuropein/die	Reduction of the sick days, i.e., acceleration of the recovery.

3.6. Cosmetic Formulations of Olive Leaf Extracts

Cosmetic products currently on the market often contain "*Olea europaea* Leaf Extract", whose composition includes the presence of TY, HT, OL, and other flavonoids, such as luteolin and apigenin. Some studies attested the strong antioxidant activity of OLE on the skin; for example, oleuropein formulations highlighted lenitive efficacy by reducing erythema, transepidermal water loss, and blood flow of about 22%, 35%, and 30%, respectively [117].

The rejuvenating effect of OLE in cosmetics was also studied on 36 people who used a particular cream containing the extract "SUPERHEAL™ O-Live Cream" (PhytoCeuticals, Inc, USA) [118]. After two months of daily applications, OLE led to an amelioration in overall skin condition concerning hydration, wrinkle state, and erythema conditions, as determined by measuring several physiological parameters, such as melanin and erythema index, transepidermal water loss, skin hydration, skin pH, sebum level, texture, and wrinkles.

Another important aspect that can be considered about a cosmetic activity is the photoprotective effect of polyphenols. This potential effect has been studied in oral and topical photoprotection. There is a lot of interest in researching natural sunscreen, also considering the low impact on the environment. An in vitro assay on sun protection factor (SPF) and molecular model studies of UV absorption supported the use of OLE as a photoprotective, antioxidant, and antimutagenic agent.

Skin cancer is one of the most common types of cancer, and it is becoming more impactful day by day. In this regard, the scientific world is trying to find a valid way of prevention that can fight even less severe reactions from sun exposure, such as erythema, photoaging, and immunosuppression [119,120]. Finding a 100% preventive photoprotective filter from natural sources—and also from waste—could be a great starting point for the development of some preventive products able to reduce the frequency of this type of chronic disease.

3.7. Secondary Metabolites and Biological Activity of Kernel and Seed Extracts

Olive stone is a lignocellulosic material, with hemicellulose, cellulose, and lignin that are the main components. Olive stones are obtained by separation of the pulp from the kernels by means of two different technologies, both before the EVOO extraction process (through the employment of the destoner [121] separating the whole kernel from the fruit) and after the EVOO extraction process (through olive pomace depicting machine). The utilization of the lignocellulosic material from olive stones in biofuel production has been recently reported [122].

Alu'datt et al. optimized various extraction conditions and characterized the phenolic olive seed compounds as well as their antioxidant activity [123]. Their research revealed that the free phenolic forms were predominant in olive seeds. In 1998 Fernández-Bolaños et al. analyzed both the water-soluble non-carbohydrate compounds obtained by steam explosion, such as sugar degradation compounds (furfural and hydroxymethylfurfural), lignin degradation compounds (vanillic acid, syringic acid, vanillin, and syringaldehyde), and phenolic olive fruit compounds (TY and HT) [124]. As a result, they observed that the concentration of hydroxytyrosol was higher than that of the other compounds. In addition, they noted that the amount of HT increased by raising both steaming temperature and time. Rodríguez et al. later confirmed olive stone as an attractive source of bioactive and valuable compounds due to the presence of polyphenols and polyols [125]. They also explored various potential uses of this EVOO by-product, such as activated carbon, furfural production, plastic filled, abrasive, cosmetics, biosorbents, animal feed, and resin, discussing the application of this material based on each component.

González-Hidalgo et al. analyzed the composition of TY, HT, OL, and tocopherol and the antioxidant activity in different fractions of the main by-product from the table olive canning industry (i.e., the stone with some residual olive flesh) [126]. The highest polyphenolic concentration (1710.0 ± 33.8 mg/kg), as well as the highest antioxidant activity (8226.9 ± 9.9 hydroxytyrosol equivalents mg/kg), were observed in the seed olive.

The highest amounts of HT (854.8 ± 66.0 mg/kg) and TY (423.6 ± 56.9 mg/kg) were registered in the whole by-product from the pepper stuffed olives, while the maximum OL content (750.2 ± 85.3 mg/kg) was reported in the stone without seed. In particular, α-tocopherol values of 79.8 ± 20.8 mg/kg and 6.2 ± 1.2 mg/kg were registered in the seed olive stone and in the whole by-product from the anchovy-stuffed olives, respectively. In light of these results, the use of table olive by-product could be a source of natural antioxidants in food, cosmetic, or pharmaceutical products. In addition, table olive by-product revaluation could help to diminish their environmental impact.

Recently, Sibel Bolek proposed to replace wheat flour with olive stone powder, rich in fiber and antioxidants derivatives, in biscuit production, to explore its effect on the rheological characteristics and quality of dough [127]. They added 0%, 5%, 10%, and 15% of olive stone powder in place of the same amounts of wheat flour. As a result, wheat flour replacement with olive stone powder increased the antioxidant activity, as well as fat and fiber content of sample biscuits. In particular, 30.44% ± 0.03% DPPH radical scavenging activity, 11.22% ± 0.09% crude fiber, and 26.32% ± 0.22% fat were quantified by substituting wheat flour with 15% olive stone powder. Furthermore, the authors showed that a replacement of wheat flour with up to 15% olive stone powder did not cause any alteration to the biscuit sensorial properties.

However, olive fruits present large variability in composition. Khadem et al. investigated the physicochemical properties and bioactive contents of whole olive stone oils extracted from six olive varieties, namely Zard, Roughani, Mari, Shengeh, Koroneiki, and Manzanilla, cultivated in the city of Fasa, Iran [128]. They analyzed fatty acids, sterols, and triacylglycerols contents, equivalent carbon number, saponification, iodine, unsaponifiable matter values, and phenolic contents, concluding that, despite the great variability in the whole olive stone oils composition among the six cultivars, whole olive stone oils could be used as a natural source of polyphenol compounds for human consumption.

Lama-Muñoz et al. proposed a multi-step process that could allow an integral use of olive stone from the point of view of a biorefinery plant [129]. They proposed an initial aqueous extraction at 130 °C for 90 min without acid addition and a solid:liquid ratio of 1:2 (w/w), useful to recover liquors with higher phenolic content and antioxidant capacity. This first step provided a double benefit: to separate phenolic compounds potentially useful in cosmetic, pharmaceutical, and food industries and to recover biomass of possible inhibitors. In a second time, olive stones were exposed to further treatment with 2% (w/v) sulfuric acid to obtain the maximum amount of fermentable sugars, mainly xylose, with a low content of compounds such as formic acid, furfural, and hydroxymethylfurfural, able to inhibit fermentative microorganisms involved in bioethanol production. The remaining olive stone was particularly rich in cellulose and lignin, and it could be subjected to enzymatic hydrolysis to achieve glucose in high yields. Glucose could be then converted into bioethanol or into other products, such as poly(3-hydroxybutyrate) and hydroxymethylfurfural. The final lignin-enriched solid could be converted into phenols, biopolymers, or fibers or directly used for energy production. The authors thus concluded that olive stone might be considered as an excellent feedstock for biorefinery plant development. A review written by Ruiz et al. in 2017 described the most recent proposals for the use of biomass derived from olive tree cultivation and olive oil production processes [130].

Spizzirri et al. obtained an ethanolic extract with antioxidant properties to be used in the food and cosmetic industry as a functional food and nutraceutical additive, starting from the olive stones discarded from the EVOO production [131]. The efficiency of the multi-step extraction method was evaluated by quantifying the recovery yield and the total phenolic compounds for a series of solvents with different polarities. Flavonoids were shown to represent about 60% of phenolic antioxidants. The antioxidant activity of the alcoholic fraction was then determined by DPPH assay, showing a good efficiency already at low concentration (IC_{30} of 0.060 mg/mL). In addition, the extract showed an interesting ability to preserve β-carotene from lipidic peroxidation (IC_{30} of 1.30 mg/mL).

4. *Olea europea* L. By-Products for Zootechnical Feeding

In addition to their use as health-promoting compounds, by-products of the olive oil industry could also represent a source of ingredients for zootechnical feeding. Feeding innovations based on the utilization of these bioactive-rich by-products can reduce enteric emissions in ruminants while improving the nutritional composition and shelf-life quality of meat and meat products, simultaneously improving environmental sustainability [132]. The by-products of olive oil production, which represent an important environmental issue in the Mediterranean area, can be valorized in the livestock sector according to the 'pyramid of the value of the bioeconomy', which favors the use of functional ingredients of high value for animal nutrition. In this regard, the content of poly-unsaturated fatty acids is improved in oils for human consumption, while saturated fatty acids are employed for animal feeding. This makes the food healthier for humans while simultaneously reducing feeding costs and the environmental impact of livestock [133,134].

Furthermore, the animal diet deeply influences the quality of the animal meat and derived products and, consequently, the quality of the human diet and health. An animal diet enriched with polyphenols olive oil waste could represent a sustainable approach both for reducing adverse environmental effects of these wastes and for improving the quality of the products of animal origin.

It is important to underline that the use of olive pomace, containing appreciable amounts of oil, has already been considered a feasible strategy to influence the quality of meat [135]. OMW has also been exploited for animal feeding. Gerasopoulos et al. separated, by means of a microfiltration method, the two liquid products from olive mill wastewater, i.e., the downstream permeate and the upstream retentate, and, after characterization, incorporated them into broilers' feed [136]. By measuring oxidative stress biomarkers in blood and tissues, they noted that broilers given OMW-supplemented feed had significantly lower levels of protein oxidation and lipid peroxidation and higher total antioxidant capacity in plasma and tissues compared to the control group. As already known, an antioxidant status able to reduce the stress level in broiler chickens could improve meat quality [137].

In order to improve growth performance and feed digestibility of pigs and pork meat quality, Paiva-Martins et al. investigated the supplementation of animal feeds with olive leaves [138]. Unfortunately, they observed that pigs fed diets with olive leaves showed a lower daily weight gain and a decrease in overall backfat compared to pigs fed by the conventional diet. However, chops from pigs fed the leaf diets had lower peroxide and conjugated diene contents, a lower drip loss, and an improved oxidative stability thanks to a significantly higher α-tocopherol concentration in intramuscular fat and backfat.

Milk quality is also affected by the introduction of by-products from the olive oil industry in animal feeding. Arco-Pérez et al. assessed the effect of the partial replacement of the forage in the diet with olive by-products in goats feeding obtaining milk with higher amounts of vaccenic, eicosadienoic, and conjugated linoleic acid, valuable molecules with several beneficial effects, with the concomitant improvement of the animal meat quality [139]. On the other hand, Branciari et al. investigated both the nutraceutical profile and quality characteristics of the cheese deriving from sheep feed with an OMW-enriched diet [140]. The polyphenol supplementation yielded TY and HT sulfate metabolites both in the obtained milk and cheese derivatives, also providing a direct antioxidant effect on cheese without modifying its chemical composition.

Kerasioti et al. studied the tissue specific effects of feeds supplemented with OMW on detoxification enzymes in sheep, which resulted in an increased glutathione S-transferase activity in the liver and spleen and a decreased γ-glutamylcysteine synthetase expression in the liver, without affecting the superoxide dismutase activity in both tissues [141]. The authors concluded that the beneficial effects of the OMW-enriched feeds were tissue- and developmental stage-specific. Instead of using OMW, Musawi et al. conducted a study to investigate the effect of ground olive leaves supplementation on milk yield and composition, as well as on some blood biochemical parameters, in goats [142]. Although the diet had no significant effect on the average animal body weight, the milk production was significantly increased in goats fed with 2% olive leaves powder. Nevertheless, milk compositions (lactose, protein, and fat percentage) and energy value, as well as blood and biochemical parameters of the ruminant, did not vary significantly from the control group.

Similar to milk and cheese, egg quality is affected by the introduction of by-products of the olive oil industry in animal feeding. Zangeneh and Torki evaluated the performance of laying hens fed with olive pulp [143]. Although the olive pulp-included diet had no significant effect on overall egg production and mass, eggshell weight was higher than that of the birds fed with the control diet, suggesting no deleterious effects on bird's performance but yielding more resistant eggs. Cayan and Erener also conducted an experiment aimed at measuring the effects of olive leaves powder on performance, egg yield, egg quality, and yolk cholesterol level of laying hens [144]. In this case, the authors noted that the supplementation had no effect on feed intake and egg weight and yield, but it significantly increased the final body weight of hens. Furthermore, the dietary olive leaves powder increased yellowness in yolk color and decreased its cholesterol content by about 10%.

5. Conclusions

It is well-known that EVOO and the by-products of its production are an important source of bioactive compounds, e.g., polyphenols and other secondary metabolites, that contribute to reducing cellular oxidative stress and inflammation, thus potentially supporting the resolution of many pathologies. Although the beneficial effects of EVOOs are recognized, e.g., in the Mediterranean Diet, currently, olive by-products are not yet properly exploited, except for a few cosmetic formulations on the market. In fact, there are many regulatory obstacles that prevent these by-products, still considered waste, from re-entering the food or nutraceutical formulations sector. Nevertheless, both olive mill wastewater and olive leaves extracts have already demonstrated peculiar properties. Similarly, kernel and seed extracts were shown to have great potential as nutraceuticals and cosmeceuticals. In addition, besides the direct exploitation for human purposes, all these by-products could be easily employed in animal feeding, thus positively affecting the quality of products for human consumption, e.g., milk, cheese, eggs, and meat. As such, their exploitation would benefit both our health and that of the environment by reducing their waste disposal. With the aim of favoring the transition from a linear to a circular economy within the olive mills, a revision of the legislation, an improvement of the environmental governance, and the identification of economic tools is needed for creating adequate incentives for adopting circular and sustainable production and consumption models, and also promoting the transition towards environmental tax reform. Although this project is quite ambitious and time-consuming, we hope that research studies devoted to demonstrating its feasibility, similarly to those reported in this review article, will contribute to its realization.

Author Contributions: Conceptualization F.C. (Filomena Corbo) and R.B.; methodology and validation M.L.C.; formal analysis, G.B. and M.M. (Matteo Micucci); data curation, F.C. (Francesca Curci); writing—original draft preparation, R.M.; writing—review and editing, C.F.; supervision, A.R.; writing—review and editing, M.M. (Marilena Muraglia) All authors have read and agreed to the published version of the manuscript.

Funding: This research was funded by 1. The AGER 2 Project, grant n. 2016-0174, AGER Foundation—Olive Tree and Oil: Competitive-Claims of olive oil to improve the market value of the product; 2. EU project 820587—OLIVE-SOUND-Ultrasound reactor—The solution for a continuous olive oil extraction process H2020-EU.2.1.—INDUSTRIAL LEADERSHIP-EIC-FTI-2018–2020-Fast Track to Innovation (FTI)—European Union's Horizon 2020 research and innovation program under grant agreement No. 820587.

Conflicts of Interest: The authors declare no conflict of interest.

References

1. Huang, C.L.; Sumpio, E.B.J. Olive Oil, the Mediterranean Diet, and Cardiovascular Health. *Am. Coll. Surg.* **2008**, *207*, 407–416. [CrossRef] [PubMed]
2. Boskou, D.; Blekas, G.; Tsimidou, M. History and characteristics of the olive tree. In *Olive Oil Chemistry and Technology*; Boskou, D., Ed.; AOCS Press: Champaign IL, USA, 1996.
3. Cicerale, S.; Lucas, L.J.; Keast, R.S.J. Antimicrobial, antioxidant and anti-inflammatory phenolic activities in extra virgin olive oil. *Curr. Opin. Biotechnol.* **2012**, *23*, 129–135. [CrossRef]
4. Marcelino, G.; Hiane, P.A.; Freitas, K.C.; Santana, L.F.; Pott, A.; Donadon, J.R.; Guimarães, R.C.A. Effects of olive oil and its minor components on cardiovascular diseases, inflammation, and gut microbiota. *Nutrients* **2019**, *11*, 1826. [CrossRef]
5. Roselli, L.; Clodoveo, M.L.; Corbo, F.; De Gennaro, B. Are health claims a useful tool to segment the category of extra-virgin olive oil? Threats and opportunities for the Italian olive oil supply chain. *Trends Food Sci. Tech.* **2017**, *68*, 176–181. [CrossRef]
6. Hanifi, S.; El Hadrami, I. Olive mill wastewaters: Diversity of the fatal product in olive oil industry and its valorisation as agronomical amendment of poor soils: A review. *J. Agron.* **2009**, *8*, 1–13. [CrossRef]
7. Jarboui, R.; Sellami, F.; Kharroubi, A.; Gharsallah, N.; Ammar, E. Olive mill wastewater stabilization in open-air ponds: Impact on clay-sandy soil. *Bioresour. Technol.* **2008**, *99*, 7699–7708. [CrossRef]
8. Chandra, R.; Takeuchi, H.; Hasegawa, T. Methane production from lignocellulosic agricultural crop wastes: A review in context to second generation of biofuel production. *Renew. Sustain. Energy Rev.* **2012**, *16*, 1462–1476. [CrossRef]
9. Demirbas, M.F.; Balat, M.; Balat, H. Biowastes-to-biofuels. *Energy Convers. Manag.* **2011**, *52*, 1815–1828. [CrossRef]
10. Romani, A.; Pinelli, P.; Ieri, F.; Bernini, R. Sustainability, innovation, and green chemistry in the production and valorization of phenolic extracts from *Olea europaea* L. *Sustainability* **2016**, *8*, 1002. [CrossRef]
11. Robert, K.W.; Parris, T.M.; Leiserowitz, A.A. What is sustainable development? Goals, indicators, values, and practice. *Environ. Sci. Policy* **2005**, *47*, 8–21. [CrossRef]
12. De Jesus, A.; Antunes, P.; Santos, R.; Mendonça, S. Eco-innovation in the transition to a circular economy: An analytical literature review. *J. Cleaner Prod.* **2018**, *172*, 2999–3018. [CrossRef]
13. Boskou, D. Olive fruit, table olives, and olive oil bioactive constituents. In *Olive and olive oil bioactive constituents*, 1st ed.; Boskou, D., Ed.; AOCS Press: Champaign IL, USA, 2015; pp. 1–30.
14. Vermerris, W.; Nicholson, R. *Phenolic Compounds Biochemistry*, 1st ed.; Springer: Dordrecht, The Netherlands, 2006; pp. 1–276.
15. Tresserra-Rimbau, A.; Lamuela-Raventos, R.M.; Moreno, J.J. Polyphenols, food and pharma. Current knowledge and directions for future research. *Biochem. Pharmacol.* **2018**, *156*, 186–195. [CrossRef] [PubMed]
16. Gambacorta, G.; Faccia, M.; Previtali, M.A.; Pati, S.; La Notte, E.; Baiano, A. Effects of olive maturation and stoning on quality indices and antioxidant content of extra virgin oils (cv. *Coratina*) during storage. *J. Food Sci.* **2010**, *75*, 229–235. [CrossRef] [PubMed]
17. Cinquanta, L.; Esti, M.; Notte, E. Evaluation of phenolic compounds in virgin olive oil during storage. *J. Am. Oil Chem. Soc.* **1997**, *74*, 1259–1264. [CrossRef]
18. Leouifoudi, I.; Harnafi, H.; Zyad, A. Olive mill waste extracts: Polyphenols content, antioxidant, and antimicrobial activities. *Adv. Pharmacol. Sci.* **2015**, *2015*, 1–11. [CrossRef]
19. Omar, S.H. Oleuropein in olive and its pharmacological effects. *Sci. Pharm.* **2010**, *78*, 133–154. [CrossRef] [PubMed]
20. Bianco, A.; Uccella, N. Biophenolic components of olives. *Food Res. Int.* **2000**, *33*, 475–485. [CrossRef]
21. Benavente-Garcıa, O.; Castillo, J.; Lorente, J.; Ortuño, A.D.R.J.; Del Rio, J.A. Antioxidant activity of phenolics extracted from *Olea europaea* L. leaves. *Food Chem.* **2000**, *68*, 457–462. [CrossRef]
22. Ragusa, A.; Centonze, C.; Grasso, M.E.; Latronico, M.F.; Mastrangelo, P.F.; Fanizzi, F.P.; Maffia, M. Composition and statistical analysis of biophenols in Apulian Italian EVOOs. *Foods* **2017**, *6*, 90. [CrossRef] [PubMed]
23. Mitjavila, M.T.; Moreno, J.J. The effects of polyphenols on oxidative stress and the arachidonic acid cascade. Implications for the prevention/treatment of high prevalence diseases. *Biochem. Pharmacol.* **2012**, *84*, 1113–1122. [CrossRef] [PubMed]
24. Giordano, E.; Dangles, O.; Rakotomanomana, N.; Baracchinia, S.; Visioli, F. 3-O-Hydroxytyrosol glucuronide and 4-O-hydroxytyrosol glucuronide reduce endoplasmic reticulum stress in vitro. *Food Funct.* **2015**, *6*, 3275–3281. [CrossRef]
25. Reboredo-Rodríguez, P.; Varela-López, A.Y.; Forbes-Hernández, T.; Gasparrini, M.; Afrin, S.; Cianciosi, D.; Zhang, J.; Manna, P.P.; Bompadre, S.; Quiles, J.L.; et al. Phenolic compounds isolated from olive oil as nutraceutical tools for the prevention and management of cancer and cardiovascular diseases. *Int. J. Mol. Sci.* **2018**, *19*, 2305. [CrossRef]
26. Zinnai, A.; Venturi, F.; Quartacci, M.F.; Sanmartin, C.; Favati, F.; Andrich, G. Solid carbon dioxide to promote the extraction of extra-virgin olive oil. *Grasas Aceites* **2016**, *67*, 121–129. [CrossRef]
27. De Santis, S.; Galleggiante, V.; Scandiffio, L.; Liso, M.; Sommella, E.; Sobolewski, A.; Spilotro, V.; Pinto, A.; Campiglia, P.; Serino, G.; et al. Secretory leukoprotease inhibitor (Slpi) expression is required for educating murine dendritic cells inflammatory response following quercetin exposure. *Nutrients* **2017**, *9*, 706. [CrossRef]
28. Venturi, F.; Sanmartin, C.; Taglieri, I.; Nari, A.; Andrich, G.; Terzuoli, E.; Donnini, S.; Nicolella, C.; Zinnai, A. Development of phenol-enriched olive oil with phenolic compounds extracted from wastewater produced by physical refining. *Nutrients* **2017**, *9*, 916. [CrossRef] [PubMed]

29. Bayram, B.; Ozcelik, B.; Grimm, S.; Roeder, T.; Schrader, C.; Ernst, I.M.; Wagner, A.E.; Grune, T.; Frank, J.; Rimbach, G. A diet rich in olive oil phenolics reduces oxidative stress in the heart of SAMP8 mice by induction of Nrf2-dependent gene expression. *Rejuvenation Res.* **2012**, *15*, 71–81. [CrossRef] [PubMed]
30. Gill, C.I.R.; Boyd, A.; McDermott, E.; McCann, M.; Servili, M.; Selvaggini, R.; Taticchi, A.; Esposto, S.; Montedoro, G.; McGlynn, H.; et al. Potential anti-cancer effects of virgin olive oil phenols on colorectal carcinogenesis models in vitro. *Int. J. Cancer* **2005**, *117*, 1–7. [CrossRef] [PubMed]
31. Rigacci, S.; Guidotti, V.; Bucciantina, M.; Parri, M.; Nediani, C.; Cerbai, E.; Stefani, M.; Berti, A.J. Oleuropein aglycon prevents cytotoxic amyloid aggregation of human amylin. *J. Nutr. Biochem.* **2010**, *21*, 725–726. [CrossRef] [PubMed]
32. Schaffer, S.; Podstawa, M.; Visioli, F.; Bogani, P.; Muller, W.E.; Eckert, G.P. Hydroxytyrosol-rich olive mill wastewater extract protects brain cells in vitro and ex vivo. *J. Agric. Food Chem.* **2007**, *55*, 5043–5049. [CrossRef] [PubMed]
33. Mitjavila, M.T.; Fandos, M.; Salas-Salvadó, J.; Covas, M.I.; Borrego, S.; Estruch, R.; Lamuela-Raventós, R.; Corella, D.; Martínez-Gonzalez, M.Á.; Sánchez, J.M.; et al. The Mediterranean diet improves the systemic lipid and DNA oxidative damage in metabolic syndrome individuals. A randomized, controlled, trial. *Clin. Nutr.* **2013**, *32*, 172–178. [CrossRef]
34. Fernandes, J.; Fialho, M.; Santos, R.; Peixoto-Plácido, C.; Madeira, T.; Sousa-Santos, N.; Virgolino, A.; Santos, O.; Vaz Carneiro, A. Is olive oil good for you? A systematic review and meta-analysis on anti-inflammatory benefits from regular dietary intake. *Nutrition* **2020**, *69*, 110559–110569. [CrossRef] [PubMed]
35. Storniolo, C.E.; Martínez-Hovelman, N.; Martínez-Huélamo, M.; Lamuela-Raventos, R.M.; Moreno, J.J. Extra virgin olive oil minor compounds modulate mitogenic action of oleic acid on colon cancer cell line. *J. Agric. Food Chem.* **2019**, *67*, 11420–11427. [CrossRef] [PubMed]
36. Storniolo, C.E.; Sacanella, I.; Lamuela-Raventos, R.M.; Moreno, J.J. Bioactive compounds of mediterranean cooked tomato sauce (Sofrito) modulate intestinal epithelial cancer cell growth through oxidative stress/arachidonic acid cascade regulation. *ACS omega* **2020**, *5*, 17071–17077. [CrossRef] [PubMed]
37. Caporaso, N.; Formisano, D.; Genovese, A. Use of phenolic compounds from olive mill wastewater as valuable ingredients for functional foods. *Crit. Rev. Food Sci. Nutr.* **2017**, *24*, 2829–2841. [CrossRef]
38. Cassano, A.; Conidi, C.; Giorno, L.; Drioli, E. Fractionation of olive mill wastewaters by membrane separation techniques. *J. Hazard. Mater.* **2013**, *248*, 185–193. [CrossRef]
39. Kim, K.; Jung, J.Y.; Kwon, J.H.; Yang, J.W. Dynamic microfiltration with a perforated disk for effective harvesting of microalgae. *J. Membr. Sci.* **2015**, *475*, 252–258. [CrossRef]
40. Díaz-Reinoso, B.; Moure, A.; Domínguez, H.; Parajó, J.C. Ultra-and nanofiltration of aqueous extracts from distilled fermented grape pomace. *J. Food Eng.* **2009**, *91*, 587–593. [CrossRef]
41. Cardinali, A.; Cicco, N.; Linsalata, V.; Minervini, F.; Pati, S.; Pieralice, M.; Tursi, N.; Lattanzio, V. Biological activity of high molecular weight phenolics from olive mill wastewater. *J. Agric. Food Chem.* **2010**, *58*, 8585–8590. [CrossRef]
42. Gurr, M.I.; Harwood, J.L.; Frayn, K.N. *Lipid Biochemistry*, 5th ed.; Blackwells Science: Oxford, UK, 2002.
43. Nawar, W.W. Chemical changes in lipids produced by thermal processing. *J. Chem.* **1984**, *61*, 299–302. [CrossRef]
44. Ghanbari, R.; Anwar, F.; Alkharfy, K.M.; Gilani, A.H.; Saari, N. Valuable nutrients and functional bioactives in different parts of olive (*Olea europaea* L.) a review. *Int. J. Mol. Sci.* **2012**, *13*, 3291–3340. [CrossRef]
45. Nadour, M.; Laroche, C.; Pierre, G.; Delattre, C.; Moulti-Mati, F.; Michaud, P. Structural characterization and biological activities of polysaccharides from olive mill wastewater. *Appl. Biochem. Biotechnol.* **2015**, *177*, 431–445. [CrossRef]
46. Delattre, C.; Pierre, G.; Gardarin, C.; Traikia, M.; Elboutachfaiti, R.; Isogai, A.; Michaud, P. Antioxidant activities of a polyglucuronic acid sodium salt obtained from TEMPO-mediated oxidation of xanthan. *Carbohydr. Polym.* **2015**, *116*, 34–41. [CrossRef]
47. Luo, A.; He, X.; Zhou, S.; Fan, Y.; Luo, A.; Chun, Z. Purification, composition analysis and antioxidant activity of the polysaccharides from *Dendrobium nobile* Lindl. *Carbohydr. Polym.* **2010**, *79*, 1014–1019. [CrossRef]
48. Wu, G.H.; Hu, T.; Li, Z.Y.; Huang, Z.L.; Jiang, J.G. In vitro antioxidant activities of the polysaccharides from *Pleurotus tuberregium* (Fr.) Sing. *Food Chem.* **2014**, *148*, 351–356. [CrossRef]
49. Xu, R.; Ye, H.; Sun, Y.; Tu, Y.; Zeng, X. Preparation, preliminary characterization, antioxidant, hepatoprotective and antitumor activities of polysaccharides from the flower of tea plant (*Camellia sinensis*). *Food Chem. Toxicol.* **2012**, *50*, 2473–2480. [CrossRef] [PubMed]
50. Chen, H.; Zhang, M.; Qu, Z.; Xie, B. Antioxidant activities of different fractions of polysaccharide conjugates from green tea (*Camellia Sinensis*). *Food Chem.* **2008**, *106*, 559–563. [CrossRef]
51. Zeng, W.C.; Zhang, Z.; Gao, H.; Jia, L.R.; Chen, W.Y. Characterization of antioxidant polysaccharides from *Auricularia auricular* using microwave-assisted extraction. *Carbohydr. Polym.* **2012**, *89*, 694–700. [CrossRef] [PubMed]
52. Dermeche, S.; Nadour, M.; Larroche, C.; Moulti-Mati, F.; Michaud, P. Olive mill wastes: Biochemical characterizations and valorization strategies. *Process Biochem.* **2013**, *48*, 1532–1552. [CrossRef]
53. Recinella, L.; Chiavaroli, A.; Orlando, G.; Menghini, L.; Ferrante, C.; Di Cesare Mannelli, L.; Ghelardini, C.; Brunetti, L.; Leone, S. Protective effects induced by two polyphenolic liquid complexes from olive (*Olea europaea*, mainly Cultivar Coratina) pressing juice in rat isolated tissues challenged with LPS. *Molecules* **2019**, *24*, 3002. [CrossRef] [PubMed]
54. Bassani, B.; Rossi, T.; Stefano, D.D.; Pizzichini, D.; Corradino, P.; Macrì, N.; Noonan, D.M.; Albini, A.; Bruno, A.J. Potential chemopreventive activities of a polyphenol rich purified extract from olive mill wastewater on colon cancer cells. *Funct. Foods* **2016**, *27*, 236–248. [CrossRef]

55. Borzì, A.M.; Biondi, A.; Basile, F.; Luca, S.; Saretto, E.; Vicari, D.; Vacante, M. Olive oil effects on colorectal cancer. *Nutrients* **2019**, *11*, 32. [CrossRef]
56. Rossi, T.; Bassani, B.; Gallo, C.; Maramotti, S.; Noonan, D.M.; Bruno, A. Effect of a purified extract of olive mill waste water on endothelial cell proliferation, apoptosis, migration and capillary-like structure in vitro and in vivo. *J. Bioanal. Biomed.* **2015**, *12*, 1–8.
57. Ramos, P.; Santos, S.A.O.; Guerraa, Â.R.; Guerreiro, O.; Felício, L.; Eliana Jerónimo, E.; Silvestrec, A.J.D.; Netoc, C.P.; Duarte, M. Valorization of olive mill residues: Antioxidant and breast cancer antiproliferative activities of hydroxytyrosol-rich extracts derived from olive oil by-products. *Ind. Crops Prod.* **2013**, *46*, 359–368. [CrossRef]
58. Cárdeno, A.; Sánchez-Hidalgo, M.; Alarcón-De-La-Lastra, C. An up-date of olive oil phenols in inflammation and cancer: Molecular mechanisms and clinical implications. *Curr. Med. Chem.* **2013**, *20*, 4758–4776. [CrossRef] [PubMed]
59. Daccache, A.; Lion, C.; Sibille, N.; Gerard, M.; Slomianny, C.; Lippens, G.; Cotelle, P. Oleuropein and derivatives from olives as Tau aggregation inhibitors. *Neurochem. Int.* **2011**, *58*, 700–707. [CrossRef]
60. Rigacci, S.; Guidotti, V.; Bucciantini, M.; Nichino, D.; Relini, A.; Berti, A.; Stefani, M. Aβ (1-42) aggregates into non-toxic amyloid assemblies in the presence of the natural polyphenol oleuropein aglycon. *Curr. Alzheimer Res.* **2011**, *8*, 841–852. [CrossRef] [PubMed]
61. Diomede, L.; Rigacci, S.; Romeo, M.; Stefani, M.; Salmona, M. Oleuropein aglycone protects transgenic C. elegans strains expressing Aβ 42 by reducing plaque load and motor deficit. *PLoS ONE* **2013**, *8*, 58893–58902. [CrossRef]
62. Grossi, C.; Rigacci, S.; Ambrosini, S.; Dami, T.E.; Luccarini, I.; Traini, C.; Failli, P.; Berti, A.; Casamenti, F.; Stefani, M. The polyphenol oleuropein aglycone protects TgCRND8 mice against Aβ plaque pathology. *PLoS ONE* **2013**, *8*, 71702–71715. [CrossRef]
63. Pantano, D.; Luccarini, I.; Nardiello, P.; Servili, M.; Stefani, M.; Casamenti, F. Oleuropein aglycone and polyphenols from olive mill waste water ameliorate cognitive deficits and neuropathology. *Br. J. Clin. Pharmacol.* **2017**, *83*, 54–62. [CrossRef] [PubMed]
64. Omar, S.H.; Kerr, P.G.; Scott, C.J.; Hamlin, A.S.; Hass, K. Olive (*Olea europaea* L.) Biophenols: A Nutriceutical against Oxidative Stress in SH-SY5Y Cells. *Molecules* **2017**, *22*, 1858. [CrossRef]
65. Moretti, P.; Massari, C.D. Fitocomplesso Polifenolico Standardizzato per la Prevenzione delle Patologie Correlate All'esposizione da Sostanze Reattive Dell'ossigeno e Relativo Metodo di Produzione. BIOENUTRA Srl, N. 102017000118607. Available online: https://www.farmaffari.it/index.php/it/companies-partner/1-2-5-integratori-e-dietetici/bioenutra-srl-1-1 (accessed on 16 January 2020).
66. Visioli, F.; Galli, C.; Bornet, F.; Mattei, A.; Patelli, R.; Galli, G.; Caruso, D. Olive oil phenolics are dose-dependently absorbed in humans. *FEBS Lett.* **2000**, *468*, 159–160. [CrossRef]
67. Storniolo, C.E.; Roselló-Catafau, J.; Pintó, X.; Mitjavila, M.T.; Moreno, J.J. Polyphenol fraction of extra virgin olive oil protects against endothelial dysfunction induced by high glucose and free fatty acids through modulation of nitric oxide and endothelin-1. *Redox Biol.* **2014**, *2*, 971–977. [CrossRef]
68. Serra, A.T.; Matias, A.A.; Nunes, A.V.M.; Leitao, M.C.; Brito, D.; Bronze, R.; Duarte, C.M. In vitro evaluation of olive- and grape-based natural extracts as potential preservatives for food. *Innov. Food Sci. Emerg. Technol.* **2008**, *9*, 311–319. [CrossRef]
69. Galanakis, C.M.; Yucetepe, A.; Kasapo, K.N.; Celik, B. High-value compounds from olive oil processing waste. In *Edible Oils Extraction, Processing, and Applications*, 1st ed.; Chemat, S., Ed.; CRC Press Taylor & Francis Group: Boca Raton, FL, USA, 2017; pp. 179–203.
70. Obied, H.K.; Bedgood, D.R., Jr.; Prenzler, P.D.; Robards, K. Effect of processing conditions, prestorage treatment, and storage conditions on the phenol content and antioxidant activity of olive mill waste. *J. Agric. Food Chem.* **2008**, *56*, 3925–3932. [CrossRef] [PubMed]
71. Galanakis, C.M.; Tornberg, E.; Gekas, V. Recovery and preservation of phenols from olive waste in ethanolic extracts. *J. Chem. Technol. Biotechnol.* **2010**, *85*, 1148–1155. [CrossRef]
72. Fki, I.; Allouche, N.; Sayadi, S. The use of polyphenolic extract, purified hydroxytyrosol and 3,4-dihydroxyphenyl acetic acid from olive mill wastewater for the stabilization of refined oils: A potential alternative to synthetic antioxidants. *Food Chem.* **2005**, *93*, 197–204. [CrossRef]
73. Troise, A.D.; Fiore, A.; Colantuono, A.; Kokkinidou, S.; Peterson, D.G.; Fogliano, V. Effect of olive mill wastewater phenol compounds on reactive carbonyl species and maillard reaction end-products in ultrahigh-temperature-treated milk. *J. Agric. Food Chem.* **2014**, *62*, 10092–10100. [CrossRef] [PubMed]
74. Servili, M.; Rizzello, C.G.; Taticchi, A.; Esposto, S.; Urbani, S.; Mazzacane, F.; Di Cagno, R. Functional milk beverage fortified with phenolic compounds extracted from olive vegetation water, and fermented with functional lactic acid bacteria. *Int. J. Food Microbiol.* **2011**, *147*, 45–52. [CrossRef]
75. Giordano, E.; Dávalos, A.; Visioli, F. Chronic hydroxytyrosol feeding modulates glutation-mediated oxido-reduction pathways in adipose tissue: A nutrigenomic study. *Nutr. Metab. Cardiovasc. Dis.* **2014**, *24*, 1144–1150. [CrossRef]
76. Giordano, E.; Dávalos, A.; Nicod, N.; Visioli, F. Hydroxytyrosol attenuates tunicamycin-induced endoplasmic reticulum stress in human hepatocarcinoma cells. *Mol. Nutr. Food Res.* **2014**, *58*, 954–962. [CrossRef] [PubMed]
77. Callaghan, T.M.; Wilhelm, K.P. A review of ageing and an examination of clinical methods in the assessment of ageing skin. Part I: Cellular and molecular perspectives of skin ageing. *Int. J. Cosmet. Sci.* **2008**, *30*, 313–322. [CrossRef] [PubMed]

78. Schwarz, K.; Bertelsen, G.; Nissen, L.R.; Gardner, P.T.; Heinonen, M.I.; Hopia, A.; Huynh-Ba, T.; Lambelet, P.; McPhail, D.; Skibsted, L.H.; et al. Investigation of plant extracts for the protection of processed foods against lipid oxidation. Comparison of antioxidant assays based on radical scavenging, lipid oxidation and analysis of the principal antioxidant compounds. *Eur. Food Res. Technol.* **2001**, *212*, 319–328. [CrossRef]
79. Zillich, O.V.; Schweiggert-Weisz, U.; Hasenkopf, K.; Eisner, P.; Kerscher, M. Antioxidant activity, lipophilicity and extractability of polyphenols from pig skin–development of analytical methods for skin permeation studies. *Biomed. Chromatogr.* **2013**, *27*, 1444–1451. [CrossRef]
80. Lee, K.K.; Cho, J.J.; Park, E.J.; Choi, J.D. Anti-elastase and anti-hyaluronidase of phenolic substance from Areca catechu as a new anti-ageing agent. *Int. J. Cosmet. Sci.* **2001**, *23*, 341–346. [CrossRef]
81. Cha, J.W.; Piao, M.J.; Kim, K.C.; Yao, C.W.; Zheng, J.; Kim, S.M.; Hyun, C.L.; Ahn, Y.S.; Hyun, J.W. The polyphenol chlorogenic acid attenuates UVB-mediated oxidative stress in human HaCaT keratinocytes. *Biomol. Ther.* **2014**, *22*, 136–142. [CrossRef] [PubMed]
82. Perez-Sanchez, A.; Barrajon-Catalan, E.; Caturla, N.; Castillo, J.; Benavente-Garcia, O.; Alcaraz, M.; Mico, V. Protective effects of citrus and rosemary extracts on UV-induced damage in skin cell model and human volunteers. *J. Photochem. Photobiol.* **2014**, *136*, 12–18. [CrossRef]
83. Shin, S.W.; Jung, E.; Kim, S.; Lee, K.E.; Youm, J.K.; Park, D. Antagonist effects of veratric acid against UVB-induced cell damages. *Molecules* **2013**, *18*, 5405–5419. [CrossRef]
84. Potapovich, A.I.; Kostyuk, V.A.; Kostyuk, T.V.; de Luca, C.; Korkina, L.G. Effects of pre- and post-treatment with plant polyphenols on human keratinocyte responses to solar UV. *Inflamm. Res.* **2013**, *62*, 773–780. [CrossRef]
85. Nunes, M.A.; Costa, A.S.; Bessada, S.; Santos, J.; Puga, H.; Alves, R.C.; Freitas, V.; Oliveira, M.B.P. Olive pomace as a valuable source of bioactive compounds: A study regarding its lipid-and water-soluble components. *Sci. Total Environ.* **2018**, *644*, 229–236. [CrossRef]
86. Goldsmith, C.D.; Vuong, Q.V.; Stathopoulos, C.E.; Roach, P.D.; Scarlett, C.J. Ultrasound increases the aqueous extraction of phenolic compounds with high antioxidant activity from olive pomace. *LWT* **2018**, *89*, 284–290. [CrossRef]
87. Ribeiro, T.; Oliveira, A.; Campos, D.; Nunes, J.; Vicente, A.A.; Pintado, M. Simulated digestion of olive pomace water-soluble ingredient: Relationship between the compounds bioaccessibility and their potential health benefits. *Food Funct.* **2020**, *11*, 2238–2254. [CrossRef] [PubMed]
88. Cea Pavez, I.; Lozano-Sánchez, J.; Borrás-Linares, I.; Nuñez, H.; Robert, P.; Segura-Carretero, A. Obtaining an extract rich in phenolic compounds from olive pomace by pressurized liquid extraction. *Molecules* **2019**, *24*, 3108. [CrossRef] [PubMed]
89. Chanioti, S.; Tzia, C. Extraction of phenolic compounds from olive pomace by using natural deep eutectic solvents and innovative extraction techniques. *Innovative Food Sci. Emerging Technol.* **2018**, *48*, 228–239. [CrossRef]
90. Vergani, L.; Vecchione, G.; Baldini, F.; Voci, A.; Ferrari, P.F.; Aliakbarian, B.; Casazza, A.A.; Perego, P. Antioxidant and hepatoprotective potentials of phenolic compounds from olive pomace. *Chem. Eng. Trans.* **2016**, *49*, 475–480.
91. Pintó, X.; Fanlo-Maresma, M.; Corbella, E.; Corbella, X.; Mitjavila, M.T.; Moreno, J.J.; Casas, R.; Estruch, R.; Corella, D.; Bulló, M.; et al. A Mediterranean diet rich in extra-virgin olive oil is associated with a reduced prevalence of nonalcoholic fatty liver disease in older individuals at high cardiovascular risk. *J. Nutr.* **2019**, *149*, 1920–1929. [CrossRef]
92. Romani, A.; Ieri, F.; Urciuoli, S.; Noce, A.; Marrone, G.; Nediani, C.; Bernini, R. Health effects of phenolic compounds found in extra-virgin olive oil, by-products, and leaf of *Olea europaea* L. *Nutrients* **2019**, *11*, 1776. [CrossRef] [PubMed]
93. Şahin, S.; Bilgin, M. Olive tree (*Olea europaea* L.) leaf as a waste by-product of table olive and olive oil industry: A review. *J. Sci. Food Agric.* **2018**, *98*, 1271–1279.
94. Ahmad-Qasem, M.H.; Cánovas, J.; Barrajón-Catalán, E.; Micol, V.; Cárcel, J.A.; García-Pérez, J.V. Kinetic and compositional study of phenolic extraction from olive leaves (var. Serrana) by using power ultrasound. *Innov. Food Sci. Emerg. Technol.* **2013**, *17*, 120–129. [CrossRef]
95. Ahmad-Qasem, M.H.; Cánovas, J.; Barrajón-Catalán, E.; Carreres, J.E.; Micol, V.; García-Pérez, J.V. Influence of olive leaf processing on the bioaccessibility of bioactive polyphenols. *J. Agric. Food Chem.* **2014**, *62*, 6190–6198. [CrossRef]
96. Ghasemi, S.; Koohi, D.E.; Emmamzadehhashemi, M.S.B.; Khamas, S.S.; Moazen, M.; Hashemi, A.K.; Amin, G.; Golfakhrabadi, F.; Yousefi, Z.; Yousefbeyk, F. Investigation of phenolic compounds and antioxidant activity of leaves extracts from seventeen cultivars of Iranian olive (*Olea europaea* L.). *J. Food Sci. Technol.* **2018**, *55*, 4600–4607. [CrossRef]
97. Guinda, Á.; Pérez Camino, M.C.; Lanzón, A. Supplementation of olis with oleanolic acid from the olive leaf (*Olea europaea*). *Eur. J. Lipid Sci. Technol.* **2004**, *106*, 22–26. [CrossRef]
98. Ranalli, A.; Contento, S.; Lucera, L.; Di Febo, M.; Marchegiani, D.; Di Fonzo, V. Factors affecting the contents of iridoid oleuropein in olive leaves (*Olea europaea* L.). *J. Agric. Food Chem.* **2006**, *54*, 434–440. [CrossRef]
99. Romani, A.; Mulas, S.; Heimler, D. Polyphenols and secoiridoids in raw material (*Olea europaea* L. leaves) and commercial food supplements. *Eur. Food Res. Technol.* **2016**, *243*, 429–435. [CrossRef]
100. Susalit, E.; Agus, N.; Effendi, I.; Tjandrawinata, R.R.; Nofiarny, D.; Perrinjaquet-Moccetti, T.; Verbruggen, M. Olive (*Olea europaea*) leaf extract effective in patients with stage-1 hypertension: Comparison with Captopril. *Phytomedicine* **2011**, *18*, 251–258. [CrossRef]

101. Storniolo, C.E.; Casillas, R.; Bulló, M.; Castañer, O.; Ros, E.; Sáez, G.T.; Toledo, E.; Estruch, R.; Ruiz-Gutiérrez, V.; Fitó, M.; et al. A Mediterranean diet supplemented with extra virgin olive oil or nuts improves endothelial markers involved in blood pressure control in hypertensive women. *Eur. J. Nutr.* **2017**, *56*, 89–97. [CrossRef] [PubMed]
102. Omar, S.H. Cardioprotective and neuroprotective roles of oleuropein in olive. *Saudi Pharm. J.* **2010**, *18*, 111–121. [CrossRef]
103. Scheffler, A.; Rauwald, H.W.; Kampa, B.; Mann, U.; Mohr, F.W.; Dhein, S. Olea europaea leaf extract exerts L-type Ca^{2+} channel antagonistic effects. *J. Ethnopharmacol.* **2008**, *120*, 233–240. [CrossRef] [PubMed]
104. Micucci, M.; Malaguti, M.; Gallina Toschi, T.; Di Lecce, G.; Aldini, R.; Angeletti, A.; Chiarini, A.; Budriesi, R.; Hrelia, S. Cardiac and vascular synergic protective effect of *Olea europea* L. leaves and *Hibiscus sabdariffa* L. flower extracts. *Oxid. Med. Cell. Longev.* **2015**, *2015*, 318125. [CrossRef] [PubMed]
105. Micucci, M.; Angeletti, A.; Cont, M.; Corazza, I.; Aldini, R.; Donadio, E.; Chiarini, A.; Budriesi, R. *Hibiscus Sabdariffa* L. flowers and *Olea Europea* L. leaves extract-based formulation for hypertension care: In vitro efficacy and toxicological profile. *J. Med. Food* **2016**, *19*, 504–512. [CrossRef]
106. Lockyer, S.; Yaqoob, P.; Spencer, J.P.E.; Rowland, I. Olive leaf phenolics and cardiovascular risk reduction: Physiological effects and mechanisms of action. *Nutr. Aging* **2012**, *1*, 125–140. [CrossRef]
107. Wang, L.; Geng, C.; Jiang, L.; Gong, D.; Liu, D.; Yoshimura, H.; Zhong, L. The anti-atherosclerotic effect of olive leaf extract is related to suppressed inflammatory response in rabbits with experimental atherosclerosis. *Eur. J. Nutr.* **2008**, *47*, 235–243. [CrossRef] [PubMed]
108. Komaki, E.; Yamaguchi, S.; Maru, I.; Kinoshita, M.; Kakehi, K.; Ohta, Y.; Tsukada, Y. Identification of anti-α-amylase components from olive leaf extracts. *Food Sci. Technol. Res.* **2003**, *9*, 35–39. [CrossRef]
109. Singh, I.; Mok, M.; Christensen, A.M.; Turner, A.H.; Hawley, J.A. The effects of polyphenols in olive leaves on platelet function. *Nutr. Metab. Cardiovasc. Dis.* **2008**, *18*, 127–132. [CrossRef] [PubMed]
110. Omar, S.H.; Scott, C.J.; Hamlin, A.S.; Obied, H.K. Olive biophenols reduces alzheimer's pathology in SH-SY5Y cells and APPswe mice. *Int. J. Mol. Sci.* **2019**, *20*, 125. [CrossRef]
111. Chiaino, E.; Micucci, M.; Cosconati, S.; Novellino, E.; Budriesi, R.; Chiarini, A.; Frosoni, M. Olive leaves and hibicus flowers extracts-based preparation protect brain from oxidative stress-induced injury. *Antioxidants* **2020**, *9*, 806. [CrossRef] [PubMed]
112. Somerville, V.; Moore, R.; Braakhuis, A. The effect of olive leaf extract on upper respiratory illness in high school athletes: A randomised control trial. *Nutrients* **2019**, *11*, 358. [CrossRef] [PubMed]
113. Castrogiovanni, P.; Trovato, F.M.; Loreto, C.; Nsir, H.; Szychlinska, M.A.; Musumeci, G. Nutraceutical supplements in the management and prevention of osteoarthritis. *Int. J. Mol. Sci.* **2016**, *17*, 2042. [CrossRef]
114. Musumeci, G.; Trovato, F.M.; Pichler, K.; Weinberg, A.M.; Loreto, C.; Castrogiovanni, P. Extra-virgin olive oil diet and mild physical activity prevent cartilage degeneration in an osteoarthritis model: An in vivo and in vitro study on lubricin expression. *J. Nutr. Biochem.* **2013**, *24*, 2064–2075. [CrossRef]
115. Ahmed, S.; Wang, N.; Lalonde, M.; Goldberg, V.M.; Haqqi, T.M. Green tea polyphenol epigallocatechin-3-gallate (EGCG) differentially inhibits interleukin-1β-induced expression of matrix metalloproteinase-1 and-13 in human chondrocytes. *J. Pharmacol. Exp. Ther.* **2004**, *308*, 767–773. [CrossRef]
116. Murakami, A.; Song, M.; Katsumata, S.I.; Uehara, M.; Suzuki, K.; Ohigashi, H. Citrus nobiletin suppresses bone loss in ovariectomized ddY mice and collagen-induced arthritis in DBA/1J mice: Possible involvement of receptor activator of NF-kappaB ligand (RANKL)-induced osteoclastogenesis regulation. *Biofactors* **2007**, *30*, 179–192. [CrossRef]
117. Perugini, P.; Vettor, M.; Rona, C.; Troisi, L.; Villanova, L.; Genta, I.; Conti, B.; Pavanetto, F. Efficacy of oleuropein against UVB irradiation: Preliminary evaluation. *Int. J. Cosmet. Sci.* **2008**, *30*, 113–120. [CrossRef] [PubMed]
118. Wanitphakdeedecha, R.; Ng, J.N.C.; Junsuwan, N.; Phaitoonwattanakij, S.; Phothong, W.; Eimpunth, S.; Manuskiatti, W. Efficacy of olive leaf extract containing cream for facial rejuvenation: A pilot study. *J. Cosmet. Dermatol.* **2020**, *19*, 1662–1666. [CrossRef] [PubMed]
119. Hussein, M.R. Ultraviolet radiation and skin cancer: Molecular mechanisms. *J. Cutan. Pathol.* **2005**, *32*, 191–205. [CrossRef] [PubMed]
120. Krutmann, J. The role of UVA rays in skin aging. *Eur. J. Dermatol.* **2001**, *11*, 170–171. [PubMed]
121. Restuccia, D.; Clodoveo, M.L.; Corbo, F.; Loizzo, M.R. De-stoning technology for improving olive oil nutritional and sensory features: The right idea at the wrong time. *Food Res. Int.* **2018**, *106*, 636–646. [CrossRef]
122. Amirante, R.; Clodoveo, M.L.; Distaso, E.; Ruggiero, F.; Tamburrano, P. A tri-generation plant fuelled with olive tree pruning residues in Apulia: An energetic and economic analysis. *Renew. Energy* **2016**, *89*, 411–421. [CrossRef]
123. Alu'datt, M.H.; Alli, I.; Ereifej, K.; Alhamad, M.N.; Alsaad, A.; Rababeh, T. Optimisation and characterisation of various extraction conditions of phenolic compounds and antioxidant activity in olive seeds. *Nat. Prod. Res.* **2011**, *25*, 876–889. [CrossRef]
124. Fernández-Bolaños, J.; Felizón, B.; Brenes, M.; Guillén, R.; Heredia, A. Hydroxytyrosol and tyrosol as the main compounds found in the phenolic fraction of steam-exploded olive stones. *J. Am. Oil Chem. Soc.* **1998**, *75*, 1643–1649. [CrossRef]
125. Rodríguez, G.; Lama, A.; Rodríguez, R.; Jiménez, A.; Guillén, R.; Fernández-Bolanos, J. Olive stone an attractive source of bioactive and valuable compounds. *Bioresour. Technol.* **2008**, *99*, 5261–5269. [CrossRef]
126. González-Hidalgo, I.; Bañón, S.; Ros, J.M. Evaluation of table olive by-product as a source of natural antioxidants. *Int. J. Food Sci. Technol.* **2012**, *47*, 674–681. [CrossRef]

127. Bolek, S. Olive stone powder: A potential source of fiber and antioxidant and its effect on the rheological characteristics of biscuit dough and quality. *Innovative Food Sci. Emerging Technol.* **2020**, *64*, 102423–102429. [CrossRef]
128. Khadem, S.; Rashidi, L.; Homapour, M. Antioxidant capacity, phenolic composition and physicochemical characteristics of whole olive stone oil extracted from different olive varieties grown in Iran. *Eur. J. Lipid Sci. Technol.* **2019**, *121*, 1800365–1800373. [CrossRef]
129. Lama-Muñoz, A.; Romero-García, J.M.; Cara, C.; Moya, M.; Castro, E. Low energy-demanding recovery of antioxidants and sugars from olive stones as preliminary steps in the biorefinery context. *Ind. Crops Prod.* **2014**, *60*, 30–38. [CrossRef]
130. Ruiz, E.; Romero-García, J.M.; Romero, I.; Manzanares, P.; Negro, M.J.; Castro, E. Olive-derived biomass as a source of energy and chemicals. *Biofuels, Bioprod. Biorefin.* **2017**, *11*, 1077–1094. [CrossRef]
131. Spizzirri, U.G.; Restuccia, D.; Chiricosta, S.; Parisi, O.I.; Cirillo, G.; Curcio, M.; Iemma, F.; Puoci, F.; Picci, N. Olive stones as a source of antioxidants for food industry. *J. Food Nutr. Res.* **2011**, *50*, 57–67.
132. Salami, S.A.; Luciano, G.; O'Grady, M.N.; Biondi, L.; Newbold, C.J.; Kerry, J.P.; Priolo, A. Sustainability of feeding plant by-products: A review of the implications for ruminant meat production. *Anim. Feed Sci. Technol.* **2019**, *251*, 37–55. [CrossRef]
133. Berbel, J.; Posadillo, A. Review and analysis of alternatives for the valorisation of agro-industrial olive oil by-products. *Sustainability* **2018**, *10*, 237. [CrossRef]
134. Makri, S.; Kafantaris, I.; Savva, S.; Ntanou, P.; Stagos, D.; Argyroulis, I.; Kotsampasi, B.; Christodoulou, V.; Gerasopoulos, K.; Petrotos, K.; et al. Novel feed including olive oil mill wastewater bioactive compounds enhanced the redox status of lambs. *In Vivo* **2018**, *32*, 291–302. [PubMed]
135. Chiofalo, V.; Liotta, L.; Lo Presti, V.; Gresta, F.; Di Rosa, A.R.; Chiofalo, B. Effect of dietary olive cake supplementation on performance, carcass characteristics, and meat quality of beef cattle. *Animals* **2020**, *10*, 1176. [CrossRef] [PubMed]
136. Gerasopoulos, K.; Stagos, D.; Kokkas, S.; Petrotos, K.; Kantas, D.; Goulas, P.; Kouretas, D. Feed supplemented with byproducts from olive oil mill wastewater processing increases antioxidant capacity in broiler chickens. *Food Chem. Toxicol.* **2015**, *82*, 42–49. [CrossRef]
137. Salami, S.A.; Majoka, M.A.; Saha, S.; Garber, A.; Gabarrou, J.F. Efficacy of dietary antioxidants on broiler oxidative stress, performance and meat quality: Science and market. *Avian Biology Research* **2015**, *8*, 65–78. [CrossRef]
138. Paiva-Martins, F.; Barbosa, S.; Pinheiro, V.; Mourão, J.L.; Outor-Monteiro, D. The effect of olive leaves supplementation on the feed digestibility, growth performances of pigs and quality of pork meat. *Meat Sci.* **2009**, *82*, 438–443. [CrossRef]
139. Arco-Pérez, A.; Ramos-Morales, E.; Yáñez-Ruiz, D.R.; Abecia, L.; Martín-García, A.I. Nutritive evaluation and milk quality of including of tomato or olive by-products silages with sunflower oil in the diet of dairy goats. *Anim. Feed Sci. Technol.* **2017**, *232*, 57–70.
140. Branciari, R.; Galarini, R.; Miraglia, D.; Ranucci, D.; Valiani, A.; Giusepponi, D.; Servili, M.; Acuti, G.; Pauselli, M.; Trabalza-Marinucci, M. Dietary Supplementation with Olive Mill Wastewater in Dairy Sheep: Evaluation of Cheese Characteristics and Presence of Bioactive Molecules. *Animals* **2020**, *10*, 1941. [CrossRef] [PubMed]
141. Kerasioti, E.; Terzopoulou, Z.; Komini, O.; Kafantaris, I.; Makri, S.; Stagos, D.; Gerasopoulos, K.; Anisimov, N.; Tsatsakis, A.; Kouretas, D. Tissue specific effects of feeds supplemented with grape pomace or olive oil mill wastewater on detoxification enzymes in sheep. *Toxicol. Rep.* **2017**, *4*, 364–372. [CrossRef]
142. Al-Musawi, J.E.; Al-Khalisy, A.F. Effect of grinded olive leave ssuplimentation in milk production and its components and some blood traits in native does. *Iraqi J. Agric. Sci.* **2016**, *47*, 1354–1359.
143. Zangeneh, S.; Torki, M. Effects of b-mannanase supplementing of olive pulp included diet on performance of laying hens, egg quality characteristics, humoral and cellular immune response and blood parameters. *Global Vet.* **2011**, *7*, 391–398.
144. Cayan, H.; Erener, G. Effect of olive leaf (*Olea europaea*) powder on laying hens performance, egg quality and egg yolk cholesterol levels. *Asian-Australas. J. Anim. Sci.* **2015**, *28*, 538–543. [CrossRef]

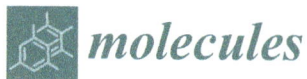

Review

Bioactive Metabolites from Marine Algae as Potent Pharmacophores against Oxidative Stress-Associated Human Diseases: A Comprehensive Review

Biswajita Pradhan [1], Rabindra Nayak [1], Srimanta Patra [2], Bimal Prasad Jit [3], Andrea Ragusa [4,5,*] and Mrutyunjay Jena [1,*]

1. Algal Biotechnology and Molecular Systematic Laboratory, Post Graduate Department of Botany, Berhampur University, Brahmapur 760007, India; pradhan.biswajita2014@gmail.com (B.P.); rabindran335@gmal.com (R.N.)
2. Cancer and Cell Death Laboratory, Department of Life Science, National Institute of Technology Rourkela, Rourkela 769001, India; 518LS2007@nitrkl.ac.in
3. Department of Biochemistry, All India Institute of Medical Science, Ansari Nagar, New Delhi 110023, India; bimaljit2019@gmail.com
4. Department of Biological and Environmental Sciences and Technologies, Campus Ecotekne, University of Salento, via Monteroni, 73100 Lecce, Italy
5. CNR-Nanotec, Institute of Nanotechnology, via Monteroni, 73100 Lecce, Italy
* Correspondence: andrea.ragusa@unisalento.it (A.R.); mj.bot@buodisha.edu.in (M.J.); Tel.: +39-0832-319-208 (A.R.)

Abstract: In addition to cancer and diabetes, inflammatory and ROS-related diseases represent one of the major health problems worldwide. Currently, several synthetic drugs are used to reduce oxidative stress; nevertheless, these approaches often have side effects. Therefore, to overcome these issues, the search for alternative therapies has gained importance in recent times. Natural bioactive compounds have represented, and they still do, an important source of drugs with high therapeutic efficacy. In the "synthetic" era, terrestrial and aquatic photosynthetic organisms have been shown to be an essential source of natural compounds, some of which might play a leading role in pharmaceutical drug development. Marine organisms constitute nearly half of the worldwide biodiversity. In the marine environment, algae, seaweeds, and seagrasses are the first reported sources of marine natural products for discovering novel pharmacophores. The algal bioactive compounds are a potential source of novel antioxidant and anticancer (through modulation of the cell cycle, metastasis, and apoptosis) compounds. Secondary metabolites in marine Algae, such as phenolic acids, flavonoids, and tannins, could have great therapeutic implications against several diseases. In this context, this review focuses on the diversity of functional compounds extracted from algae and their potential beneficial effects in fighting cancer, diabetes, and inflammatory diseases.

Keywords: marine bioactive compounds; secondary metabolites; algae; oxidative stress; ROS; cancer; diabetes; inflammation; apoptosis

Citation: Pradhan, B.; Nayak, R.; Patra, S.; Jit, B.P.; Ragusa, A.; Jena, M. Bioactive Metabolites from Marine Algae as Potent Pharmacophores against Oxidative Stress-Associated Human Diseases: A Comprehensive Review. *Molecules* **2021**, *26*, 37. https://dx.doi.org/10.3390/molecules26010037

Received: 27 November 2020
Accepted: 21 December 2020
Published: 23 December 2020

Publisher's Note: MDPI stays neutral with regard to jurisdictional claims in published maps and institutional affiliations.

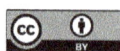

Copyright: © 2020 by the authors. Licensee MDPI, Basel, Switzerland. This article is an open access article distributed under the terms and conditions of the Creative Commons Attribution (CC BY) license (https://creativecommons.org/licenses/by/4.0/).

1. Introduction

Epidemiological studies have evidenced the dangerous effects on human health of the ever-increasing intake of junk food, alcohol, and antibiotics. This bad behavior can increase the risk of oxidative stress which, in turn, can lead to accelerated aging and inflammatory diseases, such as cardiovascular and neurodegenerative disease and many types of cancer [1]. According to reports by the WHO, more than 200 types of lethal cancer accounted approximately for 9.6 million deaths per year in 2019 globally [2]. Similarly, diabetes mellitus, a metabolic disorder, has emerged as the third foremost cause of death worldwide (1.6 million deaths per year) with several associated ill-fated diseases, such as heart attack, stroke, kidney failure, high blood pressure, blindness, and lower limb amputation [3–5]. According to WHO, the world's diabetic population will hike up to 592 million by 2035. In addition to cancer and diabetes, inflammatory diseases have tremendously increased in the recent past causing millions of deaths [6]. Unfortunately, current chemotherapeutic, anti-diabetic, and anti-inflammatory drugs often present several adverse effects, such as toxicity, drug tolerance, and metabolic impairments [1]. In this regard, natural products might provide alternative drugs with better characteristics [7]. Similarly, their regular uptake through diet or novel pharmacological formulations might help prevent oxidative stress-related diseases [8–11].

Approximately 70% of the Earth's surface is covered by oceans and it hosts an immense variety of marine organisms which represent a rich source of natural products [1,12,13]. Marine algae are among the most promising sources of novel bioactive compounds with interesting biological effects, such as antioxidant, anticancer, antibacterial, antifungal, antidiabetic, and anti-inflammatory activities [1]. Marine algae are extensively used in diet and traditional medicine in Asian countries because of the presence of minerals, dietary fiber, lipids, omega-3 fatty acids, proteins, polysaccharides, and essential amino acids [14,15]. They also contain many vitamins, such as vitamins A, B, C, and E [16]. Few marine algae-derived bioactive compounds, such as phlorotannins, polysaccharides, fucoidans, alginic acid, tripeptides, pyropheophytin, and oxylipin, have been shown to reduce the risk of cancer, diabetes, and inflammatory diseases [15]. Hence, in this review we focused our attention on the diversity of marine algal bioactive compounds and the recent findings about their molecular mode of action in potentially fighting cancer, diabetes, and inflammation (Figure 1). Furthermore, algal extracts showed potential antimicrobial activity against aerobes, psychotropic, proteolytic, and lipolytic bacteria and act as natural preservatives. Additionally, they can prevent lipid oxidation [17,18].

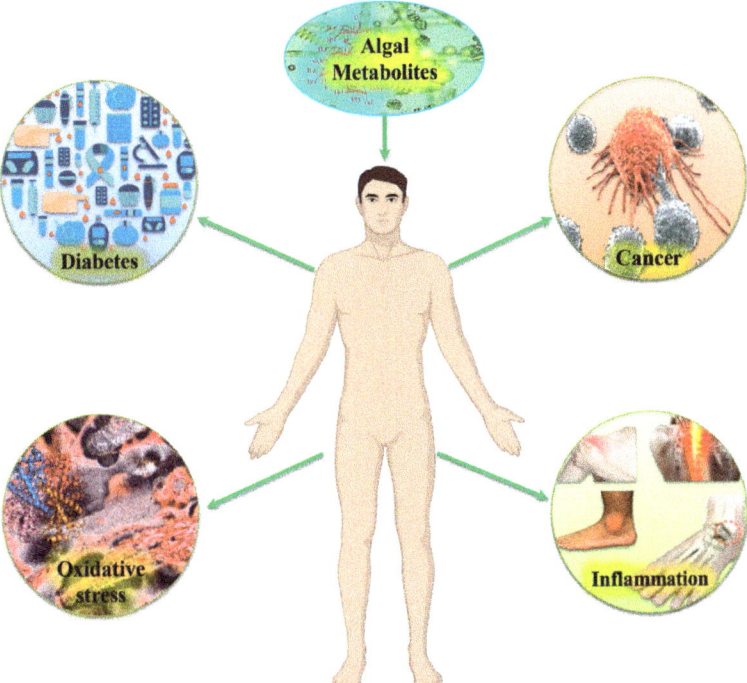

Figure 1. Potential beneficial effects of algal metabolites on human health. Secondary metabolites in marine algae could provide novel drug candidates for fighting various diseases, e.g., by reducing the α-amylase and α-glucosidase activity in diabetes; by reducing inflammation thanks to their antioxidant capacity; and inhibiting cellular proliferation in tumor cells.

2. Biological Activities of Marine Algae and Potential Health Benefits via Dietary Supplements

Diet plays an important role in disease prevention as more than 33% of diseases, such as cancer, diabetes, and inflammation-associated chronic diseases, could be avoided by changing lifestyle and food habits [19,20]. Nutritional supplements from natural sources could also play an important role in preventing diseases. Phytochemicals from marine algae, such as peptides, amino acids, lipids, fatty acids, sterols, polysaccharides, carbohydrates, polyphenols, photosynthetic pigments, vitamins, and minerals, some of which are represented in Figure 2, can act as potent antioxidants and have beneficial effects as anti-diabetic and chemotherapeutic drugs, as detailed below.

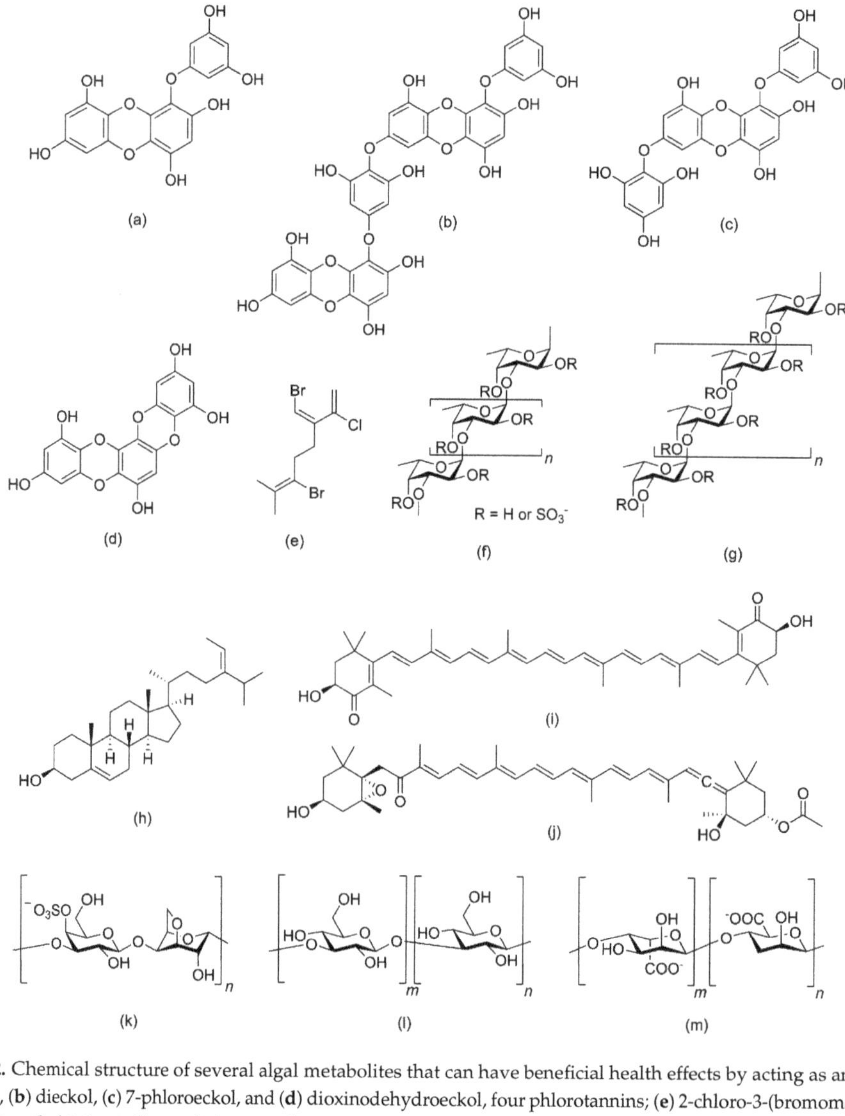

Figure 2. Chemical structure of several algal metabolites that can have beneficial health effects by acting as antioxidants: (**a**) eckol, (**b**) dieckol, (**c**) 7-phloroeckol, and (**d**) dioxinodehydroeckol, four phlorotannins; (**e**) 2-chloro-3-(bromomethylene)-6-bromo-7-methyl-1,6-octadiene, a halogenated monoterpene; (**f**) type I and (**g**) type II fucoidans; (**h**) fucosterol; (**i**) astaxanthin and (**j**) fucoxanthin; (**k**) k-carrageenan; (**l**) laminaran; and (**m**) alginate.

2.1. Peptides and Amino Acids

Hydrolysis of proteins can lead to bioactive peptides that can present beneficial health aspects and modulate the outcome of the disease. Bioactive phyto-peptides have 3 to 20 amino acid residues and display biological properties such as antioxidant, anticancer, anti-inflammation, and immunomodulation. For example, purified peptides from *Chlorella vulgaris* can prevent cellular damage and can act as potent anticancer agents [21,22].

The protein content in macro and micro algae comprises all essential amino acids which prevent cellular damage. The red alga *Palmaria palmata* is rich in Leu, Val, and Met, and their mean levels are similar to ovalbumin. Similarly, Ile and Thr concentrations are comparable to those in legume proteins. The green alga *Ulva rigida* contains Leu, Phe, and Val as major essential amino acids [23,24].

2.2. Lipids and Fatty Acids

The structural complexity of lipids and fatty acids are highly diverse and contribute to their therapeutic efficacy. It has been reported that small amounts of saturated fatty acids can help prevent cardiovascular diseases. Marine algae contain polyunsaturated fatty acids (PUFAs) and significant amounts of monounsaturated fatty acids which are beneficial to human health and could help reduce cardiovascular diseases [25].

2.2.1. Polyunsaturated Fatty Acids (PUFAs)

Humans are incapable of synthesizing PUFAs that, on the other hand, are abundant in both macro and microalgae. PUFAs in microalgae are mainly composed of omega-3 and omega-6 fatty acids (e.g., EPA and AA) [26]. PUFAs regulate blood clotting and blood pressure and modulate the function of the brain and nervous systems [27]. Moreover, they decrease the risk of several chronic diseases, such as diabetes and cancer. Additionally, they regulate inflammatory responses by producing eicosanoids, well-known inflammation mediators [27]. Omega-3 and omega-6 PUFA from macroalgae are already used as dietary supplements [28]. Red and brown algae have a high level of omega-3 fatty acids (e.g., EPA and GLA) and omega-6 fatty acids (e.g., AA and linoleic acid). Brown algae *Laminaria ochroleuca* and *Undaria pinnatifida* are a rich source of octadecatetraenoic acid, an omega-3 PUFA [29]. Green seaweed *Ulva pertusa* was found to be rich in hexadecatetraenoic (omega-3), oleic (omega-9), and palmitic acids (SFA). The lipid fraction of microalgae *C. vulgaris* contains oleic, palmitic, and linolenic acids. The green microalga *Haematococcus* sp. also contains short-chain fatty acids. Long-chain PUFAs are also used as nutritional supplements and food additives [30]. *Spirulina* sp. is a promising source of GLAs, a precursor of leukotrienes, prostaglandins, and thromboxans that regulate inflammatory, immunological, and cardiovascular disorders. Cyanobacteria and some green algae also contain bioactive fatty acids such as palmitic, oleic, and lauric acids along with DHA [22].

2.2.2. Sterols

Sterols are a class of lipids extensively found in both macro and microalgae. Sterols and some of their derivatives have potential biological, e.g., anti-inflammatory, activity. Sterols from *Spirulina* triggers the formation of the plasminogen-activating factor in vascular endothelial cells. Fucosterol, ergosterol, and chondrillasterol are found in brown algae and cholesterol has been found in red algae [22,31].

2.3. Polysaccharides and Carbohydrates

Polysaccharides are abundant in seaweeds and also found in microalgae. They generally comprise about 4% to 76% of the total dry weight of the alga. Polysaccharides are classified according to their chemical structure, such as sulfuric acid polysaccharides, sulfated xylans, and galactans (generally found in green algae). Moreover, alginic acid, fucoidan, laminarin, and sargassan are found in brown algae [32]. Agar, carrageenans, xylans, and floridean are generally found in red algae. Many algal polysaccharides present bioactivity and could become drug candidates with potential use in several human health disparities [33]. Carrageenans are sulfated galactans and they are extensively used in pharmaceutical and food industries. Soluble fibers such as fucans, alginates, and laminarans are found in brown seaweeds, whereas soluble fibers such as sulfated galactans (agars and carrageenans), xylans, and floridean starch are abundantly found in red seaweeds [34]. Green algae contain xylans, mannans, starch, and ionic sulfate group-containing polysaccharides in combination with uronic acids, rhamnose, xylose, galactose, and arabinose. Many of the polysaccharides can be regarded as dietary fibers and are classified into two groups, i.e., soluble and insoluble fibers [35,36]. Seaweeds contain about 25% to 75% dietary fibers in comparison to their dry weight, a higher percentage compared to that found in fruit and vegetables [37]. The algal dietary fiber consumption has several health benefits as they can be used as antitumor, anticancer, anticoagulant, and antiviral agents. Fucoidans are extensively found in the cell walls of brown macroalgae [38]. Fucoidans have several biological activities and act as antioxidant, antitumor, anti-inflammatory, antidiabetes, antiviral, anticoagulant, and antithrombotic agents. Additionally, they also modulate the human immune system [1]. Furthermore, laminarin is the second main source of glucan, abundantly found in brown algae, and it acts as a facilitator of intestinal metabolism [36].

Carbohydrates, such as glucose and starch, are abundantly found in microalgae [39]. Many biological functions of microalgal species are due to the presence of carbohydrates. *Chlorella pyrenoidosa* and *Chlorella ellipsoidea* contain glucose and a wide variety of combinations of galactose, mannose, rhamnose, N-acetylglucosamine, N-acetylgalactosamine, and arabinose that exert immune-modulatory and antiproliferative activity [40]. β-1,3-Glucans extracted from *Chlorella* have been shown to act as immunomodulators that can reduce blood lipids [41].

2.4. Polyphenolic Compounds

Marine algal bioactive compounds are potent antioxidant agents that protect from oxidative damage [42]. The antioxidant activity of bioactive compounds from marine algae is associated with protection against cancer, inflammatory, diabetes, and several ROS-related diseases [43]. Polyphenolic compounds are mainly found in both micro and macroalgae [42]. The phenolic components include hydroxycinnamic acids, phenolic acids, simple phenols, xanthones, coumarins, naphthoquinones, stilbenes, flavonoids, anthraquinones, and lignins [21]. The phlorotannins with potential antioxidant activity belong to polyphenolic compounds that have been screened from several brown algae. Phlorotannins are known for their chemopreventive, antibacterial, antiproliferative, and UV-protective properties [22].

2.5. Photosynthetic Pigments

Macroalgae contain chlorophylls and carotenoids as major photosynthetic pigments. Carotenoids are well known for their antioxidant properties and dietary carotenoids have high nutritional and therapeutic value [44]. Carotenoids are well known for their chemopreventive effect against several cancer subtypes. Microalgae are also the main source of antioxidants such as β-carotene and astaxanthin. β-Carotene is a natural colorant that has been conventionally used as food and drinks colorants and can act as dietary food supplements or additives with a high antioxidant capacity [45].

2.6. Vitamins and Minerals

Vitamins are micronutrients essential for human body growth and development. Seaweeds and microalgae are known to be a good source of vitamin B1, B2, and B12. Vitamin B12 (cobalamin) is extensively found in higher concentrations in green and red algae compared to brown algae [46]. Vitamin B12 is generally found in red macroalgae such as *Palmaria longat* and *Porphyra tenera*. The highest vitamin B12 content was found in red seaweed *Porphyra* sp. and green algae, such as *Enteromorpha* sp. and *Spirulina*. Cobalamin deficiency can cause health diseases, such as neuropsychiatric disorders and megaloblastic anaemia. Vitamin C (ascorbic acid) is present in all red, brown, and green seaweeds. Vitamin C has several health benefits, such as radical scavenging activity, antiaging, and immune stimulant activity. Vitamin E is a mixture of tocopherols. α Tocopherol occurs in green, red, and brown seaweeds. Phaeophyceae also contain β- and γ-tocopherols and displayed outstanding *antioxidant* activity. Vitamins C and E were also found in *Laminaria digitata* and *U. pinnatifida* [22].

Seaweeds and macroalgae are rich in minerals, trace elements, and maintain inorganic atoms in seawater. Minerals and trace elements are required for the human diet [47]. Phaeophyceae, such as *U. pinnatifida* and *Sargassum*, and rhodophyta, such as *Chondrus crispus* and *Gracilariopsis*, are considered dietary supplement that meet the recommended daily intake of some of the major minerals, such as Na, K, Ca, and Mg, as well as trace minerals, such as Fe, Zn, Mn, and Cu. In addition, seaweeds are also important sources of Ca as they reduce Ca deficiency risk in pregnant women and adolescents and they inhibit preadolescent aging [48].

3. Marine Bioactive Metabolites and Their Therapeutic Efficacy

The marine ecosystem is a source of novel natural secondary metabolites with promising biomedical applications [49]. The impact of marine algae in the area of traditional medicine is huge and they have been used as *Yunani hakim* in many countries, such as China and Egypt. Marine algae produce diverse secondary metabolites and might be the most promising sources of proteins, vitamins, omega-3, carotenoids, phenolic acids, and flavonoids, as well as other natural antioxidants [50]. These marine bioactive compounds act as free radical scavengers and prevent oxyradical formation thus reducing oxidative stress and, as such, they have great importance in the prevention of cancer, diabetes, early aging, and several other inflammatory diseases (Figure 3).

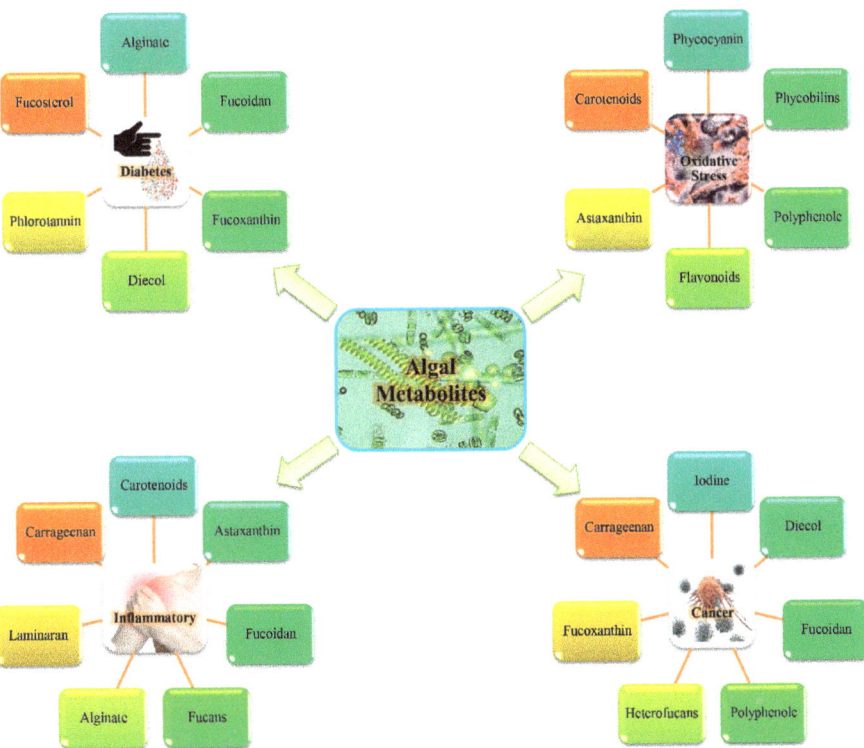

Figure 3. Potential effects of algal metabolites in different human disease.

Marine bioactive compounds, such as algal photosynthetic pigments, phycobiliproteins, carotenoids, polyphenols, terpenes, phlorotannins, and polysaccharides, have shown promising therapeutic activity in both in vitro and in vivo models [25,29,38,51].

3.1. Marine Bioactive Metabolites and Modulation of In Vitro Antioxidant Activity

Reactive oxygen species (ROS) comprise a group of oxygenic ions that are highly reactive and pose a serious threat to biological components, ultimately leading to serious disorders such as cancer, diabetes mellitus, neurodegenerative and inflammatory diseases [52]. The oxygen-containing radicals comprise of peroxyl (ROO$^\bullet$), hydroxyl (OH$^\bullet$), hydroperoxyl (HO$_2^\bullet$), superoxide (O$_2^\bullet$), alkoxyl (RO$^\bullet$), thiyl peroxyl (RSOO$^\bullet$), sulfonyl (ROS$^\bullet$), and nitric oxide (NO$^\bullet$) radical, as well as non-radical oxidizing agents such as singlet oxygen (^{1}O$_2$), hydrogen peroxide (H$_2$O$_2$), hypochlorous acid (HOCl), and organic hydroperoxides (ROOH) [52–55]. Cells can detoxify ROS as they are furnished with antioxidant defense mechanisms to maintain cellular equilibrium. Antioxidants fight against ROS and exert a positive effect on human health by protecting macromolecules such as proteins, DNA, and membrane lipids [56]. The use of synthetic antioxidants used as food additives, such as butylated hydroxyanisole, butylated hydroxytoluene, tertiary-butylhydroquinone, and propyl gallate, might represent a threat because of their side effects [57]. Hence, the development of novel antioxidants from natural sources like marine flora can represent a promising approach. Marine algae could neutralize ROS because of their antioxidant compounds, such as phycobilins, phycocyanin, carotenoids, astaxanthin, polyphenols, and vitamins, which can act against cancer, diabetes, inflammation, aging, and immune responses. The antioxidant capacity of various marine algae, such as green, red, and brown algae species, has been already extensively reported in the literature.

Antioxidant activity of marine algal compounds have been determined by several methods, such as 2,2-diphenyl-1-picrylhydrazil (DPPH) radical scavenging, ferric reducing antioxidant power (FRAP), lipid peroxide inhibition, ABTS radical scavenging, nitric oxide (NO) scavenging, hydrogen peroxide radical scavenging assays, superoxide radical and hydroxyl radical scavenging assays. The methanolic extract of blue-green algae has shown potent DPPH radical scavenging activity. In addition, phycocyanin from *Spirulina platensis* showed strong H$_2$O$_2$ scavenging activity [58]. Antioxidant properties in green algae *Ulva fasciata* and *Ulva reticulate* were characterized by free-radical-scavenging due to the presence of flavonoids [59–61]. In brown algae such as *Ecklonia cava*, *Eisenia bicyclis*, and *Ecklonia kurome* antioxidant activities were characterized by DPPH-radical scavenging [62]. Ethanolic extracts of *Gracilaria tenuistipitata* and *Callophyllis japonica* also have shown potential antioxidant activities [63,64].

3.2. Intricate Role of Algal Bioactive Metabolites as Anticancer Agents

Free radicals and ROS generally promote cancer initiation. Synthetic chemopreventive drugs often present several adverse side-effects to the tumor vicinity and bodily organs because of poor specificity and generalized biodistribution [65]. Several marine algal bioactive compounds have been designated as potent chemopreventives due to inhibition of cellular proliferation, modulation of the cell cycle, and induction of apoptosis [66,67].

3.2.1. Inhibition of Cell Proliferation

Several studies have reported that marine algal bioactive compounds have antiproliferative and inhibitory activity against several cancer subtypes in in vitro as well as in vivo [68]. Sulfated polysaccharides purified from brown seaweeds exhibited an antiproliferative effect on human leukemia and lymphoma cell lines [38]. They have also been reported to inhibit proliferation of breast (MCF-7) and cervical (HeLa) cancer cells [38]. Sulfated polysaccharides extracted from the brown seaweed *Sargassum vulgare* displayed inhibition of cell proliferation in HeLa and B16 cells without cytotoxicity in normal rabbit aortic endothelial cells [69]. Furthermore, sulfated polysaccharides from red seaweed *Amansia multifidi* inhibited the cellular viability of HeLa cells. The polysaccharides isolated from *Gracilariopsis lemaneiformis*, consisting of 3,6-anhydro-L-galactose and D-galactose and a linear structure of repeated disaccharide agarobiose units, hindered the viability of B16, A549, and MKN-28 cell lines [70]. Similarly, low-molecular-weight sulfated polysaccharides from green seaweed *Gayralia oxysperma* inhibited the cell viability of U87MG glioblastoma cells even at microgram-level concentrations (10, 100, and 1000 µg/mL) without any evident cytotoxicity [71]. Fucoidans isolated from *Undaria pinnatifida* also showed inhibition of cellular viability in SK-MEL-28, T-47, RPMI-7951, T47D, and DLD-1 cancer cell lines at microgram concentrations. Moreover, fucoidans isolated from the sporophyll of *U. pinnatifida* demonstrated to be able to inhibit cell growth in HeLa, A549, PC-3, and HepG2 cell lines, although at higher concentrations (treatment with 0.8 mg/mL for 24 h) [72]. Furthermore, in prostate cell lines (DU-145), fucoidans treatment marked a 90% reduction in cell viability [73]. Similarly, *Fucus vesiculosus* derived fucoidans were reported to reduce cell viability of human colorectal carcinoma (HCT116) cell line by 60% [74]. Fucoidan from *Ecklonia cava* have been also reported to inhibit proliferation of MDA-MB-231 cells. Moreover, the administration of fucoidan (20 mg/kg for 28 days) in a DU-145 cell-induced xenograft rat model has reduced the tumor growth by 50% [73]. Carrageenans from *Kappaphycus alvarezii* reduced the growth of liver, colon, breast, and osteosarcoma cell lines [75]. Similarly, treatment of phlorotannins (a type of polyphenol) isolated from *E. cava* has marked a reduction in cell viability in MDA-MB-231 and MCF-7 cells by 55% and 64%, respectively [76]. Similarly, phlorotannin-rich extracts from *Ascophyllum nodosum* reduced the cell viability of HT-29 colon cancer cells [77].

Halogenated monoterpenes isolated from red seaweeds *Plocamium cornutum* and *Plocamium suhrii* displayed potent antiproliferative activity as compared to anticancer drug cisplatin [78]. *U. pinnatifida* isolated fucoxanthins has a cytotoxic effect against LNCaP, DU145, PC-3, Caco-2, HT-29, DLD-1, HeLa, and Jurkat cell lines [79,80]. Moreover, fucoxanthinol displayed an anti-proliferative effect against drug-resistant HT-29-derived cells, and inhibited xenograft tumor development in a dose-dependent manner [81]. The guaiane sesquiterpene derivative guai-2-*en*-10-ol isolated from the green seaweed *Ulva fasciata*, reduced viability of breast cancer MDA-MB-231 cell line [82]. *G. tenuistipitata* aqueous extract counteracted the cellular proliferation in H1299 cells. Heterofucans from *Sargassum filipendula* exhibited anti-proliferative effects on cervical, prostate, and liver cancer cells [83]. Aqueous extracts of *Sargassum oligocystum* and *Gracilaria corticata* inhibited proliferation of human leukemic cell lines [84,85]. Ethanolic and methanolic extracts of *Gracilaria tenuistipitata* exhibited anti-proliferative effects against Ca9-22 oral cancer cells [86–88]. Several studies have reported that algae consumption modulates cancer prevention. The diets containing seaweeds decreased the growth of DU-145 human prostatic tumor cells in nude mice. Moreover, the administration of red algae *Eucheuma cottonii* extracts as dietary supplement to rats displayed tumor repression [89].

3.2.2. Cell Cycle Arrest and Inhibition of Angiogenesis

Inhibition of cell cycle hinders cancer cell proliferation for the subsequent exhibition of anticancer activity. Sulfated polysaccharides from *G. oxysperma* arrested the cell cycle [71]. Fucoidan from *Fucus vesiculosus* arrested the cell cycle at the G1 phase in HCT116 human colorectal carcinoma and HT-29 colon cancer cells [74]. Fucoxanthin arrested the cell cycle via downregulation of cyclin D1, D2, CDK4 and upregulation of p15INK4B and p27Kip1 expression [90]. Fucoxanthin from *Laminaria japonica* arrested the sub-G1 phase of the cell cycle in WiDr cancer cells [91]. Moreover, in LNCap prostate cancer cells, fucoxanthin arrested the G1 phase of the cell cycle via MAPK/ JNK and GDD45A pathways [92]. Pheophorbide a, from *G. elliptica* arrested the cell cycle in the G0/G1 phase in glioblastoma cells [93]. Aqueous extract of *G. tenuistipitata* induced G2/M arrest in the H1299 cell line [64]. Angiogenesis plays a key role in tumor growth and metastasis. Polysaccharides isolated from *S. vulgare* exhibited angiogenesis inhibitory activity. Fucoidans isolated from *U. pinnatifida* significantly reduced the expression of the angiogenesis factors VEGF-A and VEGF-162 [94]. Sulfated polysaccharides from brown seaweed *Sargassum vulgare* displayed antiangiogenic activity in HeLa and B16 cells without damage to the tumor vicinity [69]. Furthermore, dieckol decreased the expression of angiogenic markers such as PCNA, VEGF, COX-2, MMP-2, and MMP-9 to inhibit metastasis [95].

3.2.3. Induction of Apoptosis

Apoptosis (or programmed cell death, PCD) is the main goal of anticancer drugs. Several reports have demonstrated the role of algal bioactive compounds and polysaccharides as potent anticancer agents by modulating apoptosis, as schematized in Figure 4. Sulfated polysaccharides from *Phaeophyceae* act as novel chemopreventive drugs owing to their free-radical scavenging activity [1]. Sulfated polysaccharides induced apoptosis in human leukemic monocyte lymphoma cell line (U-937) [1]. Polysaccharides from *Capsosiphon fulvescens* induced apoptosis in gastric cancer cells via modulation of PI3K/Akt pathway [96]. Polysaccharides from *U. lactuca* increased the activity of antioxidant enzymes in a DMBA-induced breast cancer model via diminished lipid peroxidation as well as GSH-Px activity to restrain apoptosis [97]. Polysaccharides from red seaweed *Champia feldmannii* demonstrated in vivo antitumor effects in mice transplanted with sarcoma 180 tumors via modulation of apoptosis [98]. The polysaccharides isolated from sea lettuce *U. lactuca* displayed in vitro and in vivo anticancer activity in breast cancer via modulation of apoptosis. It also displayed a chemopreventive effect in DMBA-induced breast cancer in rat post-administration for 10 weeks and prevented breast-histological alterations and carcinogenic wounds. Additionally, it also amplified the p53 expression and inhibited the Bcl-2 expression to induce apoptosis in breast cancer cells [97].

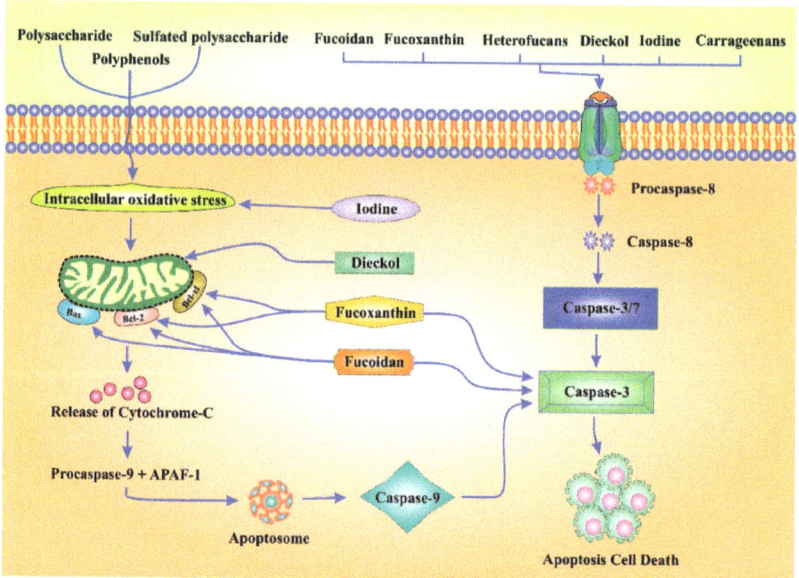

Figure 4. Apoptosis modulation by algal metabolites in cancer prevention. Polysaccharides, sulfated polysaccharides, iodine, dieckol, fucoxanthine, fucoidan, and polyphenols downregulate the expression of anti-apoptotic protein Bcl-xl, Bcl-2. Similarly, they enhance the Bax expression to aid apoptosis. Fucoidan supports the intrinsic apoptosis via regulating the cytosolic release of cytochrome C. Fucoxanthine and fucoidan induces the expression of caspase 9 and caspase 3 to induce apoptotic cell death. Moreover, fucoidan, fucoxanthine, heterofucans, dieckol, iodine, and carrageenans induce apoptosis through modulation of caspase 3 activity via death receptor-mediated apoptotic cell death in several cancer cell lines. In addition to this, they also regulate caspase 8 activity inducing extrinsic apoptosis in different cancer cells.

Fucoidans isolated from the sporophyll of *U. pinnatifida* displayed apoptosis in DU-145 cell-induced xenograft rat model via inhibition of the JAK3/STAT pathway. In addition, fucoidan (IC$_{50}$ 530 ± 3.32 mg/mL) also reduced the viability of B16 melanoma cells via activating apoptosis [99]. Fucoidan from *Fucus vesiculosus* induced p53-independent apoptosis in HCT116 human colorectal carcinoma cell line [74]. Fucoidan from *L. japonica* induced apoptosis via activation of caspase-3, poly(ADP-ribose) polymerase (PARP), and DNA degradation in HT-29 cell line [100]. Moreover, fucoidan from *E. cava* induced apoptosis in MDA-MB-231 and MCF-7 cells via induction of p53 and activation of Bax, caspases 3 and 9, and PARP with inhibition of Bcl-2 [76]. Furthermore, fucoidan from *Cladosiphon okamuranus* displayed induction of apoptosis in MCF-7 cells via activation of caspase-3 and DNA fragmentation [101]. *F. vesiculosus* extracts enhanced mitochondria membrane permeability thus inducing apoptosis via cytoplasmic release of cytochrome C and the Smac/DIABLO pathway in human colon cancer cells [102]. Similarly, fucoidan from *F. vesiculosus* treatment induced apoptosis in HT-29 colon cancer cells via decreasing the expression of Bcl-xL, Bcl-2 and upregulation of Bax, pro-caspases 3, 7, and 9. An upregulation of Rb and E2 factor proteins and Fas-regulated extrinsic apoptosis was also evident post fucoidan treatment in HT-29 colon cancer cells [103].

Fucoxanthin from *Laminaria japonica* induced apoptosis via DNA fragmentation in human colon adenocarcinoma WiDr cells [91]. Fucoxanthin from *Ishige okamurae* exhibited anticancer activity in melanoma B16F10 cells both in vitro (B16F10 cell line) and in vivo (Balb/c mice implanted with B16F10 cells) via induction of apoptosis. Moreover, fucoxanthin induced apoptosis via caspases activation and reduction of BclxL and IAP expression [90]. Laminarin from *Laminaria digitata* induced apoptosis in human colon cancer (HT-29) cells and activated ErbB2 phosphorylation. Moreover, it also inhibited cell proliferation and induced apoptosis in prostate cancer (PC-3) cells and increased the expression of P27kip1 and PTEN [104]. Dieckol from *E. cava* daily administration (40 mg/kg for 15 weeks) decreased cancer cell proliferation in albino rats via induction of apoptosis [95]. The guaiane sesquiterpene derivative guai-2-*en*-10-ol from green seaweed *Ulva fasciata* induced apoptosis in MDA-MB-231 breast cancer cell line via direct interaction with the kinase site of EGFR [82]. The halogenated monoterpene, mertensene from red alga *Pterocladiella capillacea* induced apoptosis in HT-29 and LS174 via modulation of ERK1/2, Akt, and NF B pathways [78]. Ethanolic and methanolic solvent extracts of *Gracilaria tenuistipitata* displayed apoptosis in Ca9-22 oral cancer cells via DNA damage. Furthermore, methanol extract of *Plocamium telfairiae* induced caspase-dependent apoptosis in HT-29 colon cancer cells [88]. Iodine and polyphenols from *L. japonica* induced apoptosis via inhibiting SOD activity [105]. The red alga *Porphyra yezoensis* can induce cancer cell death via apoptosis in a dose-dependent manner in in vitro cancer cell lines without exhibiting cytotoxicity towards the normal cells. Moreover, Carrageenans, heterofucans, dieckol, and iodine can induce cancer cell death via apoptosis in a dose-dependent manner in in vitro cancer cell lines without exhibiting cytotoxicity towards the normal cells. Furthermore, *L. japonica* water extracts induced apoptosis in several human breast cancer cell lines. Moreover, *Eucheuma cottonii* extract displayed the upregulation of antioxidant enzymes such as catalase (CAT), superoxide dismutase (SOD), glutathione peroxidase (GPx) in cancer-induced rats [89]. Methanolic extracts of *Fucus serratus* and *F. vesiculosus* exhibited protection of DNA damage induced by H_2O_2 in Caco-2 cells [106]. Furthermore, *Pelvetia canaliculata* inhibited H_2O_2-induced superoxide dismutase depletion in Caco-2 cells [106]. *C. japonica* ethanol extracts inhibited H_2O_2-induced apoptosis via activating cellular antioxidant enzymes [63]. *G. tenuistipitata* aqueous extract enhanced the recovery of these cells from H_2O_2-induced DNA damage in the H1299 cell line [59]. Apoptosis modulation by algal metabolites in different cancerous cell lines with molecular pathways are summarized in Table 1.

Table 1. Marine algal bioactive metabolites and their functional role in apoptosis.

	Bioactive Compounds	Algal Sources	Cell Lines/In Vivo Models Involved	Functional Involvement	Ref.
1	Sulfated polysaccharides	Brawn algae	Human leukemic monocyte lymphoma cell line (U-937)	Inhibition of cell proliferation	[1]
2	Polysaccharides	Capsosiphon fulvescens	Gastric cancer cells	Modulation of PI3K/Akt pathway	[96]
3	Polysaccharides	U. lactuca	DMBA-induced breast cancer model	Diminished lipid peroxidation also GPx activity	[97]
4	Polysaccharides	Champia feldmannii	Mice transplanted with sarcoma 180 tumors	Reduction of tumor growth	[98]
5	Polysaccharides	U. lactuca	DMBA-induced breast cancer in rat	Prevented breast-histological alterations and carcinogenic wounds	[97]
6	Polysaccharides	U. lactuca	Breast cancer cells	p53 expression and inhibited the Bcl-2 expression	[97]
7	Fucoidan	Costaria costata	DLD-1	55% (100 µg/mL)	[107]
			SK-MEL-28	20% (100 µg/mL)	[107]
8	Fucoidans	U. pinnatifida	DU-145 cell-induced xenograft rat model	Inhibition of the JAK3/STAT pathway	[99]
9	Fucoidan	Fucus vesiculosus	HCT116 human colorectal carcinoma cell line	p53-independent	[74]
10	Fucoidan	L. japonica	HT-29 cell line	Caspase-3, PARP, and DNA degradation	[100]
11	Fucoidan	E. cava	MDA-MB231 and MCF-7 cells	Induction of p53 and activation of Bax, caspases 3 and 9, and PARP with inhibition of Bcl-2	[76]
12	Fucoidan	Cladosiphon okamuranus	MCF-7 cells	Activation of caspase-3 and DNA fragmentation	[101]
13	Extracts	F. vesiculosus	Human colon cancer cells	Cytoplasmic release of cytochrome C and the Smac/DIABLO pathway	[102]
14	Fucoidan	F. vesiculosus	HT-29 colon cancer cells	Decreased expression of Bcl-xL, Bcl-2 and upregulation of Bax, pro-caspases 3, 7, and 9	[103]
15	Fucoidan	F. vesiculosus	HT-29 colon cancer cells	Upregulation of Rb and E2 factor proteins and Fas regulation	[103]
16	Fucoxanthin	Laminaria japonica	Human colon adenocarcinoma WiDr cells	DNA fragmentation	[91]
17	Fucoxanthin	Ishige okamurae	Melanoma B16F10 cells	Caspases activation and reduction of BclxL and IAP expression	[90]
18	Dieckol	E. cava	Albino rats	Decreased cancer cell proliferation	[95]

Table 1. Cont.

	Bioactive Compounds	Algal Sources	Cell Lines/In Vivo Models Involved	Functional Involvement	Ref.
19	Guaiane sesquiterpene	Ulva fasciata	MDA MB-231 breast cancer cell line	Direct interaction with kinase site of EGFR	[82]
20	Halogenated monoterpene, mertensene	Pterocladiella capillacea	HT-29 and LS174	ERK1/2, Akt, and NF B pathways	[78]
21	Ethanolic and methanolic extracts	Gracilaria tenuistipitata	Ca9-22 oral cancer cells	DNA damage	[88]
22	Methanolic extract	Plocamium telfairiae	HT-29 colon cancer cells	Induced caspase-dependent	[88]
23	Iodine and polyphenols	L. japonica	HT-29 colon cancer cells	Inhibition of SOD activity	[105]
24	Extract	Eucheuma cottonii	Cancer-induced rats	Upregulation of antioxidant enzymes, e.g., CAT, SOD, and GPx	[89]
25	Methanolic extracts	Fucus serratus and F. vesiculosus	Caco-2 cells	DNA damage	[106]
26	Methanolic extracts	Pelvetia canaliculata	Caco-2 cells	Inhibited H_2O_2-induced SOD depletion	[106]
27	Ethanol extracts	C. japonica	Caco-2 cells	Activating cellular antioxidant enzymes	[63]
28	Aqueous extract	G. tenuistipitata	H1299 cell line	Activating cellular antioxidant enzymes	[59]

3.3. Anti-Inflammatory Activity of Marine Algal Bioactive Metabolites

Inflammation is a molecular marker of carcinogenesis. Marine natural products are well-known anti-inflammatory agents due to their potent antioxidant activity. Several anti-inflammatory compounds with potential pharmacological applications have been isolated from marine algal sources. Macroalgae contain several polysaccharides, such as fucoidan, fucans, alginates, laminarin, agar, and carrageenans, which are used as prebiotic compounds and that can have potential application as anti-inflammatory agents. Marine-derived carotenoids and astaxanthin exhibit potent anti-inflammatory activity [108,109].

The anti-inflammatory activity of marine algae is due to the presence of PUFAs (e.g., omega-3) that potentiate inhibition of inflammation [27]. Several studies have demonstrated that omega-3 to 6 fatty acids reduce inflammation when taken as dietary supplements [27]. The polysaccharide extracted from *Turbinaria ornate*, *Delesseria sanguinea* exhibited anti-inflammatory potential in several in vitro systems. Sulfated polysaccharide fraction from *Gracilaria caudate*, a galactan from *Gelidium crinale*, a mucin-binding agglutinin from *Hypnea cervicornis*, lectin from *Pterocladiella capillacea*, and sulfated galactofucan from *Lobophora variegata* also exhibited anti-inflammatory potency [110]. Oral administration of marine polysaccharide in an in vivo mouse model reduced the initiation of inflammation [111].

The alga *Spirulina* had demonstrated anti-inflammatory effects when assessed using a non-alcoholic steatohepatitis model [112]. C-phycocyanin from *Spirulina platensis* blocked inflammation via inhibiting the expressions of nitric oxide synthase, cyclooxygenase-2, and production of pro-inflammatory cytokines [113,114]. Methanolic extracts of *Ulva lactuca* and *U. conglobate* have shown anti-inflammatory effects in murine hippocampal HT22 cell line [115]. Lycopene from *Chlorella marina* demonstrated anti-inflammatory effects in an arthritic rat model [116]. Phytosterols from *Dunaliella tertiolecta*, aqueous and methanolic extracts of *Caulerpa mexicana* and lectin from *Caulerpa cupressoides* exhibited anti-inflammatory activities in several in vitro models [117]. Ethanolic extract of *Ecklonia cava* inhibited LPS-induced inflammation in human endothelial cells [118]. Furthermore, *Ishige okamurae* showed anti-inflammatory effects in a few in vitro models [119]. The astaxanthin isolated from *Haematococcus pluvialis* reduced gastric inflammation in *Helicobacter pylori*-infected mice via decreasing bacterial density [120]. Moreover, astaxanthin reduced the production of pro-inflammatory mediators and cytokines such as nuclear factor-κB (NF-κB), tumor necrosis factor-α (TNF-α), and interleukin-6 (IL-6), and suppresses T lymphocyte activation in asthma patients [120]. Fucans from *Sargassum vulgare*, *Lobophora variegata*, and *Spatoglossum schroederi* also displayed anti-inflammatory effects [121]. Furthermore, Alginic acid from *Sargassum wightii* exhibited anti-inflammatory effects in vivo in a rat model [121].

Methanolic extract of *Bryothamnion triquetrum* exhibited an anti-inflammatory effect in Swiss albino mice [122]. Two fatty acids of *Gracilaria verrucosa* such as (E)-10-oxooctadec-8-enoic acid and (E)-9-oxooctadec-10-enoic acid inhibited the production of inflammatory markers, such as nitric oxide, IL-6, and TNF-α [123]. The sulfoglycolipidic isolated from the red alga *Porphyridium cruentum* exhibited an anti-inflammatory effect due to the presence of AA (6.8%), palmitic acid (26.1%), and EPA (16.6%), and omega-9 fatty acid (10.5%) [124]. Pheophytin from *Enteromorpha prolifera* has superoxide radical ($O_2^{\bullet-}$) reducing potential and inflammatory responses in mice [125,126]. A glycoprotein extracted from *Porphyra yezoensis* exhibited anti-inflammatory effects in LPS-stimulated macrophages [118]. Furthermore, phlorotannins (a polyphenol derived from *Eisenia bicyclis*, *Ecklonia cava*, and *Ecklonia kurome*), and sargachromanol G (derived from *Sargassum siliquastrum*) showed promising anti-inflammatory activity via inhibition of the production of inflammatory mediators in LPS-stimulated cells [127,128]. Moreover, methanolic extract of *Neorhodomela aculeata* inhibited ROS generation, H_2O_2-induced lipid peroxidation, and inducible nitric oxide synthase in neurological diseases via inhibition of inflammation [129].

3.4. Significance of Marine Algal Bioactive Metabolites as Anti-Diabetes Drugs

Diabetes mellitus is a chronic metabolic disorder which is characterized by high blood glucose levels that lead to renal dysfunction, cardiovascular diseases, and retinal damage [1]. Dietary management is a novel target for treating diabetes via maintaining the correct concentrations of both blood glucose and blood lipids [130]. Commercially available antidiabetic drugs exert several diseases-associated adverse side effects during treatments [131]. In this context, the identification of natural antidiabetic drugs with enhanced drug efficacy and lesser adverse effects has gained the attention of researchers in recent times. Marine algae-derived bioactive compounds exhibited antidiabetic properties furnished by regulation of various signaling pathways, such as inhibitory effect on enzymes such as α-amylase, α-glucosidase, aldose reductase, dipeptidyl peptidase-4, and protein tyrosine phosphatase 1B (PTP 1B) enzyme [132]. Enzymes like α-amylase and α-glucosidase play a significant role in the digestion of carbohydrates, leading to a delay in glucose absorption in blood and also to a reduction of glucose levels in blood plasma. Subsequently, these compounds may be exploited as potential functional food ingredients for preventing or diminishing insulin resistance and diabetes [132].

Marine algal compounds modulated the GLUT-4 and AMPK signaling pathways and triggered glucose tolerance [1]. Recent investigations displayed that fucoidan act as prebiotics and regulate the intercellular metabolism and blood sugar level [1]. Fucoidan isolated from *S. fusiforme* controlled the blood glucose level, recovered liver function, and inhibited oxidative stress in STZ-induced diabetic rats [133]. Fucoidan from *Ecklonia maxima* acted as a potent α-glucosidase inhibitor with a very low IC_{50} value (0.27–0.31 mg/mL) and regulated type II diabetes [134]. Fucoidan from *Fucus vesiculosus* displayed a robust α-glucosidase inhibitor in diabetes treatment [135]. Furthermore, low molecular weight fucoidan (LMWF) from *S. hemiphyllum* in combination with fucoxanthin displayed antidiabetic properties in type II diabetes rat model (db/db). The oral administration of LMWF in combination with fucoxanthin decreased blood glucose and fasting blood sugar levels [135]. The synergistic drug effect was more effective in the in vivo model via reduction of urinal sugar level as compared to the LMWF treatment alone. LMWF enhanced the hepatic glycogen concentration and antioxidant enzymes which were assisted by lipid metabolism. The lipid metabolism displayed the regulation of glucose transporter (GLUT), insulin receptor substrate (IRS-1), peroxisome proliferator-activated receptor-gamma (PPARγ), and uncoupling protein (UCP)-1 level with the treatment of LMWF in combination with fucoxanthin [135]. Fucoidan from *Cucumaria frondosa* amplified the expression of insulin receptor substrate 1, Glut-4, and PI3K/Akt, glucose transporter protein in insulin-resistant rats [1]. Fucoidan from *Saccarina japonica* abridged blood sugar level too [1,136].

Moreover, sulfated fucoidan isolated from *Undaria pinnatifida* inhibited hyperglycemia by eliciting insulin sensitivity in a diabetic mouse (C57BL/KSJ/db/db) model [137]. Fucoidan from *Sargassum wightii* inhibited alpha-D-glucosidase that transport glucose into the blood and reduce glucose level in blood [138]. Dieckol, fucodiphloroethol G, 6,6'-Bieckol, 7-phloroeckol, phlorofucofuroeckol A from *E. cava* and phloroglucinol, dioxinodehydroeckol, eckol from *E. stolonifera* and *E. bicyclis* displayed robust α-glucosidase activity and reduced blood sugar level [139–141]. Furthermore, dieckol-rich extract from *E. cava* improved insulin sensitivity [142]. Polyphenolic-rich extract from *I. okamurae* improved insulin sensitivity [143]. Moreover, polyphenolic-rich extract from *E. cava* inhibited glucose uptake effect in skeletal muscle [141]. Fucosterol from *Pelvetia siliquosa* reduced serum glucose concentration and inhibited sorbitol accumulation in the lenses in Sprague–Dawley diabetic rats [144]. Phlorotannin components from *Ascophyllum nodosum* displayed potential inhibition of α-amylase and α-glucosidase activities in in vitro models [145]. Sodium alginate from *Laminaria angustata* inhibited the rising blood glucose and insulin levels in Wistar rats [146]. Fucoxanthin and fucosterol from *Undaria pinnatifida* and *Ecklonia stolonifera* displayed aldose reductase inhibition [147,148]. Furthermore, pheophorbide-A, pheophytin-A also displayed aldose reductase inhibition [149]. Algal bioactive metabolites and their functional role in diabetes are summarized in Table 2.

Table 2. Marine algal bioactive metabolites and their functional role in diabetes.

	Algal Type	Algal Sources	Bioactive Metabolites	Functional Involvement	Ref.
1	Red algae	*Rhodomela confervoides*	HPN analogues	Inhibition of PTP 1B	[150]
2	Brown alga	*Ecklonia cava*	Methanolic extract	Increases phosphorylation AMP-activated protein kinase; radical scavenging property	[151]
3		*Isochrysis galbana*, *Nannochloropsis oculata*	DHA, EPA	Regulates glucose and lipid metabolism	[152]
4		*Palmaria*, *Ascophyllum*, *Alaria*	Phenol rich extract	Inhibitory of α-amylase and α-glucosidase	[145]
5	Brown algae		Polyphenols/Phlorotannins	Inhibition of α-glucosidase and α-amylase; increases skeletal muscle glucose uptake; inhibition of PTP 1B enzyme; increases insulin sensitivity.	[153]
6	Brown algae	*E. cava*	Dieckol	α-Glucosidase inhibitor [20]; postprandial hyperglycemia-lowering effect [7]; glucose uptake effect in skeletal muscle [40]; PTP 1B inhibition [10]; protective effect against diabetes complication	[139,140,154,155]
7	Brown algae	*E. cava*	Fucodiphloroethol G	α-Glucosidase inhibitor	[140]
8	Brown algae	*E. cava*	6,6′-Bieckol	α-Glucosidase inhibitor	[140]
9	Brown algae	*E. cava*	7-Phloroeckol	α-Glucosidase inhibitor; PTP 1B inhibition	[139,140]
10	Brown algae	*E. cava*	Phlorofucofuroeckol A	α-Glucosidase inhibitor; PTP 1B inhibition	[139,140]
11	Brown algae	*E. stolonifera* *E. bicyclis*	Phloroglucinol	α-Glucosidase inhibitor; PTP 1B inhibition	[139]
12	Brown algae	*E. stolonifera* *E. bicyclis*	Dioxinodehydroeckol	α-Glucosidase inhibitor; PTP 1B inhibition	[139]
13	Brown algae	*I. okamurae*	Diphlorethohydroxycarmalol	α-Glucosidase inhibitor; postprandial hyperglycemia-lowering effect; protective effect against diabetes complication	[156]
14	Brown algae	*E. stolonifera* *E. bicyclis*	Eckol	α-Glucosidase inhibitor; PTP 1B inhibition	[139]
15	Brown algae	*I. foliacea*	Octaphlorethol A	Glucose uptake effect in skeletal muscle	[142]
16	Brown algae	*A. nodosum* *F. vesiculosus*	Polyphenolic-rich extract	α-Glucosidase inhibitor; postprandial hyperglycemia-lowering effect	[145]
17	Brown algae	*E. cava*	Polyphenolic-rich extract	Glucose uptake effect in skeletal muscle	[141]
18	Brown algae	*E. cava*	Dieckol-rich extract	Improvement of insulin sensitivity	[142]
19	Brown algae	*I. okamurae*	Polyphenolic-rich extract	Improvement of insulin sensitivity	[143]
20	Brown algae	*Ulva rigida*	Ethanolic extract	Decreased blood glucose concentrations in Wistar diabetic rats	[157]
21		*Petретia siliquosa*	Fucosterol	Reduction of serum glucose levels and inhibition of sorbitol accumulation in the lenses in Sprague–Dawley diabetic rats	[144]
22	Brown algae	*Ecklonia cava*	Methanolic extract	Reduction in plasma glucose levels and increased insulin concentration; activation of AMPK/ACC and PI3/Akt signaling pathways in Sprague–Dawley diabetic rats	[141]

Table 2. Cont.

	Algal Type	Algal Sources	Bioactive Metabolites	Functional Involvement	Ref.
23	Green algae and Diatoms	*Chlorella* sp., *Nitzschia laevis*	Microalgal extracts	Inhibition of advanced glycation endproducts (AGEs) formation in in vitro models	[158]
24	Brown algae	*Ascophyllum nodosum*	Phlorotannin components	Inhibition of α-amylase and α-glucosidase activities in vitro	[145]
25	Brown algae	*Laminaria angustata*	Sodium alginate	Inhibition of rising blood glucose and insulin levels in Wistar rats	[146]
26	Brown algae	*Eisenia bicyclis*	Dioxinodehydroeckol	α-Glucosidase inhibitor	[159]
27	Brown algae	*Eisenia bicyclis*	7-Phloroeckol	PTP 1B inhibition; α-glucosidase inhibitor	[159]
28	Brown algae	*Eisenia bicyclis*	Fucoxanthin	Aldose reductase inhibition	[148]
29	Brown algae	*Ecklonia cava*	Dieckol	α-Glucosidase inhibitor	[160]
30	Brown algae	*Ecklonia cava*	Fucodiphloroethol G	α-Amylase inhibitor	[160]
31	Brown algae	*Ecklonia cava*	6,6′-Bieckol	PTP 1B inhibition	[160]
32	Brown algae	*Ecklonia cava*	7-Phloroeckol	ACE inhibitor	[160]
33	Brown algae	*Ecklonia cava*	2-Phloroeckol	α-Glucosidase inhibitor; α-glucosidase inhibitor; PTP 1B inhibition; aldose reductase inhibition; aldose reductase inhibition	[139,161]
34	Brown algae	*Ecklonia cava*	Phlorofucofuroeckol A	α-glucosidase inhibitor; PTP 1B inhibition; ACE inhibitor; AGEs inhibition; Aldose reductase inhibition	[139,162]
35	Brown algae	*Ecklonia stolonifera*	Phloroglucinol	α-glucosidase inhibitor	[153]
36	Brown algae	*Ecklonia stolonifera*	Eckol	PTP 1B inhibition α-glucosidase inhibitor	[153]
37	Brown algae	*Ecklonia stolonifera*	Dieckol	α-Amylase inhibitor; ACE inhibitor; PTP 1B inhibition; α-glucosidase inhibitor	[144,160]
38	Brown algae	*Ecklonia stolonifera*	Phlorofucofuroeckol A	α-Amylase inhibitor; PTP 1B inhibition; ACE inhibitor; α-glucosidase inhibitor	[144,160]
39	Brown algae	*Ecklonia stolonifera*	Fucosterol	PTP 1B inhibition; aldose reductase inhibition	[147]
40	Brown algae	*Ishige okamurae*	Diphlorethohydroxycarmalol	α-Glucosidase inhibitor; α-amylase inhibitor	[163]
41	Brown algae	*Myagropsis myagroides*	Eckol	α-Glucosidase inhibitor; α-amylase inhibitor	[153]
42	Brown algae	*Sargassum serratifolium*	Sargahydroquinoic acid	ACE inhibitor; PTP 1B inhibition	[164]
43	Brown algae	*Ascophyllum nodosum*	Methanol extract	α-Glucosidase inhibitor; α-amylase inhibitor	[145]
44	Brown algae	*Saccharina japonica*	Pheophorbide-A	Aldose reductase inhibition	[149]
45	Brown algae	*Saccharina japonica*	Pheophytin-A	Aldose reductase inhibition	[149]
46	Brown algae	*Undaria pinnatifida*	Fucoxanthin	Aldose reductase inhibition	[148]

4. Algal Metabolites as Prebiotics for Human Health with Special References to Fucoidan

Algal metabolite consumption, such as polysaccharides, sulfated polysaccharides, fucoidans, chlorophylls, phycobilins, fucoxanthins, carotenoids, polyphenols, and omega-3 fatty acids, decreases blood pressure and sugar level, and it can have antiviral, anti-inflammatory, anticancer, and neuroprotective effects, as well as act as immune boost-up. The immunomodulatory potential of prebiotics modulates immune fitness via several metabolic processes and interactions with the gut microbiota in humans [165]. The gut microbiota produces short-chain fatty acids (SCFA) such as propionate, acetate and butyrate by breaking down prebiotics and modulating the immune response [165]. Intravenous use of acetate amplified the activity of NK cells in cancer patients. In addition, it activated G protein-coupled receptors (GPR41 and GPR43) in rats, thus triggering mitogen-activated protein kinase (MAPK) signaling and modulating the transcription factors activity [166]. Acetate also increased the production of IL-10 in rats and prevented the inhibitory activity of butyrate on IL-2 production [167]. Daily administration of fucoidans from *A. nodosum* increased in *Lactobacillus* and *Ruminococcus* in the intestine of mice [168].

Fucoidan possesses a wide range of immune-modulation effects by stimulating activation of natural killer (NK) cells, dendritic cells (DCs), and T cells and increasing anti-tumor and anti-viral responses [169]. Fucoidan enhanced immune modulation via activation of macrophage facilitated by membrane receptors, such as TLR4, cluster of differentiation 14 (CD14), competent receptor-3 (CR-3), and scavenging receptor (SR). This led to signal transduction via MAPK and activation of transcription factors, and it also induced cytokines production, which regulates activation of NK cells and T lymphocytes [170]. In this regard, treatment of C57BL/6 rats with fucoidan extracted from *Fucus vesiculosus* up-regulated pro-inflammatory cytokines (IL-6, IL-12, and TNF-α) in serum and spleenocytes after 3 h of administration [171]. Furthermore, fucoidan from *L. cichorioides*, *L. Japonica*, and *F. evanescens* served as TLR ligands and their interaction with TLR-2 and TLR-4 receptors in vitro activated NF-jB. Furthermore, it also controlled the expression of the defense mechanisms of intrinsic immunity, such as secretion of chemokines, cytokines, and manifestation of MHC class I and II particles [1]. These are essential for the defense against foreign attackers and for activating adaptive immune systems. A clinical trial based on the diet supplementation of 1 g/day of fucoidan from *Undaria pinnatifida* on adult male and female volunteers for 24 weeks showed modulation of the immunity to seasonal influenza vaccine by antibody production [172]. Based on these reports, there are several evidences that fucoidan acts as a potent prebiotic and that it is able to modulate immunity. This is achieved by interacting with intestinal cells of the gut microbiota and direct motivation of immune cells through TLRs.

5. Conclusions and Future Perspectives

Natural extracts have been used since ancient times for treating various illnesses. Products from natural products have also provided a large number of pharmaceuticals, or their prototypes, in recent times. Among the many natural sources, marine algae can still play a pivotal role in human health and disease because of the need for novel drug candidates. Their extracts are already well-known in traditional medicine and more recent studies investigated the many beneficial effects of their secondary metabolites, such as reduction of oxidative stress and modulation of apoptosis, and the main findings of these researches are summarized in this review. The exploitation of these results might lead to the development of novel algal dietary supplements and pharmaceuticals for preventing and treating chronic malfunctions and other age-associated chronic diseases. For example, sulfated fucoidans have been shown to be potential candidates as new pharmaceuticals in fighting cancer and diabetes. However, despite the extensive use of algae-derived compounds and extracts in the food industry, there are still no FDA-approved anticancer, antioxidant, anti-inflammatory, and antidiabetic drugs. Technology transfer from the preclinical results to the clinical application of secondary metabolites extracted from marine algae is still in its infancy and not fully exploited and more clinical studies are needed to really evaluate the pharmaceutical efficacy algal compounds.

In conclusion, marine algae offer a great variety of bioactive molecules with potential health benefits. Several types of marine algae are already consumed as food additives and nutritional supplements, potentially exerting their beneficial effects through diet. There is, however, an impelling necessity of considering the algal bioactive compounds in new drug discovery programs and to investigate their biological effects in deeper detail in order to find new pharmaceuticals with preventive and therapeutic efficacy.

Author Contributions: Writing—original draft preparation, B.P., R.N., and S.P.; visualization, B.P. and B.P.J.; review and editing, A.R. and M.J. All authors have read and agreed to the published version of the manuscript.

Funding: This research was partially funded by "Tecnopolo per la medicina di precisione" (TecnoMed Puglia)—Regione Puglia: DGR n.2117 del 21/11/2018, CUP: B84I18000540002 and "Tecnopolo di Nanotecnologia e Fotonica per la medicina di precisione" (TECNOMED)—FISR/MIUR-CNR: delibera CIPE n.3449 del 7-08-2017, CUP: B83B17000010001.

Acknowledgments: The authors are thankful to Berhampur University for providing the necessary facilities to carry out this work. We are also thankful to Pradyot Kumar Behera for helping to draw the molecular structure of algal metabolites.

Conflicts of Interest: The authors declare no conflict of interest.

References

1. Pradhan, B.; Patra, S.; Nayak, R.; Behera, C.; Dash, S.R.; Nayak, S.; Sahu, B.B.; Bhutia, S.K.; Jena, M. Multifunctional role of fucoidan, sulfated polysaccharides in human health and disease: A journey under the sea in pursuit of potent therapeutic agents. *Int. J. Biol. Macromol.* **2020**, *164*, 4263–4278. [CrossRef] [PubMed]
2. World Health Organization. *Global Status Report on Alcohol and Health 2018*; World Health Organization: Geneve, Switzerland, 2018.
3. Balakumar, P.; Maung-U, K.; Jagadeesh, G. Prevalence and prevention of cardiovascular disease and diabetes mellitus. *Pharmacol. Res.* **2016**, *113*, 600–609. [CrossRef] [PubMed]
4. Adeloye, D.; Ige, J.O.; Aderemi, A.V.; Adeleye, N.; Amoo, E.O.; Auta, A.; Oni, G. Estimating the prevalence, hospitalisation and mortality from type 2 diabetes mellitus in Nigeria: A systematic review and meta-analysis. *BMJ Open* **2017**, *7*, e015424. [CrossRef]
5. Niemeijer, M.N.; van den Berg, M.E.; Leening, M.J.; Hofman, A.; Franco, O.H.; Deckers, J.W.; Heeringa, J.; Rijnbeek, P.R.; Stricker, B.H.; Eijgelsheim, M. Declining incidence of sudden cardiac death from 1990–2010 in a general middle-aged and elderly population: The Rotterdam Study. *Heart Rhythm* **2015**, *12*, 123–129. [CrossRef]
6. Wepner, B.; Giesecke, S. Drivers, trends and scenarios for the future of health in Europe. Impressions from the FRESHER project. *Eur. J. Futures Res.* **2018**, *6*, 2. [CrossRef]
7. Azab, A.; Nassar, A.; Azab, A.N. Anti-Inflammatory Activity of Natural Products. *Molecules* **2016**, *21*, 1321. [CrossRef] [PubMed]
8. Ragusa, A.; Centonze, C.; Grasso, M.E.; Latronico, M.F.; Mastrangelo, P.F.; Fanizzi, F.P.; Maffia, M. Composition and Statistical Analysis of Biophenols in Apulian Italian EVOOs. *Foods* **2017**, *6*, 90. [CrossRef]
9. Ragusa, A.; Centonze, C.; Grasso, M.E.; Latronico, M.F.; Mastrangelo, P.F.; Sparascio, F.; Fanizzi, F.P.; Maffia, M. A Comparative Study of Phenols in Apulian Italian Wines. *Foods* **2017**, *6*, 24. [CrossRef]
10. Ragusa, A.; Centonze, C.; Grasso, M.E.; Latronico, M.F.; Mastrangelo, P.F.; Sparascio, F.; Maffia, M. HPLC Analysis of Phenols in Negroamaro and Primitivo Red Wines from Salento. *Foods* **2019**, *8*, 45. [CrossRef]
11. Zafar, M.S.; Quarta, A.; Marradi, M.; Ragusa, A. Recent Developments in the Reduction of Oxidative Stress through Antioxidant Polymeric Formulations. *Pharmaceutics* **2019**, *11*, 505. [CrossRef]
12. Patra, S.; Praharaj, P.P.; Panigrahi, D.P.; Panda, B.; Bhol, C.S.; Mahapatra, K.K.; Mishra, S.R.; Behera, B.P.; Jena, M.; Sethi, G.; et al. Bioactive compounds from marine invertebrates as potent anticancer drugs: The possible pharmacophores modulating cell death pathways. *Mol. Biol. Rep.* **2020**, *47*, 7209–7228. [CrossRef] [PubMed]
13. Maharana, S.; Pradhan, B.; Jena, M.; Misra, M.K. Diversity of Phytoplankton in Chilika Lagoon, Odisha, India. *Environ. Ecol.* **2019**, *37*, 737–746.
14. Suleria, H.A.R.; Osborne, S.; Masci, P.; Gobe, G. Marine-based nutraceuticals: An innovative trend in the food and supplement industries. *Mar. Drugs* **2015**, *13*, 6336–6351. [CrossRef] [PubMed]
15. Tanna, B.; Mishra, A. Metabolites unravel nutraceutical potential of edible seaweeds: An emerging source of functional food. *Compr. Rev. Food Sci. Food Saf.* **2018**, *17*, 1613–1624. [CrossRef] [PubMed]
16. Mohanty, S.; Pradhan, B.; Patra, S.; Behera, C.; Nayak, R.; Jena, M. Screening for nutritive bioactive compounds in some algal strains isolated from coastal Odisha. *J. Adv. Plant Sci.* **2020**, *10*, 1–8.

17. Miranda, J.M.; Trigo, M.; Barros-Velázquez, J.; Aubourg, S.P. Effect of an icing medium containing the alga Fucus spiralis on the microbiological activity and lipid oxidation in chilled megrim (Lepidorhombus whiffiagonis). *Food Control* **2016**, *59*, 290–297. [CrossRef]
18. Barros-Velázquez, J.; Miranda, J.M.; Ezquerra-Brauer, J.M.; Aubourg, S.P. Impact of icing systems with aqueous, ethanolic and ethanolic-aqueous extracts of alga Fucus spiralis on microbial and biochemical quality of chilled hake (Merluccius merluccius). *Int. J. Food Sci. Technol.* **2016**, *51*, 2081–2089. [CrossRef]
19. Conlon, M.A.; Bird, A.R. The impact of diet and lifestyle on gut microbiota and human health. *Nutrients* **2015**, *7*, 17–44. [CrossRef]
20. Patra, S.; Pradhan, B.; Nayak, R.; Behera, C.; Rout, L.; Jena, M.; Efferth, T.; Bhutia, S.K. Chemotherapeutic efficacy of curcumin and resveratrol against cancer: Chemoprevention, chemoprotection, drug synergism and clinical pharmacokinetics. *Semin. Cancer Biol.* **2020**. [CrossRef]
21. Ibañez, E.; Herrero, M.; Mendiola, J.A.; Castro-Puyana, M. Extraction and characterization of bioactive compounds with health benefits from marine resources: Macro and micro algae, cyanobacteria, and invertebrates. In *Marine Bioactive Compounds*; Springer: Boston, MA, USA, 2012; pp. 55–98.
22. Lordan, S.; Ross, R.P.; Stanton, C. Marine bioactives as functional food ingredients: Potential to reduce the incidence of chronic diseases. *Mar. Drugs* **2011**, *9*, 1056–1100. [CrossRef]
23. Bocanegra, A.; Bastida, S.; Benedí, J.; Rodenas, S.; Sanchez-Muniz, F.J. Characteristics and nutritional and cardiovascular-health properties of seaweeds. *J. Med. Food* **2009**, *12*, 236–258. [CrossRef] [PubMed]
24. Taboada, C.; Millán, R.; Míguez, I. Composition, nutritional aspects and effect on serum parameters of marine algae Ulva rigida. *J. Sci. Food Agric.* **2010**, *90*, 445–449. [PubMed]
25. Ruxton, C.; Reed, S.C.; Simpson, M.; Millington, K. The health benefits of omega-3 polyunsaturated fatty acids: A review of the evidence. *J. Hum. Nutr. Diet.* **2004**, *17*, 449–459. [CrossRef] [PubMed]
26. Zheng, J.-S.; Hu, X.-J.; Zhao, Y.-M.; Yang, J.; Li, D. Intake of fish and marine n-3 polyunsaturated fatty acids and risk of breast cancer: Meta-analysis of data from 21 independent prospective cohort studies. *BMJ* **2013**, *346*, f3706. [CrossRef] [PubMed]
27. Wall, R.; Ross, R.P.; Fitzgerald, G.F.; Stanton, C. Fatty acids from fish: The anti-inflammatory potential of long-chain omega-3 fatty acids. *Nutr. Rev.* **2010**, *68*, 280–289. [CrossRef]
28. Fleurence, J.; Gutbier, G.; Mabeau, S.; Leray, C. Fatty acids from 11 marine macroalgae of the French Brittany coast. *J. Appl. Phycol.* **1994**, *6*, 527–532. [CrossRef]
29. Sánchez-Machado, D.; López-Cervantes, J.; Lopez-Hernandez, J.; Paseiro-Losada, P. Fatty acids, total lipid, protein and ash contents of processed edible seaweeds. *Food Chem.* **2004**, *85*, 439–444. [CrossRef]
30. Rodríguez-Meizoso, I.; Jaime, L.; Santoyo, S.; Señoráns, F.J.; Cifuentes, A.; Ibáñez, E. Subcritical water extraction and characterization of bioactive compounds from Haematococcus pluvialis microalga. *J. Pharm. Biomed. Anal.* **2010**, *51*, 456–463. [CrossRef]
31. Bouzidi, N.; Viano, Y.; Ortalo-Magne, A.; Seridi, H.; Alliche, Z.; Daghbouche, Y.; Culioli, G.; El Hattab, M. Sterols from the brown alga Cystoseira foeniculacea: Degradation of fucosterol into saringosterol epimers. *Arab. J. Chem.* **2019**, *12*, 1474–1478. [CrossRef]
32. Menshova, R.V.; Ermakova, S.P.; Anastyuk, S.D.; Isakov, V.V.; Dubrovskaya, Y.V.; Kusaykin, M.I.; Um, B.-H.; Zvyagintseva, T.N. Structure, enzymatic transformation and anticancer activity of branched high molecular weight laminaran from brown alga Eisenia bicyclis. *Carbohydr. Polym.* **2014**, *99*, 101–109. [CrossRef]
33. Pereira, L.; Bahcevandziev, K.; Joshi, N.H. *Seaweeds as Plant Fertilizer, Agricultural Biostimulants and Animal Fodder*; CRC Press: Boca Raton, FL, USA, 2019.
34. Mohamed, S.; Hashim, S.N.; Rahman, H.A. Seaweeds: A sustainable functional food for complementary and alternative therapy. *Trends Food Sci. Technol.* **2012**, *23*, 83–96. [CrossRef]
35. Lahaye, M. Marine algae as sources of fibres: Determination of soluble and insoluble dietary fibre contents in some 'sea vegetables'. *J. Sci. Food Agric.* **1991**, *54*, 587–594. [CrossRef]
36. Mišurcová, L.; Škrovánková, S.; Samek, D.; Ambrožová, J.; Machů, L. Health benefits of algal polysaccharides in human nutrition. In *Advances in Food and Nutrition Research*; Elsevier: Amsterdam, The Netherlands, 2012; Volume 66, pp. 75–145.
37. Jiménez-Escrig, A.; Sánchez-Muniz, F. Dietary fibre from edible seaweeds: Chemical structure, physicochemical properties and effects on cholesterol metabolism. *Nutr. Res.* **2000**, *20*, 585–598. [CrossRef]
38. Wijesinghe, W.; Jeon, Y.-J. Biological activities and potential industrial applications of fucose rich sulfated polysaccharides and fucoidans isolated from brown seaweeds: A review. *Carbohydr. Polym.* **2012**, *88*, 13–20. [CrossRef]
39. Becker, W. Microalgae in human and animal nutrition. In *Handbook of Microalgal Culture: Biotechnology and Applied Phycology*; Richmond, A., Ed.; Wiley Online Library: Hoboken, NJ, USA, 2004; pp. 312–351.
40. Pugh, N.; Ross, S.A.; ElSohly, H.N.; ElSohly, M.A.; Pasco, D.S. Isolation of three high molecular weight polysaccharide preparations with potent immunostimulatory activity from Spirulina platensis, Aphanizomenon flos-aquae and Chlorella pyrenoidosa. *Planta Med.* **2001**, *67*, 737–742. [CrossRef]
41. Shao, B.; Wang, Z.; Liu, X.; Yu, J.; Lan, J.; Wang, J.; Ma, L.; Chen, Z. Breeding of a Chlorella strain with high yield of polysaccharide and its effect on growth and immunoregulation of Litopenaeus vannamei. *J. Nucl. Agric. Sci.* **2013**, *27*, 168–172.
42. Bravo, L. Polyphenols: Chemistry, dietary sources, metabolism, and nutritional significance. *Nutr. Rev.* **1998**, *56*, 317–333. [CrossRef]

43. Fernando, I.S.; Kim, M.; Son, K.-T.; Jeong, Y.; Jeon, Y.-J. Antioxidant activity of marine algal polyphenolic compounds: A mechanistic approach. *J. Med. Food* **2016**, *19*, 615–628. [CrossRef]
44. Faulks, R.M.; Southon, S. Challenges to understanding and measuring carotenoid bioavailability. *Biochim. Biophys. Acta (BBA) Mol. Basis Dis.* **2005**, *1740*, 95–100. [CrossRef]
45. Matos, J.; Cardoso, C.; Bandarra, N.; Afonso, C. Microalgae as healthy ingredients for functional food: A review. *Food Funct.* **2017**, *8*, 2672–2685. [CrossRef]
46. Kim, S.-K.; Taylor, S. *Marine Medicinal Foods: Implications and Applications, Macro and Microalgae*; Academic Press: Cambridge, MA, USA, 2011; Volume 64.
47. Circuncisão, A.R.; Catarino, M.D.; Cardoso, S.M.; Silva, A. Minerals from macroalgae origin: Health benefits and risks for consumers. *Mar. Drugs* **2018**, *16*, 400. [CrossRef]
48. Rupérez, P. Mineral content of edible marine seaweeds. *Food Chem.* **2002**, *79*, 23–26. [CrossRef]
49. Kini, S.; Divyashree, M.; Mani, M.K.; Mamatha, B.S. Algae and cyanobacteria as a source of novel bioactive compounds for biomedical applications. In *Advances in Cyanobacterial Biology*; Elsevier: Amsterdam, The Netherlands, 2020; pp. 173–194.
50. Shahidi, F. Functional foods: Their role in health promotion and disease prevention. *J. Food Sci.* **2004**, *69*, R146–R149. [CrossRef]
51. Sharma, N.; Khanra, A.; Rai, M.P. Potential applications of antioxidants from algae in human health. In *Oxidative Stress: Diagnostic Methods and Applications in Medical Science*; Springer: Berlin, Germany, 2017; pp. 153–168.
52. Bayr, H. Reactive oxygen species. *Crit. Care Med.* **2005**, *33*, S498–S501. [CrossRef] [PubMed]
53. Halliwell, B. Free radicals and other reactive species in disease. *eLS* **2001**. [CrossRef]
54. Storz, P. Reactive oxygen species in tumor progression. *Front. Biosci.* **2005**, *10*, 1881–1896. [CrossRef] [PubMed]
55. Halliwell, B. Reactive species and antioxidants. Redox biology is a fundamental theme of aerobic life. *Plant Physiol.* **2006**, *141*, 312–322. [CrossRef]
56. Gechev, T.S.; Van Breusegem, F.; Stone, J.M.; Denev, I.; Laloi, C. Reactive oxygen species as signals that modulate plant stress responses and programmed cell death. *Bioessays* **2006**, *28*, 1091–1101. [CrossRef]
57. Ribeiro, J.S.; Santos, M.J.M.C.; Silva, L.K.R.; Pereira, L.C.L.; Santos, I.A.; da Silva Lannes, S.C.; da Silva, M.V. Natural antioxidants used in meat products: A brief review. *Meat Sci.* **2019**, *148*, 181–188. [CrossRef]
58. Estrada, J.P.; Bescós, P.B.; Del Fresno, A.V. Antioxidant activity of different fractions of *Spirulina platensis* protean extract. *IL Farmaco* **2001**, *56*, 497–500. [CrossRef]
59. Chakraborty, K.; Paulraj, R. Sesquiterpenoids with free-radical-scavenging properties from marine macroalga Ulva fasciata Delile. *Food Chem.* **2010**, *122*, 31–41. [CrossRef]
60. Meenakshi, S.; Gnanambigai, D.M.; Mozhi, S.T.; Arumugam, M.; Balasubramanian, T. Total flavanoid and in vitro antioxidant activity of two seaweeds of Rameshwaram coast. *Glob. J. Pharm.* **2009**, *3*, 59–62.
61. Balaji Raghavendra Rao, H.; Sathivel, A.; Devaki, T. Antihepatotoxic nature of Ulva reticulata (Chlorophyceae) on acetaminophen-induced hepatoxicity in experimental rats. *J. Med. Food* **2004**, *7*, 495–497. [CrossRef] [PubMed]
62. Shibata, T.; Ishimaru, K.; Kawaguchi, S.; Yoshikawa, H.; Hama, Y. Antioxidant activities of phlorotannins isolated from Japanese Laminariaceae. In Proceedings of the Nineteenth International Seaweed Symposium, Kobe, Japan, 26–31 March 2007; Borowitzka, M.A., Critchley, A.T., Kraan, S., Peters, A., Sjøtun, K., Notoya, M., Eds.; Springer: Amsterdam, The Netherlands, 2009; pp. 255–261.
63. Kang, K.A.; Bu, H.D.; Park, D.S.; Go, G.M.; Jee, Y.; Shin, T.; Hyun, J.W. Antioxidant activity of ethanol extract of Callophyllis japonica. *Phytother. Res.* **2005**, *19*, 506–510. [CrossRef] [PubMed]
64. Yang, J.-I.; Yeh, C.-C.; Lee, J.-C.; Yi, S.-C.; Huang, H.-W.; Tseng, C.-N.; Chang, H.-W. Aqueous extracts of the edible Gracilaria tenuistipitata are protective against H2O2-induced DNA damage, growth inhibition, and cell cycle arrest. *Molecules* **2012**, *17*, 7241–7254. [CrossRef]
65. Avendaño, C.; Menendez, J.C. *Medicinal Chemistry of Anticancer Drugs*; Elsevier: Amsterdam, The Netherlands, 2015.
66. Kalimuthu, S.; Se-Kwon, K. Cell survival and apoptosis signaling as therapeutic target for cancer: Marine bioactive compounds. *Int. J. Mol. Sci.* **2013**, *14*, 2334–2354. [CrossRef]
67. Pradhan, B.; Patra, S.; Behera, C.; Nayak, R.; Patil, S.; Bhutia, S.K.; Jena, M. Enteromorpha compressa extract induces anticancer activity through apoptosis and autophagy in oral cancer. *Mol. Biol. Rep.* **2020**. [CrossRef]
68. Talero, E.; García-Mauriño, S.; Ávila-Román, J.; Rodríguez-Luna, A.; Alcaide, A.; Motilva, V. Bioactive compounds isolated from microalgae in chronic inflammation and cancer. *Mar. Drugs* **2015**, *13*, 6152–6209. [CrossRef]
69. Dore, C.M.P.G.; Alves, M.G.C.F.; Santos, N.D.; Cruz, A.K.M.; Câmara, R.B.G.; Castro, A.J.G.; Alves, L.G.; Nader, H.B.; Leite, E.L. Antiangiogenic activity and direct antitumor effect from a sulfated polysaccharide isolated from seaweed. *Microvasc. Res.* **2013**, *88*, 12–18. [CrossRef]
70. Kang, Y.; Wang, Z.-J.; Xie, D.; Sun, X.; Yang, W.; Zhao, X.; Xu, N. Characterization and potential antitumor activity of polysaccharide from Gracilariopsis lemaneiformis. *Mar. Drugs* **2017**, *15*, 100. [CrossRef]
71. Ropellato, J.; Carvalho, M.M.; Ferreira, L.G.; Noseda, M.D.; Zuconelli, C.R.; Gonçalves, A.G.; Ducatti, D.R.; Kenski, J.C.; Nasato, P.L.; Winnischofer, S.M. Sulfated heterorhamnans from the green seaweed Gayralia oxysperma: Partial depolymerization, chemical structure and antitumor activity. *Carbohydr. Polym.* **2015**, *117*, 476–485. [CrossRef] [PubMed]
72. Synytsya, A.; Kim, W.-J.; Kim, S.-M.; Pohl, R.; Synytsya, A.; Kvasnička, F.; Čopíková, J.; Park, Y.I. Structure and antitumour activity of fucoidan isolated from sporophyll of Korean brown seaweed Undaria pinnatifida. *Carbohydr. Polym.* **2010**, *81*, 41–48. [CrossRef]

73. Rui, X.; Pan, H.-F.; Shao, S.-L.; Xu, X.-M. Anti-tumor and anti-angiogenic effects of Fucoidan on prostate cancer: Possible JAK-STAT3 pathway. *BMC Complement. Altern. Med.* **2017**, *17*, 378. [CrossRef] [PubMed]
74. Park, H.Y.; Park, S.-H.; Jeong, J.-W.; Yoon, D.; Han, M.H.; Lee, D.-S.; Choi, G.; Yim, M.-J.; Lee, J.M.; Kim, D.-H. Induction of p53-independent apoptosis and G1 cell cycle arrest by fucoidan in HCT116 human colorectal carcinoma cells. *Mar. Drugs* **2017**, *15*, 154. [CrossRef] [PubMed]
75. Suganya, A.M.; Sanjivkumar, M.; Chandran, M.N.; Palavesam, A.; Immanuel, G. Pharmacological importance of sulphated polysaccharide carrageenan from red seaweed Kappaphycus alvarezii in comparison with commercial carrageenan. *Biomed. Pharmacother.* **2016**, *84*, 1300–1312. [CrossRef]
76. Kong, C.-S.; Kim, J.-A.; Yoon, N.-Y.; Kim, S.-K. Induction of apoptosis by phloroglucinol derivative from Ecklonia cava in MCF-7 human breast cancer cells. *Food Chem. Toxicol.* **2009**, *47*, 1653–1658. [CrossRef]
77. Corona, G.; Coman, M.; Spencer, J.; Rowland, I. Digested and fermented seaweed phlorotannins reduce DNA damage and inhibit growth of HT-29 colon cancer cells. *Proc. Nutr. Soc.* **2014**, *73*, E31. [CrossRef]
78. Antunes, E.M.; Afolayan, A.F.; Chiwakata, M.T.; Fakee, J.; Knott, M.G.; Whibley, C.E.; Hendricks, D.T.; Bolton, J.J.; Beukes, D.R. Identification and in vitro anti-esophageal cancer activity of a series of halogenated monoterpenes isolated from the South African seaweeds Plocamium suhrii and Plocamium cornutum. *Phytochemistry* **2011**, *72*, 769–772. [CrossRef]
79. Hosokawa, M.; Kudo, M.; Maeda, H.; Kohno, H.; Tanaka, T.; Miyashita, K. Fucoxanthin induces apoptosis and enhances the antiproliferative effect of the PPARγ ligand, troglitazone, on colon cancer cells. *Biochim. Biophys. Acta (BBA) Gen. Subj.* **2004**, *1675*, 113–119. [CrossRef]
80. Ishikawa, C.; Tafuku, S.; Kadekaru, T.; Sawada, S.; Tomita, T.; Okudaira, T.; Nakazato, T.; Toda, T.; Uchihara, J.N.; Taira, N. Antiadult T-cell leukemia effects of brown algae fucoxanthin and its deacetylated product, fucoxanthinol. *Int. J. Cancer* **2008**, *123*, 2702–2712. [CrossRef]
81. Terasaki, M.; Maeda, H.; Miyashita, K.; Tanaka, T.; Miyamoto, S.; Mutoh, M. A marine bio-functional lipid, fucoxanthinol, attenuates human colorectal cancer stem-like cell tumorigenicity and sphere formation. *J. Clin. Biochem. Nutr.* **2017**, 16–112. [CrossRef]
82. Lakshmi, T.P.; Vajravijayan, S.; Moumita, M.; Sakthivel, N.; Gunasekaran, K.; Krishna, R. A novel guaiane sesquiterpene derivative, guai-2-en-10α-ol, from Ulva fasciata Delile inhibits EGFR/PI3K/Akt signaling and induces cytotoxicity in triple-negative breast cancer cells. *Mol. Cell. Biochem.* **2018**, *438*, 123–139. [CrossRef]
83. Lee, J.-C.; Hou, M.-F.; Huang, H.-W.; Chang, F.-R.; Yeh, C.-C.; Tang, J.-Y.; Chang, H.-W. Marine algal natural products with anti-oxidative, anti-inflammatory, and anti-cancer properties. *Cancer Cell Int.* **2013**, *13*, 1–7. [CrossRef]
84. Zandi, K.; Tajbakhsh, S.; Nabipour, I.; Rastian, Z.; Yousefi, F.; Sharafian, S.; Sartavi, K. In vitro antitumor activity of Gracilaria corticata (a red alga) against Jurkat and molt-4 human cancer cell lines. *Afr. J. Biotechnol.* **2010**, *9*, 6787–6790.
85. Zandi, K.; Ahmadzadeh, S.; Tajbakhsh, S.; Rastian, Z.; Yousefi, F.; Farshadpour, F.; Sartavi, K. Anticancer activity of Sargassum oligocystum water extract against human cancer cell lines. *Eur. Rev. Med Pharmacol. Sci.* **2010**, *14*, 669–673.
86. Yeh, C.-C.; Tseng, C.-N.; Yang, J.-I.; Huang, H.-W.; Fang, Y.; Tang, J.-Y.; Chang, F.-R.; Chang, H.-W. Antiproliferation and induction of apoptosis in Ca9-22 oral cancer cells by ethanolic extract of Gracilaria tenuistipitata. *Molecules* **2012**, *17*, 10916–10927. [CrossRef]
87. Yeh, C.-C.; Yang, J.-I.; Lee, J.-C.; Tseng, C.-N.; Chan, Y.-C.; Hseu, Y.-C.; Tang, J.-Y.; Chuang, L.-Y.; Huang, H.-W.; Chang, F.-R. Anti-proliferative effect of methanolic extract of Gracilaria tenuistipitata on oral cancer cells involves apoptosis, DNA damage, and oxidative stress. *BMC Complement. Altern. Med.* **2012**, *12*, 142. [CrossRef]
88. Kim, J.-Y.; Yoon, M.-Y.; Cha, M.-R.; Hwang, J.-H.; Park, E.; Choi, S.-U.; Park, H.-R.; Hwang, Y.-I. Methanolic extracts of Plocamium telfairiae induce cytotoxicity and caspase-dependent apoptosis in HT-29 human colon carcinoma cells. *J. Med. Food* **2007**, *10*, 587–593. [CrossRef]
89. Namvar, F.; Mohamed, S.; Fard, S.G.; Behravan, J.; Mustapha, N.M.; Alitheen, N.B.M.; Othman, F. Polyphenol-rich seaweed (Eucheuma cottonii) extract suppresses breast tumour via hormone modulation and apoptosis induction. *Food Chem.* **2012**, *130*, 376–382. [CrossRef]
90. Kim, K.-N.; Ahn, G.; Heo, S.-J.; Kang, S.-M.; Kang, M.-C.; Yang, H.-M.; Kim, D.; Roh, S.W.; Kim, S.-K.; Jeon, B.-T. Inhibition of tumor growth in vitro and in vivo by fucoxanthin against melanoma B16F10 cells. *Environ. Toxicol. Pharmacol.* **2013**, *35*, 39–46. [CrossRef]
91. Das, S.K.; Hashimoto, T.; Shimizu, K.; Yoshida, T.; Sakai, T.; Sowa, Y.; Komoto, A.; Kanazawa, K. Fucoxanthin induces cell cycle arrest at G0/G1 phase in human colon carcinoma cells through up-regulation of p21WAF1/Cip1. *Biochim. Biophys. Acta (BBA) Gen. Subj.* **2005**, *1726*, 328–335. [CrossRef] [PubMed]
92. Satomi, Y. Fucoxanthin induces GADD45A expression and G1 arrest with SAPK/JNK activation in LNCap human prostate cancer cells. *Anticancer Res.* **2012**, *32*, 807–813. [PubMed]
93. Cho, M.; Park, G.-M.; Kim, S.-N.; Amna, T.; Lee, S.; Shin, W.-S. Glioblastoma-specific anticancer activity of pheophorbide a from the edible red seaweed Grateloupia elliptica. *J. Microbiol. Biotechnol.* **2014**, *24*, 346–353. [CrossRef]
94. Koyanagi, S.; Tanigawa, N.; Nakagawa, H.; Soeda, S.; Shimeno, H. Oversulfation of fucoidan enhances its anti-angiogenic and antitumor activities. *Biochem. Pharmacol.* **2003**, *65*, 173–179. [CrossRef]
95. Sadeeshkumar, V.; Duraikannu, A.; Ravichandran, S.; Kodisundaram, P.; Fredrick, W.S.; Gobalakrishnan, R. Modulatory efficacy of dieckol on xenobiotic-metabolizing enzymes, cell proliferation, apoptosis, invasion and angiogenesis during NDEA-induced rat hepatocarcinogenesis. *Mol. Cell. Biochem.* **2017**, *433*, 195–204. [CrossRef]

96. Xue, M.; Ji, X.; Xue, C.; Liang, H.; Ge, Y.; He, X.; Zhang, L.; Bian, K.; Zhang, L. Caspase-dependent and caspase-independent induction of apoptosis in breast cancer by fucoidan via the PI3K/AKT/GSK3β pathway in vivo and in vitro. *Biomed. Pharmacother.* **2017**, *94*, 898–908. [CrossRef] [PubMed]
97. Abd-Ellatef, G.-E.F.; Ahmed, O.M.; Abdel-Reheim, E.S.; Abdel-Hamid, A.-H.Z. Ulva lactuca polysaccharides prevent Wistar rat breast carcinogenesis through the augmentation of apoptosis, enhancement of antioxidant defense system, and suppression of inflammation. *Breast Cancer Targets Ther.* **2017**, *9*, 67.
98. Lins, K.O.; Bezerra, D.P.; Alves, A.P.N.; Alencar, N.M.; Lima, M.W.; Torres, V.M.; Farias, W.R.; Pessoa, C.; de Moraes, M.O.; Costa-Lotufo, L.V. Antitumor properties of a sulfated polysaccharide from the red seaweed Champia feldmannii (Diaz-Pifferer). *J. Appl. Toxicol.* **2009**, *29*, 20–26. [CrossRef]
99. Wang, Z.-J.; Xu, W.; Liang, J.-W.; Wang, C.-S.; Kang, Y. Effect of fucoidan on B16 murine melanoma cell melanin formation and apoptosis. *Afr. J. Tradit. Complement. Altern. Med.* **2017**, *14*, 149–155. [CrossRef]
100. Kang, Y.; Li, H.; Wu, J.; Xu, X.; Sun, X.; Zhao, X.; Xu, N. Transcriptome profiling reveals the antitumor mechanism of polysaccharide from marine algae Gracilariopsis lemaneiformis. *PLoS ONE* **2016**, *11*, e0158279. [CrossRef]
101. Teruya, T.; Konishi, T.; Uechi, S.; Tamaki, H.; Tako, M. Anti-proliferative activity of oversulfated fucoidan from commercially cultured Cladosiphon okamuranus TOKIDA in U937 cells. *Int. J. Biol. Macromol.* **2007**, *41*, 221–226. [CrossRef] [PubMed]
102. Kim, E.J.; Park, S.Y.; Lee, J.-Y.; Park, J.H.Y. Fucoidan present in brown algae induces apoptosis of human colon cancer cells. *BMC Gastroenterol.* **2010**, *10*, 96. [CrossRef] [PubMed]
103. Kim, I.H.; Kwon, M.J.; Nam, T.J. Differences in cell death and cell cycle following fucoidan treatment in high-density HT-29 colon cancer cells. *Mol. Med. Rep.* **2017**, *15*, 4116–4122. [CrossRef] [PubMed]
104. Park, H.-K.; Kim, I.-H.; Kim, J.; Nam, T.-J. Induction of apoptosis and the regulation of ErbB signaling by laminarin in HT-29 human colon cancer cells. *Int. J. Mol. Med.* **2013**, *32*, 291–295. [CrossRef] [PubMed]
105. Jung, H.A.; Jung, H.J.; Jeong, H.Y.; Kwon, H.J.; Ali, M.Y.; Choi, J.S. Phlorotannins isolated from the edible brown alga Ecklonia stolonifera exert anti-adipogenic activity on 3T3-L1 adipocytes by downregulating C/EBPα and PPARγ. *Fitoterapia* **2014**, *92*, 260–269. [CrossRef]
106. O'sullivan, A.; O'callaghan, Y.; O'grady, M.; Queguineur, B.; Hanniffy, D.; Troy, D.; Kerry, J.; O'brien, N. In vitro and cellular antioxidant activities of seaweed extracts prepared from five brown seaweeds harvested in spring from the west coast of Ireland. *Food Chem.* **2011**, *126*, 1064–1070. [CrossRef]
107. Ermakova, S.; Sokolova, R.; Kim, S.-M.; Um, B.-H.; Isakov, V.; Zvyagintseva, T. Fucoidans from brown seaweeds Sargassum hornery, Eclonia cava, Costaria costata: Structural characteristics and anticancer activity. *Appl. Biochem. Biotechnol.* **2011**, *164*, 841–850. [CrossRef]
108. Abad, M.J.; Bedoya, L.M.; Bermejo, P. Natural marine anti-inflammatory products. *Mini Rev. Med. Chem.* **2008**, *8*, 740–754. [CrossRef]
109. D'Orazio, N.; Gammone, M.A.; Gemello, E.; De Girolamo, M.; Cusenza, S.; Riccioni, G. Marine bioactives: Pharmacological properties and potential applications against inflammatory diseases. *Mar. Drugs* **2012**, *10*, 812–833. [CrossRef]
110. Chaves, L.d.S.; Nicolau, L.A.D.; Silva, R.O.; Barros, F.C.N.; Freitas, A.L.P.; Aragão, K.S.; Ribeiro, R.d.A.; Souza, M.H.L.P.; Barbosa, A.L.d.R.; Medeiros, J.-V.R. Antiinflammatory and antinociceptive effects in mice of a sulfated polysaccharide fraction extracted from the marine red algae Gracilaria caudata. *Immunopharmacol. Immunotoxicol.* **2013**, *35*, 93–100. [CrossRef]
111. Ananthi, S.; Raghavendran, H.R.B.; Sunil, A.G.; Gayathri, V.; Ramakrishnan, G.; Vasanthi, H.R. In vitro antioxidant and in vivo anti-inflammatory potential of crude polysaccharide from Turbinaria ornata (Marine Brown Alga). *Food Chem. Toxicol.* **2010**, *48*, 187–192. [CrossRef] [PubMed]
112. Ku, C.S.; Pham, T.X.; Park, Y.; Kim, B.; Shin, M.S.; Kang, I.; Lee, J. Edible blue-green algae reduce the production of pro-inflammatory cytokines by inhibiting NF-κB pathway in macrophages and splenocytes. *Biochim. Biophys. Acta (BBA) Gen. Subj.* **2013**, *1830*, 2981–2988. [CrossRef] [PubMed]
113. Romay, C.; Armesto, J.; Remirez, D.; Gonzalez, R.; Ledon, N.; Garcia, I. Antioxidant and anti-inflammatory properties of C-phycocyanin from blue-green algae. *Inflamm. Res.* **1998**, *47*, 36–41. [CrossRef] [PubMed]
114. Shih, C.-M.; Cheng, S.-N.; Wong, C.-H.; Kuo, Y.-L.; Chou, T.-C. Antiinflammatory and antihyperalgesic activity of C-phycocyanin. *Anesth. Analg.* **2009**, *108*, 1303–1310. [CrossRef]
115. Jin, D.-Q.; Lim, C.S.; Sung, J.-Y.; Choi, H.G.; Ha, I.; Han, J.-S. Ulva conglobata, a marine algae, has neuroprotective and anti-inflammatory effects in murine hippocampal and microglial cells. *Neurosci. Lett.* **2006**, *402*, 154–158. [CrossRef]
116. Renju, G.; Muraleedhara Kurup, G.; Saritha Kumari, C. Anti-inflammatory activity of lycopene isolated from Chlorella marina on Type II Collagen induced arthritis in Sprague Dawley rats. *Immunopharmacol. Immunotoxicol.* **2013**, *35*, 282–291. [CrossRef]
117. Caroprese, M.; Albenzio, M.; Ciliberti, M.G.; Francavilla, M.; Sevi, A. A mixture of phytosterols from Dunaliella tertiolecta affects proliferation of peripheral blood mononuclear cells and cytokine production in sheep. *Vet. Immunol. Immunopathol.* **2012**, *150*, 27–35. [CrossRef]
118. Shin, E.-S.; Hwang, H.-J.; Kim, I.-H.; Nam, T.-J. A glycoprotein from Porphyra yezoensis produces anti-inflammatory effects in liposaccharide-stimulated macrophages via the TLR4 signaling pathway. *Int. J. Mol. Med.* **2011**, *28*, 809–815.
119. Kim, M.M.; Rajapakse, N.; Kim, S.K. Anti-inflammatory effect of Ishige okamurae ethanolic extract via inhibition of NF-κB transcription factor in RAW 264.7 cells. *Phytother. Res. Int. J. Devoted Pharmacol. Toxicol. Eval. Nat. Prod. Deriv.* **2009**, *23*, 628–634.

120. Kim, S.H.; Lim, J.W.; Kim, H. Astaxanthin inhibits mitochondrial dysfunction and interleukin-8 expression in Helicobacter pylori-infected gastric epithelial cells. *Nutrients* **2018**, *10*, 1320. [CrossRef]
121. Dore, C.M.P.G.; Alves, M.G.d.C.F.; Will, L.S.E.P.; Costa, T.G.; Sabry, D.A.; de Souza Rêgo, L.A.R.; Accardo, C.M.; Rocha, H.A.O.; Filgueira, L.G.A.; Leite, E.L. A sulfated polysaccharide, fucans, isolated from brown algae Sargassum vulgare with anticoagulant, antithrombotic, antioxidant and anti-inflammatory effects. *Carbohydr. Polym.* **2013**, *91*, 467–475. [CrossRef] [PubMed]
122. Cavalcante-Silva, L.H.A.; Barbosa Brito da Matta, C.; De Araújo, M.V.; Barbosa-Filho, J.M.; Pereira de Lira, D.; de Oliveira Santos, B.V.; De Miranda, G.E.C.; Alexandre-Moreira, M.S. Antinociceptive and anti-inflammatory activities of crude methanolic extract of red alga Bryothamnion triquetrum. *Mar. Drugs* **2012**, *10*, 1977–1992. [CrossRef] [PubMed]
123. Lee, H.-J.; Kang, G.-J.; Yang, E.-J.; Park, S.-S.; Yoon, W.-J.; Jung, J.H.; Kang, H.-K.; Yoo, E.-S. Two enone fatty acids isolated from Gracilaria verrucosa suppress the production of inflammatory mediators by down-regulating NF-κB and STAT1 activity in lipopolysaccharide-stimulated Raw 264.7 cells. *Arch. Pharmacal Res.* **2009**, *32*, 453–462. [CrossRef] [PubMed]
124. Bergé, J.; Debiton, E.; Dumay, J.; Durand, P.; Barthomeuf, C. In vitro anti-inflammatory and anti-proliferative activity of sulfolipids from the red alga Porphyridium cruentum. *J. Agric. Food Chem.* **2002**, *50*, 6227–6232. [CrossRef] [PubMed]
125. Song, W.; Wang, Z.; Zhang, X.; Li, Y. Ethanol extract from Ulva prolifera prevents high-fat diet-induced insulin resistance, oxidative stress, and inflammation response in mice. *BioMed Res. Int.* **2018**, *2018*, 1374565. [CrossRef] [PubMed]
126. Pangestuti, R.; Kim, S.-K. Biological activities and health benefit effects of natural pigments derived from marine algae. *J. Funct. Foods* **2011**, *3*, 255–266. [CrossRef]
127. Yoon, W.-J.; Heo, S.-J.; Han, S.-C.; Lee, H.-J.; Kang, G.-J.; Kang, H.-K.; Hyun, J.-W.; Koh, Y.-S.; Yoo, E.-S. Anti-inflammatory effect of sargachromanol G isolated from Sargassum siliquastrum in RAW 264.7 cells. *Arch. Pharmacal Res.* **2012**, *35*, 1421–1430. [CrossRef] [PubMed]
128. Kim, M.-M.; Kim, S.-K. Effect of phloroglucinol on oxidative stress and inflammation. *Food Chem. Toxicol.* **2010**, *48*, 2925–2933. [CrossRef]
129. Lim, C.S.; Jin, D.-Q.; Sung, J.-Y.; Lee, J.H.; Choi, H.G.; Ha, I.; Han, J.-S. Antioxidant and anti-inflammatory activities of the methanolic extract of Neorhodomela aculeate in hippocampal and microglial cells. *Biol. Pharm. Bull.* **2006**, *29*, 1212–1216. [CrossRef]
130. Riccardi, G.; Rivellese, A.A. Effects of dietary fiber and carbohydrate on glucose and lipoprotein metabolism in diabetic patients. *Diabetes Care* **1991**, *14*, 1115–1125. [CrossRef]
131. Gupta, P.; Bala, M.; Gupta, S.; Dua, A.; Dabur, R.; Injeti, E.; Mittal, A. Efficacy and risk profile of anti-diabetic therapies: Conventional vs traditional drugs—A mechanistic revisit to understand their mode of action. *Pharmacol. Res.* **2016**, *113*, 636–674. [CrossRef] [PubMed]
132. Unnikrishnan, P.S.; Jayasri, M.A. Marine algae as a prospective source for antidiabetic compounds–A brief review. *Curr. Diabetes Rev.* **2018**, *14*, 237–245. [CrossRef] [PubMed]
133. Cheng, Y.; Sibusiso, L.; Hou, L.; Jiang, H.; Chen, P.; Zhang, X.; Wu, M.; Tong, H. Sargassum fusiforme fucoidan modifies the gut microbiota during alleviation of streptozotocin-induced hyperglycemia in mice. *Int. J. Biol. Macromol.* **2019**, *131*, 1162–1170. [CrossRef] [PubMed]
134. Daub, C.D.; Mabate, B.; Malgas, S.; Pletschke, B.I. Fucoidan from Ecklonia maxima is a powerful inhibitor of the diabetes-related enzyme, α-glucosidase. *Int. J. Biol. Macromol.* **2020**, *151*, 412–420. [CrossRef]
135. Kim, K.-T.; Rioux, L.-E.; Turgeon, S.L. Alpha-amylase and alpha-glucosidase inhibition is differentially modulated by fucoidan obtained from Fucus vesiculosus and Ascophyllum nodosum. *Phytochemistry* **2014**, *98*, 27–33. [CrossRef]
136. Wang, D.; Zhao, X.; Liu, Y. Hypoglycemic and hypolipidemic effects of a polysaccharide from flower buds of Lonicera japonica in streptozotocin-induced diabetic rats. *Int. J. Biol. Macromol.* **2017**, *102*, 396–404. [CrossRef]
137. Kim, K.-J.; Yoon, K.-Y.; Lee, B.-Y. Fucoidan regulate blood glucose homeostasis in C57BL/KSJ m+/+ db and C57BL/KSJ db/db mice. *Fitoterapia* **2012**, *83*, 1105–1109. [CrossRef]
138. Kumar, T.V.; Lakshmanasenthil, S.; Geetharamani, D.; Marudhupandi, T.; Suja, G.; Suganya, P. Fucoidan–A α-d-glucosidase inhibitor from Sargassum wightii with relevance to type 2 diabetes mellitus therapy. *Int. J. Biol. Macromol.* **2015**, *72*, 1044–1047. [CrossRef]
139. Moon, H.E.; Islam, M.N.; Ahn, B.R.; Chowdhury, S.S.; Sohn, H.S.; Jung, H.A.; Choi, J.S. Protein tyrosine phosphatase 1B and α-glucosidase inhibitory phlorotannins from edible brown algae, Ecklonia stolonifera and Eisenia bicyclis. *Biosci. Biotechnol. Biochem.* **2011**, *75*, 1472–1480. [CrossRef]
140. Lee, S.H.; Karadeniz, F.; Kim, M.M.; Kim, S.K. α-Glucosidase and α-amylase inhibitory activities of phloroglucinal derivatives from edible marine brown alga, Ecklonia cava. *J. Sci. Food Agric.* **2009**, *89*, 1552–1558. [CrossRef]
141. Kang, C.; Jin, Y.B.; Lee, H.; Cha, M.; Sohn, E.-T.; Moon, J.; Park, C.; Chun, S.; Jung, E.-S.; Hong, J.-S. Brown alga Ecklonia cava attenuates type 1 diabetes by activating AMPK and Akt signaling pathways. *Food Chem. Toxicol.* **2010**, *48*, 509–516. [CrossRef] [PubMed]
142. Lee, S.-H.; Min, K.-H.; Han, J.-S.; Lee, D.-H.; Park, D.-B.; Jung, W.-K.; Park, P.-J.; Jeon, B.-T.; Kim, S.-K.; Jeon, Y.-J. Effects of brown alga, Ecklonia cava on glucose and lipid metabolism in C57BL/KsJ-db/db mice, a model of type 2 diabetes mellitus. *Food Chem. Toxicol.* **2012**, *50*, 575–582. [CrossRef]
143. Min, K.-H.; Kim, H.-J.; Jeon, Y.-J.; Han, J.-S. Ishige okamurae ameliorates hyperglycemia and insulin resistance in C57BL/KsJ-db/db mice. *Diabetes Res. Clin. Pract.* **2011**, *93*, 70–76. [CrossRef] [PubMed]

144. Lee, Y.S.; Shin, K.H.; Kim, B.-K.; Lee, S. Anti-Diabetic activities of fucosterol fromPelvetia siliquosa. *Arch. Pharmacal Res.* **2004**, *27*, 1120–1122. [CrossRef] [PubMed]
145. Nwosu, F.; Morris, J.; Lund, V.A.; Stewart, D.; Ross, H.A.; McDougall, G.J. Anti-proliferative and potential anti-diabetic effects of phenolic-rich extracts from edible marine algae. *Food Chem.* **2011**, *126*, 1006–1012. [CrossRef]
146. Kimura, Y.; Watanabe, K.; Okuda, H. Effects of soluble sodium alginate on cholesterol excretion and glucose tolerance in rats. *J. Ethnopharmacol.* **1996**, *54*, 47–54. [CrossRef]
147. Jung, H.A.; Yoon, N.Y.; Woo, M.-H.; Choi, J.S. Inhibitory activities of extracts from several kinds of seaweeds and phlorotannins from the brown alga Ecklonia stolonifera on glucose-mediated protein damage and rat lens aldose reductase. *Fish. Sci.* **2008**, *74*, 1363–1365. [CrossRef]
148. Peng, J.; Yuan, J.-P.; Wu, C.-F.; Wang, J.-H. Fucoxanthin, a marine carotenoid present in brown seaweeds and diatoms: Metabolism and bioactivities relevant to human health. *Mar. Drugs* **2011**, *9*, 1806–1828. [CrossRef]
149. Jung, H.A.; Islam, M.N.; Lee, C.M.; Oh, S.H.; Lee, S.; Jung, J.H.; Choi, J.S. Kinetics and molecular docking studies of an anti-diabetic complication inhibitor fucosterol from edible brown algae Eisenia bicyclis and Ecklonia stolonifera. *Chem. Biol. Interact.* **2013**, *206*, 55–62. [CrossRef]
150. Shi, D.; Guo, S.; Jiang, B.; Guo, C.; Wang, T.; Zhang, L.; Li, J. HPN, a synthetic analogue of bromophenol from red alga Rhodomela confervoides: Synthesis and anti-diabetic effects in C57BL/KsJ-db/db mice. *Mar. Drugs* **2013**, *11*, 350–362. [CrossRef]
151. Yamazaki, H.; Nakazawa, T.; Sumilat, D.A.; Takahashi, O.; Ukai, K.; Takahashi, S.; Namikoshi, M. Euryspongins A–C, three new unique sesquiterpenes from a marine sponge Euryspongia sp. *Bioorg. Med. Chem. Lett.* **2013**, *23*, 2151–2154. [CrossRef]
152. Nuño, K.; Villarruel-López, A.; Puebla-Pérez, A.; Romero-Velarde, E.; Puebla-Mora, A.; Ascencio, F. Effects of the marine microalgae Isochrysis galbana and Nannochloropsis oculata in diabetic rats. *J. Funct. Foods* **2013**, *5*, 106–115. [CrossRef]
153. Lee, S.-H.; Jeon, Y.-J. Anti-diabetic effects of brown algae derived phlorotannins, marine polyphenols through diverse mechanisms. *Fitoterapia* **2013**, *86*, 129–136. [CrossRef] [PubMed]
154. Guan, J.; Cui, Z.; Lee, D.; Lee, Y.; Park, D. Effect of dieckol from Ecklonia cava on glucose transport in L6 muscle cells. *Planta Med.* **2011**, *77*, PH3. [CrossRef]
155. Lee, S.-H.; Park, M.-H.; Heo, S.-J.; Kang, S.-M.; Ko, S.-C.; Han, J.-S.; Jeon, Y.-J. Dieckol isolated from Ecklonia cava inhibits α-glucosidase and α-amylase in vitro and alleviates postprandial hyperglycemia in streptozotocin-induced diabetic mice. *Food Chem. Toxicol.* **2010**, *48*, 2633–2637. [CrossRef] [PubMed]
156. Heo, S.-J.; Hwang, J.-Y.; Choi, J.-I.; Han, J.-S.; Kim, H.-J.; Jeon, Y.-J. Diphlorethohydroxycarmalol isolated from Ishige okamurae, a brown algae, a potent α-glucosidase and α-amylase inhibitor, alleviates postprandial hyperglycemia in diabetic mice. *Eur. J. Pharmacol.* **2009**, *615*, 252–256. [CrossRef] [PubMed]
157. Celikler, S.; Tas, S.; Vatan, O.; Ziyanok-Ayvalik, S.; Yildiz, G.; Bilaloglu, R. Anti-hyperglycemic and antigenotoxic potential of Ulva rigida ethanolic extract in the experimental diabetes mellitus. *Food Chem. Toxicol.* **2009**, *47*, 1837–1840. [CrossRef]
158. Sun, Z.; Peng, X.; Liu, J.; Fan, K.-W.; Wang, M.; Chen, F. Inhibitory effects of microalgal extracts on the formation of advanced glycation endproducts (AGEs). *Food Chem.* **2010**, *120*, 261–267. [CrossRef]
159. Abdelsalam, S.S.; Korashy, H.M.; Zeidan, A.; Agouni, A. The role of protein tyrosine phosphatase (PTP)-1B in cardiovascular disease and its interplay with insulin resistance. *Biomolecules* **2019**, *9*, 286. [CrossRef]
160. Lee, J.Y.; Kim, S.M.; Jung, W.-S.; Song, D.-G.; Um, B.-H.; Son, J.-K.; Pan, C.-H. Phlorofucofuroeckol-A, a potent inhibitor of aldo-keto reductase family 1 member B10, from the edible brown alga Eisenia bicyclis. *J. Korean Soc. Appl. Biol. Chem.* **2012**, *55*, 721–727. [CrossRef]
161. Gunathilaka, M.; Ranasinghe, P.; Samarakoon, K.; Peiris, L. In-vitro anti-diabetic activity of polyphenole-rich extract from marine brown algae Choonospora minima (Hering 1841). In Proceedings of the 12th International Conference of KDU, General Sri John Kotelawala University, Kandawala, Sri Lanka, 11–12 September 2019; p. 185.
162. Son, Y.K.; Jin, S.E.; Kim, H.-R.; Woo, H.C.; Jung, H.A.; Choi, J.S. Inhibitory activities of the edible brown alga Laminaria japonica on glucose-mediated protein damage and rat lens aldose reductase. *Fish. Sci.* **2011**, *77*, 1069–1079. [CrossRef]
163. Yang, H.-W.; Fernando, K.; Oh, J.-Y.; Li, X.; Jeon, Y.-J.; Ryu, B. Anti-obesity and anti-diabetic effects of Ishige okamurae. *Mar. Drugs* **2019**, *17*, 202. [CrossRef] [PubMed]
164. Ali, M.; Kim, D.H.; Seong, S.H.; Kim, H.-R.; Jung, H.A.; Choi, J.S. α-Glucosidase and protein tyrosine phosphatase 1B inhibitory activity of plastoquinones from marine brown alga Sargassum serratifolium. *Mar. Drugs* **2017**, *15*, 368. [CrossRef] [PubMed]
165. Lopez-Santamarina, A.; Miranda, J.M. Potential Use of Marine Seaweeds as Prebiotics: A Review. *Molecules* **2020**, *25*, 1004. [CrossRef] [PubMed]
166. Kim, M.H.; Kang, S.G.; Park, J.H.; Yanagisawa, M.; Kim, C.H. Short-chain fatty acids activate GPR41 and GPR43 on intestinal epithelial cells to promote inflammatory responses in mice. *Gastroenterology* **2013**, *145*, 396–406.e1-10. [CrossRef]
167. Cavaglieri, C.R.; Nishiyama, A.; Fernandes, L.C.; Curi, R.; Miles, E.A.; Calder, P.C. Differential effects of short-chain fatty acids on proliferation and production of pro-and anti-inflammatory cytokines by cultured lymphocytes. *Life Sci.* **2003**, *73*, 1683–1690. [CrossRef]
168. Sun, Y.; Liu, Y.; Ai, C.; Song, S.; Chen, X. Caulerpa lentillifera polysaccharides enhance the immunostimulatory activity in immunosuppressed mice in correlation with modulating gut microbiota. *Food Funct.* **2019**, *10*, 4315–4329. [CrossRef]
169. Zhang, W.; Oda, T.; Yu, Q.; Jin, J.-O. Fucoidan from Macrocystis pyrifera has powerful immune-modulatory effects compared to three other fucoidans. *Mar. Drugs* **2015**, *13*, 1084–1104. [CrossRef]

170. Ale, M.T.; Maruyama, H.; Tamauchi, H.; Mikkelsen, J.D.; Meyer, A.S. Fucoidan from Sargassum sp. and Fucus vesiculosus reduces cell viability of lung carcinoma and melanoma cells in vitro and activates natural killer cells in mice in vivo. *Int. J. Biol. Macromol.* **2011**, *49*, 331–336. [CrossRef]
171. Jin, J.-O.; Zhang, W.; Du, J.-Y.; Wong, K.-W.; Oda, T.; Yu, Q. Fucoidan can function as an adjuvant in vivo to enhance dendritic cell maturation and function and promote antigen-specific T cell immune responses. *PLoS ONE* **2014**, *9*, e99396. [CrossRef]
172. Negishi, H.; Mori, M.; Mori, H.; Yamori, Y. Supplementation of elderly Japanese men and women with fucoidan from seaweed increases immune responses to seasonal influenza vaccination. *J. Nutr.* **2013**, *143*, 1794–1798. [CrossRef] [PubMed]

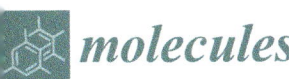

Article

Potent Activity of a High Concentration of Chemical Ozone against Antibiotic-Resistant Bacteria

Karyne Rangel [1,2,*], Fellipe O. Cabral [3], Guilherme C. Lechuga [1,2], João P. R. S. Carvalho [1,2,4], Maria H. S. Villas-Bôas [3], Victor Midlej [5] and Salvatore G. De-Simone [1,2,4,*]

1. Center for Technological Development in Health (CDTS), National Institute of Science and Technology for Innovation in Neglected Population Diseases (INCT-IDPN), FIOCRUZ, Rio de Janeiro 21040-900, Brazil; gclechuga@gmail.com (G.C.L.); joaopedrorsc@gmail.com (J.P.R.S.C.)
2. Laboratory of Epidemiology and Molecular Systematics (LESM), Oswaldo Cruz Institute, FIOCRUZ, Rio de Janeiro 21040-900, Brazil
3. Microbiology Department, National Institute for Quality Control in Health (INCQS), FIOCRUZ, Rio de Janeiro 21040-900, Brazil; fellipe.cabral@incqs.fiocruz.br (F.O.C.); maria.villas@incqs.fiocruz.br (M.H.S.V.-B.)
4. Post-Graduation Program in Science and Biotechnology, Department of Molecular and Cellular Biology, Biology Institute, Federal Fluminense University, Niterói 22040-036, Brazil
5. Laboratory of Cellular and Ultrastructure, Oswaldo Cruz Institute, FIOCRUZ, Rio de Janeiro 21040-900, Brazil; victor.midlej@ioc.fiocruz.br
* Correspondence: karyne.rangelk@gmail.com (K.R.); salvatore.simone@fiocruz.br or dsimone@cdts.fiocruz.br (S.G.D.-S.); Tel.: +55-2138658182 (K.R. & S.G.D.-S.)

Abstract: Background: Health care-associated infections (HAIs) are a significant public health problem worldwide, favoring multidrug-resistant (MDR) microorganisms. The SARS-CoV-2 infection was negatively associated with the increase in antimicrobial resistance, and the ESKAPE group had the most significant impact on HAIs. The study evaluated the bactericidal effect of a high concentration of O_3 gas on some reference and ESKAPE bacteria. Material and Methods: Four standard strains and four clinical or environmental MDR strains were exposed to elevated ozone doses at different concentrations and times. Bacterial inactivation (growth and cultivability) was investigated using colony counts and resazurin as metabolic indicators. Scanning electron microscopy (SEM) was performed. Results: The culture exposure to a high level of O_3 inhibited the growth of all bacterial strains tested with a statistically significant reduction in colony count compared to the control group. The cell viability of *S. aureus* (MRSA) (99.6%) and *P. aeruginosa* (XDR) (29.2%) was reduced considerably, and SEM showed damage to bacteria after O_3 treatment Conclusion: The impact of HAIs can be easily dampened by the widespread use of ozone in ICUs. This product usually degrades into molecular oxygen and has a low toxicity compared to other sanitization products. However, high doses of ozone were able to interfere with the growth of all strains studied, evidencing that ozone-based decontamination approaches may represent the future of hospital cleaning methods.

Keywords: ozone; pathogenic bacteria; antimicrobial resistance; SEM; ESKAPE pathogens; antimicrobial activity

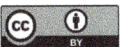

1. Introduction

Health care-associated infections (HAI) are a significant public health problem worldwide, especially in developing countries where the frequency can be at least three times higher than that of resource-rich countries [1]. It is estimated that approximately four million people acquire HAIs in the European Union (EU) and that some 37,000 persons die due to resistant infections acquired in hospital environments. Most of these deaths (67.6%) are caused by multidrug-resistant (MDR) bacteria to antimicrobials [2]. The 2016 European Annual Report recorded the incidence density (DI) for ventilator-associated pneumonia (VAP) of 3.9/1000 days, central catheter-associated bloodstream infections

(CCAB) of 1.7/1000 days, and infections of the urinary tract related to a catheter (ITURC) of 2.1/1000 days [2], while in Brazil, the DI of device-related HAIs in the year 2016 indicated VAP of 13.6/1000 days, primary clinical bloodstream infection associated with central vascular catheter (CBIACC) of 4.6/1000 days, and catheter-related urinary tract infections (CRUTI) of 5.1/1000 days [3]. The increasing burden of HAIs stemming from poor infection monitoring and control practices are among the drivers of antimicrobial resistance. Evidence indicates a strong relationship between antimicrobial resistance and HAIs [4], with MDR pathogens being a common cause [5,6]. Although they are frequent adverse events with high morbidity and mortality rates and costs, HAIs are recognized as preventable in up to 70% of cases [7].

Antimicrobial resistance (AMR) results from bacteria's natural evolution and adaptation processes. However, selection pressure has accelerated it, originating from the inadequate or excessive use of antimicrobials, favoring MDR microorganisms' appearance and rapid spread [8–10]. The problem is highlighted in the ICU, where patients have higher risk factors for nosocomial infections. In addition, the cost of antimicrobial resistance in these infections is very high, as diseases caused by these pathogens have worse clinical outcomes, prolonged hospital stays, and increased mortality rates [11]. More than 700,000 deaths are associated with AMR [12,13], and by 2050, the number of lives lost annually could reach 10 million [14]. The COVID-19 pandemic was declared by the World Health Organization (WHO) on 12 March 2020 [15–17]; at that time, the disease had been spreading rapidly since the first detection of the SARS-CoV-2 coronavirus in Wuhan, China, in December 2019 [18]. The SARS-CoV-2 infection had a negative association with the increase in antimicrobial resistance for reasons related mainly to the rise in the practical use of antimicrobials, the overcrowding of health systems, a lack of management measures, and a decrease in the pace of activity of laboratories in surveillance cultures and diagnostic tests to detect antimicrobial-resistant organisms.

On the other hand, the lower impact on the development of antimicrobial resistance may be associated with increased infection control measures adopted to prevent the contamination of healthcare professionals with SARS-CoV-2, including hand hygiene and the use of individual protective equipment and devices to decontaminate the air and surfaces [19]. According to some studies, up to 5% of patients infected with SARS-CoV-2 had to be admitted to the ICU [20,21]. In addition, it has been documented that up to 50% of these patients may have had secondary bacterial infections or superinfections, mainly bacteremia and urinary tract infections [22,23]. Undoubtedly, the dramatic increase in COVID-19 deaths includes HAI coinfection cases. Furthermore, the hospitalization length increases the risk of being affected by HAIs, which may even exacerbate a severe morbidity condition, further leading to the patient's death, particularly if with comorbidity [24]. A study in Lombardy, the Italian region with the most COVID-19 deaths, revealed that most HAIs occurred in ICUs [25]. Other authors reported the high prevalence of HAIs in ICUs in Italy and associated such infections with the use of a urinary catheter, surgical drainage, intravascular catheters, and mechanical ventilation [26,27]. These infections are more prevalent in terminally ill patients and are primarily due to the spread of MDR pathogens.

Among the MDR pathogens, those from the ESKAPE group have the most significant impact on HAIs. Also called "super bacteria", they group six pathogens that can escape the biocidal activity of antimicrobials: *Enterococcus faecium*, *Staphylococcus aureus*, *Klebsiella pneumoniae*, *Acinetobacter baumannii*, *Pseudomonas aeruginosa*, and *Enterobacter* spp. [28,29]. The inefficiency of antimicrobials against these pathogens is due to several resistance mechanisms, such as drug inactivation, modification of drug binding sites/targets, changes in cell permeability, and mutation [30]. As a result, these pathogens can survive in the hospital environment for extended periods and be transported from one individual to another, thus spreading in the community and hospital [31].

A priority list of antimicrobial-resistant bacteria was described in 2017 by WHO to support renewed efforts in researching and developing new antimicrobials, diagnostics, vaccines, and other tools [32]. Most ESKAPE pathogens appear on this list of the most problematic microbial species, which appeals to focus research efforts on this topic [33]. The European Centre for Disease Prevention and Control (ECDC) and the US Centers for Disease Control and Prevention (CDC) provided the following standardized definitions for MDR, extensively drug-resistant (XDR), and pan-drug resistant (PDR) bacteria. MDR bacteria are defined as those with acquired resistance to at least one agent in three or more categories of antimicrobials. XDRs are not susceptible to at least one agent in all classes of antimicrobials except two or fewer types (i.e., they remain sensitive to only one or two categories). Bacteria resistance to all agents in all antimicrobial types is called PDR [34]. The environment plays a central role in transmitting hospital-acquired pathogens and the pathogenesis of HAIs.

Many bacteria, especially MDR, can survive in the hospital environment for several months, particularly in areas close to patients. Among the factors that favor the contamination of the health services environment, we can mention the hands of health professionals in contact with surfaces; maintenance of damp, wet, and dusty surfaces; precarious conditions of coatings; and maintenance of organic matter [35]. The presence of dirt, mainly organic matter of human origin, can serve as a substrate for the proliferation of microorganisms or favor the presence of vectors, which can passively carry these agents. This indicates the importance of rapid cleaning and disinfection of any area with organic matter, regardless of the hospital area [33]. The effective disinfection of surfaces and the environment is considered one of the primary measures to control the spread of HAIs. Unfortunately, many studies have concluded that current cleaning methods are microbiologically ineffective. This failure concerns daily cleaning and final cleaning after the patient is discharged. Improvements in environmental cleanliness are associated with a decrease in hospital-acquired pathogens and HAIs [36]. Last year, a new global emergency introduced the requirement for further disinfection and sanitization procedures to optimize the quality of care and work safety in professional environments [37,38].

According to all this and considering the increasing prevalence of MDR microorganisms in hospitals, which has become a severe threat to public health, the need for safe and validated technologies capable of ensuring the disinfection of air environments, room surfaces, and sanitary materials has become evident against the current pandemic or future events. In this sense, the study of alternative methods and/or agents for disinfection and sanitization should receive special attention, and ozone (O_3) can be a valid option with different objectives [39]. Ozone is a blue-colored gas with a characteristic odor, presented in the triatomic form of oxygen (O_3), and is partially soluble in water and highly unstable, decomposing quickly into oxygen. Therefore, it cannot be produced in large quantities without being continuously [40]. With an oxidative potential superior to most commercial disinfectants and a faster reaction faster than O_2, it has been studied for decades in medicine and biological sciences, becoming a versatile therapeutic agent which helps treat several diseases [41]. The exposure to ozone, also known as the time concentration value (mg L-1 min), is the most important operational parameter in O_3 disinfection, representing the time-integrated ozone concentration in its most general form. Medium temperature also has a strong influence [42,43]. The humidity is also a key parameter when ozone is applied in the gas phase, requiring high relative humidity conditions to obtain a significant inactivation of target microorganisms [44,45]. The chemical composition of the surface to be treated and its shape and texture could also be important factors.

Gaseous disinfectants are proven to be effective because, in addition to the antimicrobial effect, gas can reach surfaces difficult to get by conventional cleaning [46,47]. For example, ozone gas in the concentration of 25 ppm caused a significant reduction in the number of viable bacteria and the total biomass of *K. pneumoniae* biofilm [48]. Furthermore, ozone seems to be very effective against planktonic bacteria, which are susceptible to ozone action and are often significantly reduced or completely eradicated from the surfaces with smaller concentrations [49–52]. Currently, with the COVID-19 pandemic, ozone has been investigated as a possible preventive measure for the spread of infection [53], in hospital hygiene for disinfecting rooms [54], in viability on different surfaces [55], and as a therapeutic option in the treatment of patients [24,56].

Ozone acts first on the cell membrane as a disinfectant, reacting with glycoproteins, glycolipids, and nucleic acids. Then, microorganisms are inactivated by cell disruption due to the action of molecular ozone or free radicals during the decomposition of the gas [57]. Studies show that ozone influences the global polarity of the bacterial surface [58], involving mechanisms of lipid peroxidation [59] and the degradation of transmembrane proteins that control the flow of ions. Thus, cells rupture with a subsequent leakage of ions between the media, resulting in the microorganism's death [60].

Despite having been used in the hospital environment for some time, little is known about the potential of this agent, especially in the Brazilian context, where studies on the subject are scarce. Therefore, from this perspective and due to the aspects reported, there was an interest in evaluating the bactericidal action of high concentration ozone gas on some reference bacteria used in the process of assessing the bactericidal activity of disinfectants and some bacteria from the ESKAPE group that have a high antimicrobial resistance profile.

2. Materials and Methods

2.1. Bacterial Strains

Standard strains (*Staphylococcus aureus* (ATCC 6538), *Salmonella enterica* subsp. enterica serovar *choleraesuis* (ATCC 10708), *Escherichia coli* (ATCC 25922), and *Pseudomonas aeruginosa* (ATCC 15442)) were obtained from the American Type Culture Collection (ATCC) (Plast Labor Ind. Com. EH Lab. Ltd.a, Rio de Janeiro, Brazil). Representative MDR strains of the ESKAPE group were also used, with four clinical strains isolated from HAIs, which were: methicillin-resistant *S. aureus* (MRSA), carbapenemase-producing *K. pneumoniae* (KPC+), *A. baumannii* PDR carrying the bla_{OXA-23} gene and representing one of the genotypes disseminated in Brazil (ST15/CC15), and an environmental strain of *P. aeruginosa* (XDR) from hospital effluent. These strains were kindly provided by Dr. Maria H. S. Villas-Bôas (National Institute for Quality Control in Health of the Oswaldo Cruz Foundation—INCQS/FIOCRUZ) and Dra. Catia Chaia de Miranda (Interdisciplinary Medical Research Laboratory, LIPMED, FIOCRUZ). These bacterial strains were initially cultivated according to the instructions of the ATCC, aliquoted, and stored in cryotubes containing tryptic soy broth (TSB, Difco) with 20% glycerol (v/v) and kept at $-20\ °C$ for later use.

2.2. Ozone Generating and Monitoring

The ozone generating equipment (SANITECH O3-80-Sanitization, Astech Serv. and Fabrication Ltd.a., Petrópolis, Brazil) is adjustable from 10 to 80 ppm, and the capacity to treat the room air up to 1000 m^3 (not habitable) was used. The environmental concentration of O_3 emitted was monitored and measured using two portable electrochemical ozone detection modules (model ZE14-O3) (Zhengzhou Winsen Electronics Technology Co., Ltd., Honā, Zhengzhou, China). In addition, this equipment was coupled to a module containing a digital temperature and relative humidity sensor (model AM2302) (Guangzhou ASAIR Electronic Co., Ltd., Guangzhou, China). The ZE14-O3/AM2302 modules constantly monitored these three parameters during the experiment, with 2–3 s detection and simultaneous recording on a computer. The measurement was made with the ZE14-O3/AM2302 (Sensors 1 and 2) inserted directly inside each container, always on the first shelf.

2.3. Inoculation of the Test Surface

The strains were removed from the freezer stock culture for bacterial reactivation, sown in TSB, and incubated at 37 °C for 24 h. After the microorganisms were suspended in sterile 0.85% saline, the concentration of 10^8 colony-forming units (CFU) mL^{-1} was determined with a densitometer (Densichek Plus, BioMérieux, Rio de Janeiro, Brazil). The successive dilutions (10^5 and 10^4 CFU mL^{-1}) were made in the brain–heart infusion broth (BHI). One hundred microliter aliquots of each bacterial suspension (*S. aureus*, *S. enterica*,

E. coli, P. aeruginosa, S. aureus (MRSA), K. pneumoniae (KPC+), A. baumannii (PDR), and P. aeruginosa (XDR)) in different concentrations (10^5 and 10^4 CFU mL^{-1}) were plated in triplicate by spread plate on Triptona Soy Agar (TSA; DIFCO Laboratories Inc., Detroit, MI, USA) and incubated at 37 °C for 24 h.

2.4. Ozone Treatment

The ozone generated was infused into two hermetically sealed containers, with a volume of approximately 1 m^3 each (Figure S1). The plates inoculated with the different microorganisms were placed on each container's shelves. After closing the lid of each container, we started the exposure to ozone using only one SANITECH O3-80-Sanitization ozone generator, producing ozone at a concentration of 80 ppm (maximum) (Figure S1). ATCC strains were exposed to ozone for 1, 10, 20, 30, and 40 min. According to the results obtained with the reference strains, we verified that the initial concentration of the inoculum (10^4 or 10^5 CFU/mL) had no significant interference in the colony count results, but rather the time of exposure to ozone presented the best impact at 40 min. As a result, the other strains (ESKAPE) were exposed to ozone at 10^5 CFU/mL/40 min. The ozone-generating equipment takes time to reach its maximum concentration (ppm). For this reason, for each exposure time determined, a 2 min addition to the readings was considered after this initial time. After the exposure time, the container was opened, and the plates were closed and incubated at 37 °C for 24 h. As a positive control for the assay, we used plates with TSA containing the same bacterial suspensions but without exposure to ozone. These plates remained at room temperature and were incubated at 37 °C for 24 h, with the plates exposed to ozone. A plate containing only TSA was used as a negative control. The test was performed in triplicate. Colony counting was performed only on plates with many colonies from 0 to 300.

2.5. Cell Viability

The cell viability was measured on a selected bacterial suspension of 10^5 CFU mL^{-1} after 40 min exposure to O_3 based on previous results (cell count—CFU mL^{-1}). The entire previous experiment was performed again (at the defined concentration and time), and after 24 h of incubation, three distinct colonies from each plate were inoculated separately in a test tube containing TSB broth (Difco). As a positive control of the assay, we performed the same procedure with the plates that were not exposed to O_3, where three distinct colonies of each dish were inoculated separately in a test tube containing TSB broth (Difco). Afterward, 100 µL of the bacterial suspension of each colony was transferred, in triplicate, to the wells of the 96-well microplate, which was incubated at 37 °C for 24 h. Each strain was tested in duplicate and bacterial growth was detected by adding 0.02% resazurin (7-hydroxyphenoxazin-3-one 10-oxide; Sigma-Merck, St. Louis, MO, USA) with 1 h incubation [61]. Resazurin is a non-toxic, non-fluorescent blue reagent that, after enzymatic reduction, becomes highly fluorescent. This conversion occurs only in viable cells; as such, the amount of resorufin produced is proportional to the number of viable cells in the sample [62–64]. As a negative control, we used TSB broth, and the measurement at 590 nm was conducted on an ELISA plate reader (Flex Station 3; Molecular Devices, San José, CA, USA).

The collected data were analyzed using the program R (version 3.6.0) (Vienna, Austria) and R Studio, where the paired t-test was applied to compare the statistical significance between the two samples (with and without treatment with O_3) with ≤ 0.01. Each experiment was repeated three times for each microorganism treated with O_3.

2.6. Scanning Electron Microscopy (SEM)

SEM visualizes morphological changes in the bacteria species. For analysis, control cells under O_3 treatment were fixed for 1 h with 2.5% glutaraldehyde in 0.1 M cacodylate buffer. After fixation, the cells were washed three times in PBS for 5 min, post-fixed for 15 min in 1% osmium tetroxide (OsO4), and rewashed three times in PBS for 5 min. Next, the samples were dehydrated in an ascending series of ethanol (7.5, 15, 30, 50, 70, 90, and

100% ethanol) for 15 min each step, critical point dried with CO_2, sputter-coated with a 15 nm thick layer of gold, and examined in a Jeol JSM 6390 (Tokyo, Japan) scanning electron microscope.

3. Results

3.1. Monitoring of Ozone Concentration

Monitoring the O_3 concentration inside each container showed that the average ozone emission from the equipment (1 to 40 min) ranged from 21.1 ppm to 71.7 ppm, with the average of all measurements being 43.9 ppm (Figure 1). The mean ozone concentration in the 40 min time chosen for testing with the MDR strains was 30.8 ppm (Figure 2). The ambient temperature ranged from 22.5 °C to 24.3 °C, with an average of 23.4 °C. Regarding the relative humidity of the air, it went from 71.4% RH to 75.5% RH, with an average of 74.2% RH (Table 1, Figure 2).

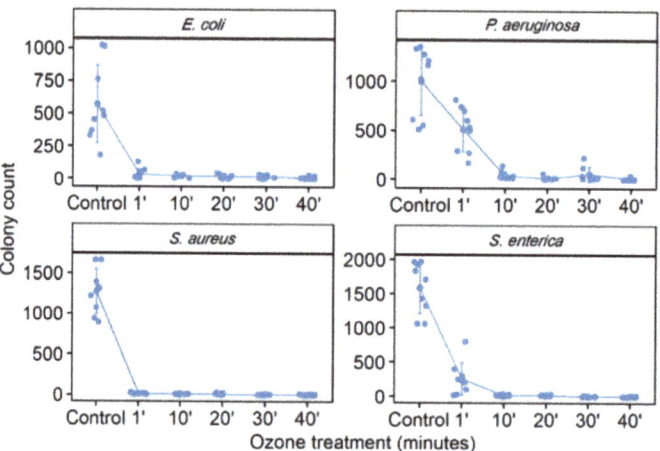

Figure 1. The number of colony-forming units (CFU) in different bacterial strains (*S. aureus* (ATCC 6538), *P. aeruginosa* (ATCC 15442), *S. enterica* (ATCC 10708), and *E. coli* (ATCC 25922)) was counted. CFU counting was performed in the control group (no treatment) and bacterial suspensions (10^5 CFU/mL) after exposure to ozone for 1, 10, 20, 30, and 40 min.

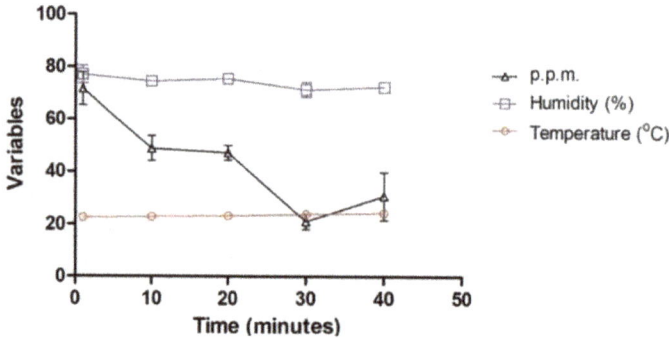

Figure 2. Average temperature, relative humidity, and ozone concentration at times of 1, 10, 20, 30, and 40 min with ATCC (*S. aureus* (ATCC 6538), *P. aeruginosa* (ATCC 15442), *S. enterica* (ATCC) strains 10708), and *E. coli* (ATCC 25922)) and multidrug-resistant *S. aureus* (MRSA), *P. aeruginosa* (XDR), *A. baumannii* (PDR), and *K. pneumoniae* (KPC+).

Table 1. Monitoring ozone concentration, temperature, and humidity of different bacterial strains after exposure to ozone.

Ozone Exposure Time (Minutes)	Evaluated Parameters		
	Temperature (°C)	Relative Humidity of Air (% RH)	Ozone Concentration (ppm)
1	22.5	77.2	71.7
10	22.8	74.6	48.8
20	23.7	75.5	47.2
30	23.9	71.4	21.1
40	24.3	72.4	30.8
Mean	23.4	74.2	43.9

3.2. Ozone Treatment

The culture exposure at different times (1 to 40 min) with a high level of gaseous O_3 was able to inhibit the in vitro growth of all bacterial strains tested (Figures 1 and 2) with a statistically significant reduction in colony count compared to the control group (not treated with ozone) (Table 2). Among the ATCC strains (10^5 CFU/mL), *P. aeruginosa* (ATCC 15442) was the only one that did not significantly reduce the CFU count with only 1 min of ozone exposure, with a reduction of only 17.5% CFU. The other strains significantly reduced the number of colonies, with the most significant reduction being for *S. enterica* (ATCC 10708) (90.4%), followed by *E. coli* (ATCC 25922) and *S. aureus* (ATCC 6538) (both 98%). After 10 min of exposure to ozone, all ATCC strains showed a significant reduction in the number of counted CFU: *S. aureus* (ATCC 6538), 99.4%; *P. aeruginosa* (ATCC 15442), 93.2%; and *S. enterica* (ATCC 10708), 95.1%. *E. coli* (ATCC 25922) maintained the same percentage reduction of 98%. From 20 min to 40 min of exposure to ozone, all ATCC strains showed higher percentages of reduction in the number of CFU counts, ranging from 97.2% to 99.7%. In the MDR strains (10^5 CFU/mL), a significant reduction in the number of counted CFU in 40 min was observed: *S. aureus* (MRSA) with a reduction of 99.99%, *P. aeruginosa* (XDR) with 99.7%, *A. baumannii* (PDR) with 99.5%, and *K. pneumoniae* (KPC+) with 95.5%.

Table 2. Count and percentage reduction in the number of CFU in ATCC (*S. aureus* (ATCC 6538), *P. aeruginosa* (ATCC 15442), *S. enterica* (ATCC 10708), and *E. coli* (ATCC 25922)) strains and multidrug-resistant *S. aureus* (MRSA), *P. aeruginosa* (XDR), *A. baumannii* (PDR), and *K. pneumoniae* (KPC+). ATCC strains (10^5 CFU/mL) after exposure to ozone (1, 10, 20, 30, and 40 min) and in bacterial suspensions of multi-resistant strains (10^5 CFU/mL) after exposure to ozone (40 min).

Bacterial Strains	Ozone Exposure Times					
	C	1′	10′	20′	30′	40′
		Count Number CFU/% of Reduction				
S. aureus (ATCC 6538)	6287	123.1/98	36/99.4	31.9/99.5	27.2/99.6	20.4/99.7
P. aeruginosa (ATCC 15442)	3767	3109/17.5	256/93.2	105.2/97.2	65.33/98.3	57.8/98.5
S. enterica (ATCC 10708)	7391	711.3/90.4	360.8/95.1	69.7/99.1	63.11/99.2	53.9/99.3
E. coli (ATCC 25922)	3090	62/98	66.1/98	57.2/98.1	31.2/99	30.3/99

Table 2. Cont.

Bacterial Strains	Ozone Exposure Times					
	C	1′	10′	20′	30′	40′
		Count Number CFU/% of Reduction				
S. aureus (MRSA)	4041	-	-	-	-	0.1/99.99
P. aeruginosa (XDR)	1946	-	-	-	-	6.33/99.7
A. baumannii (PDR)	3228	-	-	-	-	16.6/99.5
K. pneumoniae (KPC+)	1894	-	-	-	-	86/95.5

C: control not exposed to ozone; CFU: colony-forming units.

3.3. Cell Viability

Ozone treatment significantly reduced bacterial growth in *S. aureus* (MRSA), leading to an inhibition of about 99.6%, followed by *P. aeruginosa* XDR (29.2%) (Figure 3). No difference was found in bacterial viability after ozone treatment in strains of *S. aureus* (ATCC 6538), *P. aeruginosa* (ATCC 15442), *S. enterica* (ATCC 10708), *E. coli* (ATCC 25922), *A. baumannii* (PDR), and *K. pneumoniae* (KPC+) (Figures 3 and 4).

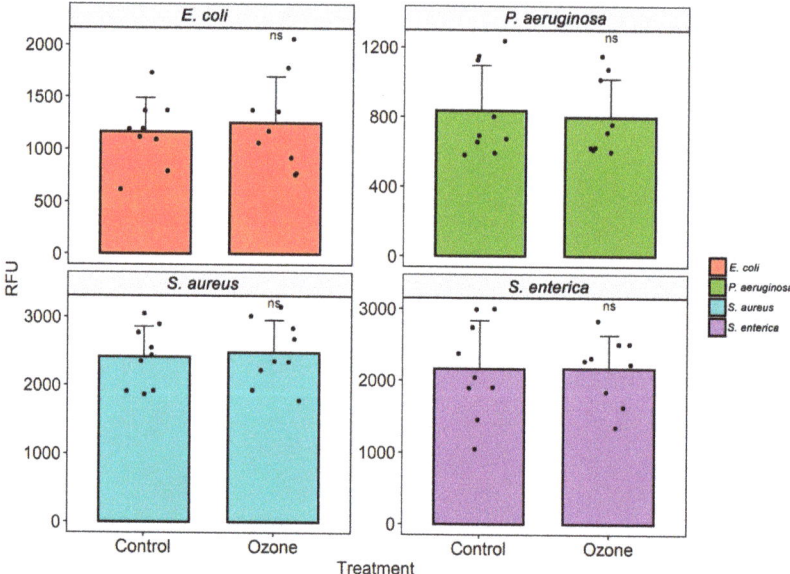

Figure 3. Analysis of cell viability after ozone treatment in different bacterial strains (*S. aureus* (ATCC 6538), *S. enterica* (ATCC 10708), *E. coli* (ATCC 25922), and *P. aeruginosa* (ATCC 15442)). The measurement of fluorescence intensity (relative fluorescence units, RFU) after the conversion of resazurin to resofurin by viable bacteria was performed in the control group (no treatment) and bacterial suspensions (10^5 CFU/mL) after exposure to ozone for 40 min. Results represent values from 3 randomly chosen colonies in the control group (no treatment) and after treatment with ozone. The black dots represent the values of fluorescence emission after addition of resazurin.

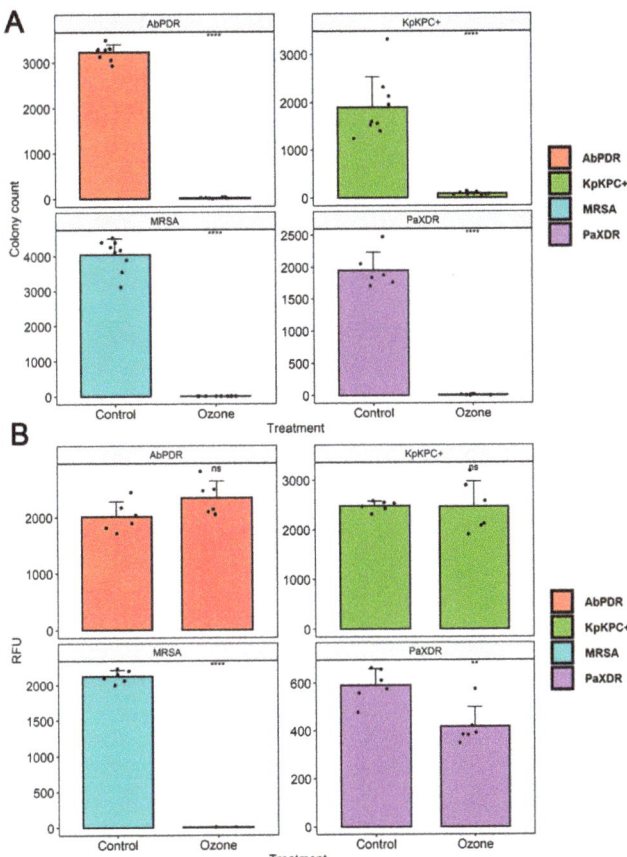

Figure 4. (**A**) The number of colony-forming units (CFU) in different bacterial strains (*S. aureus* (MRSA), *P. aeruginosa* (XDR), *A. baumannii* (PDR), and *K. pneumoniae* (KPC+)) were counted. The number of CFU in the control group (no treatment) and bacterial suspensions (10^5 CFU/mL) after exposure to ozone for 40 min was quantified. The black dots represent the number of CFU count of the different strains. (**B**) Analysis of cell viability after ozone treatment in different bacterial strains (*S. aureus* (MRSA), *P. aeruginosa* (XDR), *A. baumannii* (PDR), and *K. pneumoniae* (KPC+)). The measurement of fluorescence intensity (Relative fluorescence units, RFU) after the conversion of resazurin to resofurin by viable bacteria was performed in the control group (no treatment) and bacterial suspensions (10^5 CFU/mL) after exposure to ozone for 40 min. Results represent three randomly chosen colonies in the control group (no treatment) and after ozone treatment. The black dots show cell viability values through fluorescence emission after the addition of resazurin. ** Statistically significant ($p < 0.01$); **** statistically significant ($p < 0.001$).

3.4. Scanning Electron Microscopy (SEM)

Scanning electron microscopy was performed to confirm membrane damage to bacterial species. Morphological analysis showed that *S. aureus* (MRSA) and *P. aeruginosa* (XDR) present membrane alterations after O_3 treatment. All bacterial controls showed smooth and homogeneous surfaces. The therapy produced some cell wall protrusions (Figure 5).

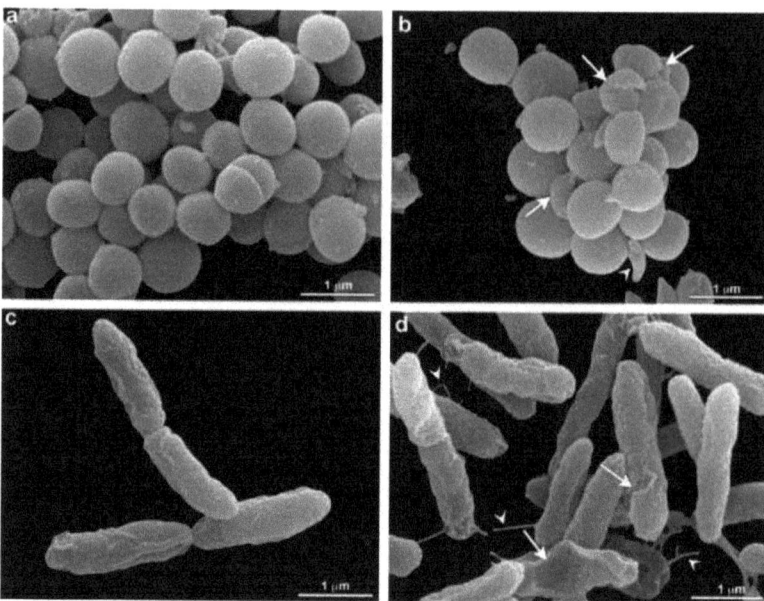

Figure 5. Morphological analysis of O_3 treatment by electron microscopy. *S. aureus* (MRSA) (**a,b**) and *P. aeruginosa* (XDR) (**c,d**) are seen without (**a,c**) and under O_3 treatment (**b,d**). An alteration in *S. aureus* (MRSA) shape is seen (arrowhead) in b. Damage in bacteria is observed after treatment (arrows) (**b**). Note that control cells are rounded and present in a homogeneous surface (**a**). Damaged cells are observed after treatment in *P. aeruginosa* (XDR) (arrows) (**d**). Some cell wall protrusions are observed in treated cells (arrowhead) (**d**). These aspects were not verified in control cells (**c**).

4. Discussion

Ozone generating equipment is already used as an easy and effective method of disinfection and sanitization to prevent the spread of MDR microorganisms in hospital wards. Furthermore, the portable characteristic of the equipment makes the mobile sanitation process viable for application in specific hospital areas [50,65,66]. Its high efficiency has been evaluated against many microorganisms, such as bacteria, fungi, and viruses, both on the surface and suspended in the air [45], and, for this reason, it has also been validated by several international organizations [67]. The practical applicability of ozone gas in the hospital environment can improve the microbiological condition, preventing and contributing to reducing HAI rates. For this reason, in this in vitro study, we used gaseous ozone, which has a greater disinfectant capacity due to its distribution and uniform penetration. Thus, we can inactivate microorganisms that may be present both on the surfaces and under the covers of hospital furniture [38].

Although few studies have investigated the relationship between ozone concentration and the microclimate conditions of different environments [68], some experiments have demonstrated that ozone concentration and relative humidity values played an important role in ozone efficiency and antimicrobial effect [69]. Humidity is an important parameter and must be considered because, in arid environmental conditions, the disinfection procedure may require a considerably longer exposure time. In addition, microorganisms die more quickly with increasing humidity, which favors the formation of free radicals [69]. Hudson and colleagues evaluated the effect of concentration, exposure time, and relative humidity in a study using 12 viruses. This work showed a reduction of three orders of magnitude, concerning the initial virus titer, at a concentration of 25 ppm of ozone per 15 min exposure to >90% RH [70]. Another study suggested that ozone sterilization was more effective with no air movement (no fans) at low temperature and humidity than at high temperature and humidity [71]. Finally, a recent study analyzed the influence of microclimate on the effectiveness of ozone indoors, showing that different temperature conditions, relative humidity, and distance from the ozone generator did not reduce microbial load [38]. The current study's parameters were satisfactory, with relative humidity ranging from 71.4% RH to 77.2% RH and an average temperature of around 23.4 °C.

The total ozone dose has been considered an essential factor for biocidal activity and is calculated as the product of exposure time and concentration [72]. In 2008, Tseng and Li [73] reported that the ozone dosage required for 99% viral inactivation should be calculated as ppm × min (i.e., a product of the ozone gas concentration multiplied by the duration), obtaining a value of 114 min [ppm] at 55% relative humidity to inactivate the dsDNA virus (T7). Although it has not been tested for antiviral action on pathogenic viruses or their substitutes, Pironti et al. [38] evaluated ozone's effectiveness in Gram-negative bacteria as an indicator of microbial contamination. By calculating the mean concentration (1.6 ppm) and the exposure time (70 min), the value of 112 min [ppm], which was very close to that suggested by others to inactivate the viruses, was obtained [73]. As stated in the literature, the critical factor for the inactivation of microorganisms in the total ozone dose is calculated as the product of the exposure time and the concentration. However, considering this calculation, our values will be higher as we use higher ozone concentrations and exposure times with large variation intervals (10 in 10 min). According to our measurements, the average ozone concentration recorded reached 43.9 ppm, reaching the minimum average value of 21.1 ppm and the maximum average value of 71.1 ppm, with the complete disappearance of the ozone after 30 min. Short exposure time to ozone was able to interfere with bacterial growth, showing that in 1 min, ozone inhibited colony growth by 90% (1 $\log_{10}$) for *S. enterica* ATCC 10708 and 98% (~2 $\log_{10}$) for *S. aureus* ATCC 6538 and *E. coli* ATCC 25922, respectively. *P. aeruginosa* ATCC 15442 was an exception, showing an inhibition rate of 17.5% with 1 min exposure to ozone. Conversely, at 10 min of exposure, its bacterial growth inhibition rate increased to approximately 95%. After exposure to ozone for 10 min, *S. aureus* ATCC 6538 showed a reduced rate in colony growth (CFU/mL) around 99% (2 $\log_{10}$). The same was verified for *S. enterica* (ATCC 10708) at 20 min and *E. coli* ATCC 25922 at 30 min. The longest exposure time used in this study was 40 min, and among the ATCC strains tested, *P. aeruginosa* ATCC 15442, despite a high value, had the lowest rate of reduction in colony growth (98.5%) in comparison to others. In the MDR strains of the ESKAPE group, ozone was able to reduce the increase by 99.99% (3 $\log_{10}$) of the colonies, followed by *P. aeruginosa* (XDR) with 99.7% (~3 $\log_{10}$), *A. baumannii* (PDR) with 99.5%, and *K. pneumoniae* (KPC+) with 95.5% (~1.5 $\log_{10}$). Our results agree with previous studies that demonstrated a reduction in colony number (CFU/mL) by around three $\log_{10}$ bacteria known to cause hospital-acquired infections [47,49,74]. One of the studies used an ozone dose of 25 ppm for 20 min, with a short period of excess moisture (90% RH) and was able to inactivate more than 3 $\log_{10}$ in most bacteria, including *A. baumannii*, *Clostridium difficile*, and methicillin-resistant *S. aureus*, both in a laboratory test system and under simulated field conditions [49]. Another study obtained the same reduction by applying the exact ozone dosage at different exposure times and 75–95% [74]. According to Moat et al., the increase in ozone concentration can lead to disinfectant efficacy [47]. Zoutman et al. showed that it could only achieve a greater than six $\log_{10}$ reduction for MRSA at an ozone concentration of 500 ppm (exposure time 90 min) at a relative humidity of 80%, produced by a separate humidifier [75].

Reduced cell viability is one of the highly reliable biomarkers of cytotoxicity [76]. Several tests allow evaluating cell viability after a toxicity study in cultured cells. In our study, the method used to assess cell viability was the resazurin reduction assay, one of the most frequently used tests. Resazurin (7-hydroxy-3H-phenoxazin-3-one 10-oxide) is a redox dye indicator of metabolic activity in cell cultures and has numerous applications, such as toxicity, proliferation, and cell viability studies [64]. Resazurin is a non-fluorescent blue reagent that, by the action of the dehydrogenase enzyme found in metabolically active cells, is reduced to resorufin, which is highly fluorescent and has a pink color. This conversion only occurs in viable cells; as such, the amount of resorufin produced is proportional to the number of viable cells in the sample [64]. Resazurin is not toxic to cells, and the occurrence of cell death is not necessary to obtain the measurements. It is a simple and fast test that can be measured either by colorimetry or fluorimetry [62], and the amount of resorufin produced is proportional to the number of viable cells [63]. According to our results, we observed that ozone significantly reduced the in vitro growth of bacteria.

Conversely, when we investigated its metabolic capacity through resazurin, we found a significant reduction in values only for two strains, showing that ozone was able to interfere with the cell viability of S. aureus (MRSA), which showed inhibition of about 99.6%, followed by P. aeruginosa XDR (29.2%). Curiously, in a recent study using the same strains, we showed that ozone at low concentrations did not interfere with bacterial growth, but it could significantly inhibit cell viability [51]. Interestingly, all species' reference strains (ATCC) were less susceptible to ozone treatment. Similarly, a study demonstrated that the antibiotic resistance of the isolates was not correlated to a higher ozone tolerance [77]. The increased susceptibility of PaXDR and MRSA to ozone may be due to a metabolic cost associated with antibiotic resistance that decreases fitness and reduces the ecological versatility of resistant strains [78].

Although not as pronounced, the effectiveness of ozone as a disinfectant varies significantly between different types of bacteria, even at the strain level [79,80], and depends on several factors such as the growth stage, the cell envelope, the efficiency of repair mechanisms, and the type of viability indicator used [81–83]. In addition, some factors can reduce the ozone stability or protect microorganisms from its effects, thus decreasing the disinfection efficiency, such as concentration and type of dissolved organic material or the presence of flakes or particles [84–86]. Yet, ozone decomposition results in superoxide, hydroperoxyl, and hydroxyl radicals [87,88]. Microorganisms, through detoxification enzymes, can develop mechanisms such as the production of superoxide dismutases, reductases, peroxides, and catalases to neutralize the lethal effects of reactive oxygen species [58,89,90]. In *E. coli*, two of these mechanisms' (*SoxR* and *OxyR*) responsive redox transcription regulators have already been well described [91]. Both regulators are induced in the presence of radicals [92] and activate several genes such as *soxS* and *sod*, which, in turn, protect against these radicals through DNA repair or removal of the radicals [91]. *DnaK* and *RpoS* are two general stress gene regulators that, although not dedicated mechanisms of protection against oxidative radicals, have previously been shown to confer protection against them [93–95]. *S. aureus* uses the expression of several of these detoxification proteins, including catalase (*katA*), superoxide dismutase (*sodA*, *sodM*), thioredoxin reductase (*trxB*), thioredoxin (*trxA*), alkyl hydroperoxide reductase (*ahpC*, *ahpF*) enzymes, and glutathione peroxidase (*gpxA*) [96]. Similar radicals are produced during ozone treatments; therefore, these genes are expected to play an important role in protecting cells against this technology in different bacteria that could also justify interfering with cell viability.

The disinfectant potential of ozone is attributed to its ability to promote cell wall disturbance and extravasation of ions and intracellular molecules, triggering cell death [96]. The primary cellular targets for ozone are nucleic acids, where damage can range from base lesions to single- and double-strand breaks [80]. Lesions can lead to more or less compromising point mutations, whereas massive DNA breakage is lethal if not repaired [96–99]. Many studies prove that the cell envelope is also affected during ozonation, even before severe DNA damage [100–102]. Ozone can influence the global polarity of the bacterial surface [58], involving mechanisms of lipid peroxidation [59,103] and the degradation of transmembrane proteins that control the flow of ions. As a result, the cells will rupture with a subsequent leakage of ions between the media, resulting in the death of the microorganism [60]. In addition, the high oxidative potential of ozone contributes to changes in the zeta potential. A physical property is applied to assess the degree of peripheral electronegativity on the cell surface when suspended in a fluid [104]. In a study by Feng et al. (2018), as the ozone dose increased, the zeta potential tended to decrease, becoming hostile and causing greater bacterial instability in the medium [58,105]. Ozone is a gas that can oxidize glycoproteins, glycolipids, and cell wall amino acids, destroying sulfhydryl groups in enzymes and causing the breakdown of cell enzymatic activity [106,107].

Our study expands on and corroborates what is already known about the gas since the analysis of the inhibition of microbial growth and/or reduction of the CFU count in plates exposed to ozone, containing both reference strains and clinical and environmental strains highly resistant to antimicrobials, compared to the control group, proved its effectiveness as a chemical compound in microbial control processes. The practical applicability of gaseous ozone in hospital environments can improve the microbiological condition, preventing and contributing to HAI rates. It is exciting and unprecedented evidence of the potential for ozone disinfection because, in natural indoor environments, it is possible to disinfect surfaces not typically disinfected with hand-applied liquid disinfectants. In this sense, it can eliminate MDR organisms with a significant advantage compared to mechanical disinfection methods with liquid disinfectants of environmental surfaces in health care establishments, including the hospital environment, where it is common to use other chemical compounds in liquid form.

5. Conclusions

HAIs represent the most common adverse event in ICUs and are usually caused by MDR bacteria. As a result, preventing the transmission of MDR bacteria has become increasingly important to limit the spread of these infections, and a correct sanitization protocol is particularly crucial. Given the prolonged hospital stays and increased treatment costs seen in patients who develop HAIs, ozone-based decontamination approaches that have low toxicity compared to other sanitization products may represent the future of hospital cleaning methods as a highly cost-effective and promising intervention capable of being used as an additional procedure for terminal cleaning, in addition to the "classic" terminal cleaning (by current biocides). Our results evidenced the antimicrobial potential of gaseous ozone in bacteria that are currently a significant problem worldwide. In the future, this resource may be a part of the protocol for the disinfection of hospital environments and surfaces, ensuring the control of microbial development.

Supplementary Materials: The following supporting information can be downloaded at: https://www.mdpi.com/article/10.3390/molecules27133998/s1, Figure S1: SANITECH O3-80-Sanitization equipment ozone generator coupled to two containers of approximately 1 m^3 each, used for exposing samples to ozone.

Author Contributions: Conceptualization, K.R.; formal analysis, K.R., G.C.L., V.M., F.O.C. and J.P.R.S.C.; data curation, M.H.S.V.-B.; writing—review and editing, K.R. and S.G.D.-S.; visualization, K.R. and S.G.D.-S.; supervision, K.R.; funding acquisition, S.G.D.-S. All authors have read and agreed to the published version of the manuscript.

Funding: This research was funded by the Carlos Chagas Filho Foundation for Research Support of the State of Rio de Janeiro (FAPERJ—n° E-26 110.198-13; E26 202.841-2018) and the Brazilian Council for Scientific Research (CNPq—n° 467.488.2014-2; 3075732011; 3013322015-0).

Institutional Review Board Statement: Not applicable.

Informed Consent Statement: Not applicable.

Data Availability Statement: The data presented in this study are available upon request from the corresponding author.

Acknowledgments: We thank the Rudolf Barth Electron Microscopy Platform of the Oswaldo Cruz Institute/FIOCRUZ for the use of electron microscopy analysis facilities. K.R. and G.C.L. are post-doc fellows from CAPES/CDTS. J.P.R.S.C is a CAPES/MSci fellow from the Science and Biotechnology Post Graduation program of the Federal Fluminense University.

Conflicts of Interest: The authors declare no conflict of interest.

References

1. Allegranzi, B.; Bagheri Nejad, S.; Combescure, C.; Graafmans, W.; Attar, H.; Donaldson, L.; Pittet, D. Burden of endemic health-care-associated infection in developing countries: Systematic review and meta-analysis. *Lancet* **2011**, *337*, 228–241. [CrossRef]
2. ECDC. European Centre for Disease Prevention and Control Annual Epidemiological Report 2016- Healthcare-Associated Infections Acquired in Intensive Care Units. 2017. Available online: https://www.ecdc.Europa.eu/en/publications-data/healthcare-associated-infections-intensive-care-units-annualepidemiological-0 (accessed on 20 August 2021).
3. Brasil. Boletim Segurança do Paciente e Qualidade em Serviços de Saúde n° 16: Avaliação dos indicadores nacionais das Infecções Relacionadas à Assistência à Saúde (IRAS) e Resistência microbiana do ano de 2016. 2017. Available online: https://www20.Anvisa.gov.br/segurancadopaciente/index.php/publicacoes/item/boletim-seguranca-do-paciente-e-qualidade-em-servicos-de-saude-n-16-avaliacaoods-indicadores-nacionais-das-infeccoes-relacionadas-a-assistencia-a-saudeiras-e-resistenciamicrobiana-do-ano-de-2016 (accessed on 20 August 2021).
4. Jenks, J.; Duse, A.; Wattal, C.; Zaidi, A.K.; Wertheim, H.F.; Sumpradit, N.; Vlieghe, E.; Hara, G.L.; Gould, I.M.; Goossens, H.; et al. Antibiotic resistance needs global solutions. *Lancet Infect. Dis.* **2014**, *14*, 550. [CrossRef]
5. WHO (World Health Organization). *The Burden of Healthcare-Associated Infection Worldwide: A Summary*; World Health Organization: Lisboa, Portugal, 2011; Volume 3. Available online: http://www.who.int/gpsc/countrywork/summary20100430em.pdf (accessed on 20 August 2021).
6. Ali, S.; Birhane, M.; Bekele, S.; Kibru, G.; Teshager, L.; Yilma, Y.; Ahmed, Y.; Fentahun, N.; Assefa, H.; Gashaw, M.; et al. Healthcare-associated infection and its risk factors among patients admitted to a tertiary hospital in Ethiopia: A longitudinal study. *Antimicrob. Resist. Infect. Control* **2018**, *7*, 2. [CrossRef] [PubMed]
7. Umscheid, C.; Mitchell, M.D.; Doshi, J.A.; Agarwal, R.; Williams, K.; Brennan, P.J. Estimating the proportion of healthcare-associated infections that are reasonably preventable and the associated mortality and costs. *Infect. Control Hosp. Epidemiol.* **2011**, *32*, 101–114. [CrossRef] [PubMed]
8. Gatt, Y.E.; Margalit, H. Common adaptive strategies underlie within-host evolution of bacterial pathogens. *Mol. Biol. Evol.* **2021**, *38*, 1101–1121. [CrossRef] [PubMed]
9. Santajit, S.; Indrawattana, N. Mechanisms of antimicrobial resistance in ESKAPE pathogens. *Biomed. Res. Int.* **2016**, *2016*, 2475067. [CrossRef] [PubMed]
10. Georgescu, M.; Gheorghe, I.; Curutiu, C.; Lazar, V.; Bleotu, C.; Chifiriuc, M.C. Virulence and resistance features of *Pseudomonas aeruginosa* strains isolated from chronic leg ulcers. *BMC Infect. Dis.* **2016**, *16*, 92. [CrossRef] [PubMed]
11. Coelho, F.; Coelho, M.; Diniz, A.; Vicente, G.; Vieira, C. Velhos Problemas, novos desafios. *Rev. Technol. Hospitalar.* **2011**, *43*, 30–32.
12. Tadesse, B.T.; Ashley, E.A.; Ongarello, S.; Havumaki, J.; Wijegoonewardena, M.; Gonzalez, I.J.; Dittrich, S. Antimicrobial resistance in Africa: A systematic review. *BMC Infect. Dis.* **2017**, *17*, 616. [CrossRef] [PubMed]
13. Gajdács, M.; Albericio, F. Antibiotic resistance: From the bench to patients. *Antibiotics* **2019**, *8*, 129. [CrossRef] [PubMed]
14. Bocé, M.; Tassé, M.; Mallet-Ladeira, S.; Pillet, F.; Da Silva, C.; Vicendo, P.; Lacroix, P.G.; Malfant, I.; Rols, M.P. Effect of trans(NO, OH)-[RuFT(Cl)(OH)NO](PF(6)) ruthenium nitrosyl complex on methicillin-resistant *Staphylococcus epidermidis*. *Sci. Rep.* **2019**, *9*, 4867. [CrossRef] [PubMed]
15. Andersen, K.G.; Rambaut, A.; Lipkin, W.I.; Holmes, E.C.; Garry, R.F. The proximal origin of SARS-CoV-2. *Nat. Med.* **2020**, *26*, 450–452. [CrossRef]
16. Park, S.E. Epidemiology, virology, and clinical features of severe acute respiratory syndrome -coronavirus-2 (SARS-CoV-2; Coronavirus Disease-19). *Clin. Exp. Pediatr.* **2020**, *63*, 119–124. [CrossRef]
17. Cucinotta, D.; Vanelli, M. WHO Declares COVID-19 a Pandemic. *Acta Biomed.* **2020**, *91*, 157–160. [CrossRef] [PubMed]
18. Zhu, N.; Zhang, D.; Wang, W.; Li, X.; Yang, B.; Song, J.; Zhao, X.; Huang, B.; Shi, W.; Lu, R.; et al. China novel coronavirus investigating and research team. A novel coronavirus from patients with pneumonia in China, 2019. *N. Engl. J. Med.* **2020**, *382*, 727–733. [CrossRef] [PubMed]
19. Canto, N.R.; Ruiz-Garbajosa, P. Co-resistance: An opportunity for the bacteria and resistance genes. *Curr. Opin. Pharmacol.* **2011**, *11*, 477–485. [CrossRef] [PubMed]
20. Clancy, C.J.; Nguyen, M.H. Coroviruses disease 2019, superinfections, and antimicrobial development. What can we expect? *Clin. Infect. Dis.* **2020**, *71*, 2736–2743. [CrossRef] [PubMed]
21. Bengoechea, J.Á.; Bamford, C.G.G. SARS-CoV-2, bacterial coinfections, and AMR: The deadly trio in COVID-19? *EMBO Mol. Med.* **2020**, *26*, e12560. [CrossRef]
22. Fu, Y.; Yang, Q.; Xu, M.; Kong, H.; Chen, H.; Fu, Y.; Yao, Y.; Zhou, H.; Zhou, J. Secondary bacterial infections in critically ill patients with coronavirus disease 2019. *Open Forum Infect. Dis.* **2020**, *5*, ofaa220. [CrossRef] [PubMed]
23. Rawson, T.M.; Moore, L.S.P.; Zhu, N.; Ranganathan, N.; Skolimowska, K.; Gilchrist, M.; Satta, G.; Cooke, G.; Holmes, A. Bacterial and fungal coinfection in individuals with coronavirus: A rapid review to support COVID-19 antimicrobial prescribing. *Clin. Infect. Dis.* **2020**, *71*, 2459–2468. [CrossRef] [PubMed]
24. Chirumbolo, S.; Simonetti, V.; Franzini, M.; Valdenassi, L.; Bertossi, D.; Pandolfi, S. Estimating coronavirus disease 2019 (COVID19)-caused deaths in hospitals and healthcare units: Do hospital-acquired infections play a role? Comments with a proposal. *Infect. Control. Hosp. Epidemiol.* **2021**, *19*, 1–2. [CrossRef]

25. Lizioli, A.; Privitera, G.; Alliata, E.; Banfi, E.M.A.; Boselli, L.; Panceri, M.L.; Perna, M.C.; Porretta, A.D.; Santini, M.G.; Carreri, V. Prevalence of nosocomial infections in Italy: Result from the Lombardy survey in 2000. *J. Hosp. Infect.* **2003**, *54*, 141–148. [CrossRef]
26. Nicastri, E.; Petrosillo, N.; Martini, L.; Larosa, M.; Gesu, G.P.; Ippolito, G.; INF-NOS Study Group. Prevalence of nosocomial infections in 15 Italian hospitals: First point prevalence study for the INF-NOS project. *Infection* **2003**, *71*, 10–15. [PubMed]
27. Zotti, C.M.; Ioli, G.M.; Charrier, L.; Arditi, G.; Argentero, P.A.; Biglino, A.; Farina, E.C.; Ruggenini, A.M.; Reale, R.; Romagnoli, S.; et al. Hospital-acquired infections in Italy: A region wide prevalence study. *J. Hosp. Infect.* **2004**, *56*, 142–149. [CrossRef] [PubMed]
28. Mulani, M.S.; Kamble, E.E.; Kumkar, S.N.; Tawre, M.S.; Pardesi, K.R. Emerging strategies to combat eskape pathogens in the era of antimicrobial resistance: A review. *Front. Microbiol.* **2019**, *10*, 539. [CrossRef]
29. De Oliveira, D.M.P.; Forde, B.M.; Kidd, T.J.; Harris, P.N.A.; Schembri, M.A.; Beatson, S.A.; Paterson, D.L.; Walker, M.J. Antimicrobial resistance in ESKAPE pathogens. *Clin. Microbiol. Rev.* **2020**, *33*, e00181-19. [CrossRef]
30. Munita, J.M.; Arias, C.A. Mechanisms of antibiotic resistance. *Microbiol. Spectr.* **2016**, *4*, 10. [CrossRef]
31. Miller, W.R.; Munita, J.M.; Arias, C.A. Mechanisms of antibiotic resistance in enterococci. *Expert. Rev. Anti. Infect. Ther.* **2014**, *12*, 1221–1236. [CrossRef]
32. WHO (World Health Organization). *Global Priority List of Antibiotic-Resistant Bacteria to Guide Research, Discovery, and Development of New Antibiotics*; World Health Organization: Geneva, Switzerland, 2017. Available online: https://www.who.int/medicines/publications/WHO-PPL-Short_Summary_25Feb-ET_NM_WHO.pdf (accessed on 15 August 2021).
33. Fernandes, A.T.; Fernandes, M.O.V.; Ribeiro Filho, N.; Graziano, K.U.; Gabrielloni, M.C.; Cavalcante, N.J.F.; Lacerda, R.A. *Infecção Hospitalar e Suas Interfaces na Área da Saúde*, 1st ed.; Atheneu: São Paulo, Brazil, 2000; p. 1795.
34. Magiorakos, A.P.; Srinivasan, A.; Carey, R.B.; Carmeli, Y.; Falagas, M.E.; Giske, C.G.; Harbarth, S.; Hindler, J.F.; Kahlmeter, G.; Olsson-Liljequist, B.; et al. Multidrug-resistant, extensively drug-resistant and pan drug-resistant bacteria: An international expert proposal for interim standard definitions for acquired resistance. *Clin. Microbiol. Infect.* **2012**, *18*, 268–281. [CrossRef]
35. Oliveira, A.C. *Infecções Hospitalares, Epidemiologia, Prevenção e Controle*, 1st ed.; Guanabara Koogan—Grupo Gen: Rio de Janeiro, Brazil, 2005; p. 710.
36. Stephanie, J.D. Controlling hospital-acquired infection: Focus on the role of the environment and new technologies for decontamination. *Clin. Microbiol. Rev.* **2014**, *27*, 665–690. [CrossRef]
37. Moccia, G.; Motta, O.; Pironti, C.; Proto, A.; Capunzo, M.; De Caro, F. An alternative approach for the decontamination of hospital settings. *J. Infect. Public Health* **2020**, *13*, 2038–2044. [CrossRef] [PubMed]
38. Pironti, C.; Motta, O.; Proto, A. Development of a new vapor phase methodology for textiles disinfection. *Clean. Engin. Technol.* **2021**, *4*, 100170. [CrossRef]
39. Bayarri, B.; Cruz-Alcalde, A.; López-Vinent, N.; Micó, M.M.; Sans, C.J. Can ozone inactivate SARS-CoV-2? A review of mechanisms and performance on viruses. *J. Hazard. Mater.* **2021**, *415*, 125658. [CrossRef] [PubMed]
40. Nascente, E.P.; Chagas, S.R.; Pessoa, A.V.C.; Matos, M.P.C.; Andrade, M.A.; Pascoal, L.M. Potencial antimicrobiano do ozônio: Aplicações e perspectivas em medicina veterinária. *Pubvet* **2019**, *13*, 130. [CrossRef]
41. Bocci, V. *Ozone: A New Medical Drug*, 2nd ed.; Springer: Berlin/Heidelberg, Germany, 2010; p. 336. [CrossRef]
42. Wickramanayake, G.B.; Sproul, O.J. Ozone concentration and temperature effects on disinfection kinetics. *Ozone Sci. Eng.* **1988**, *10*, 123–135. [CrossRef]
43. Wolf, C.; Von Gunten, U.; Kohn, T. Kinetics of inactivation of waterborne enteric viruses by ozone. *Environ. Sci. Technol.* **2018**, *52*, 2170–2177. [CrossRef]
44. Blanchard, E.L.; Lawrence, J.D.; Noble, J.A.; Xu, M.; Joo, T.; Ng, N.L.; Schmidt, B.E.; Santangelo, P.J.; Finn, M.G.G. Enveloped virus inactivation on personal protective equipment by exposure to ozone. *medRxiv* **2020**. [CrossRef]
45. Dubuis, M.E.E.; Dumont-Leblond, N.; Lalibert'e, C.; Veillette, M.; Turgeon, N.; Jean, J.; Duchaine, C. Ozone efficacy for the control of airborne viruses: Bacteriophage and norovirus models. *PLoS ONE* **2020**, *15*, e0231164. [CrossRef]
46. Davies, A.; Pottage, T.; Bennett, A.; Walker, J. Gaseous and air decontamination technologies for *Clostridium difficile* in the healthcare environment. *J. Hosp. Infect.* **2011**, *77*, 199–203. [CrossRef]
47. Moat, J.; Cargill, J.; Shone, J.; Upton, M. Application of a novel decontamination process using gaseous ozone. *Canad. J. Microbiol.* **2009**, *55*, 928–933. [CrossRef]
48. Piletić, K.; Kovač, B.; Perčić, M.; Žigon, J.; Broznić, D.; Karleuša, L.; Blagojević, S.L.; Oder, M.; Gobin, I. Disinfectin action of gaseous ozone on OXA-48-producing *Klebsiella pneumoniae* biofilm in vitro. *Int. J. Environ. Res. Public Health* **2022**, *19*, 6177. [CrossRef] [PubMed]
49. Sharma, M.; Hudson, J.B. Ozone gas is an effective and practical antibacterial agent. *Am. J. Infect. Control* **2008**, *36*, 559–563. [CrossRef] [PubMed]
50. Moccia, G.; De Caro, F.; Pironti, C.; Boccia, G.; Capunzo, M.; Borrelli, A.; Motta, O. Development and improvement of an effective method for air and surfaces disinfection with ozone gas as a decontaminating agent. *Medicina* **2020**, *56*, 578. [CrossRef] [PubMed]
51. Rangel, K.; Cabral, F.O.; Lechuga, G.C.; Carvalho, J.P.R.S.C.; Villas-Bôas, M.H.S.; Midlej, V.; De-Simone, S.G. Detrimental effect of ozone on pathogenic bacteria. *Microorganisms* **2022**, *10*, 40. [CrossRef] [PubMed]
52. Fontes, B.; Heimbecker, A.M.C.; de Souza Brito, G.; Costa, S.F.; van der Heijden, I.M.; Levin, A.S.; Rasslan, S. Effect of low-dose gaseous ozone on pathogenic bacteria. *BMC Infect. Dis.* **2012**, *12*, 358. [CrossRef]

53. Merks, P.; Religioni, U.; Bilmin, K.; Bogusz, J.; Juszczyk, G.; Barańska, A.; Kuthan, R.; Drelich, E.; Jakubowska, M.; Świeczkowski, D.; et al. Ozone disinfection of community pharmacies during the COVID-19 pandemic as a possible preventive measure for infection spread. *Med. Pr.* **2021**, *72*, 529–534. [CrossRef] [PubMed]
54. Franke, G.; Knobling, B.; Brill, F.H.; Becker, B.; Klupp, E.M.; Belmar Campos, C.; Pfefferle, S.; Lütgehetmann, M.; Knobloch, J.K. An automated room disinfection system using ozone is highly active against surrogates for SARS-CoV-2. *J. Hosp. Infect.* **2021**, *112*, 108–113. [CrossRef]
55. Percivalle, E.; Clerici, M.; Cassaniti, I.; Nepita, E.V.; Marchese, P.; Olivati, D.; Catelli, C.; Berri, A.; Baldanti, F.; Marone, P.; et al. SARS-CoV-2 viability on different surfaces after gaseous ozone treatment: A preliminary evaluation. *J. Hosp. Infect.* **2021**, *110*, 33–36. [CrossRef]
56. Radvar, S.; Karkon-Shayan, S.; Motamed-Sanaye, A.; Majidi, M.; Hajebrahimi, S.; Taleschian-Tabrizi, N.; Pashazadeh, F.; Sahebkar, A. Using ozone therapy as an option for treatment of COVID-19 Patients: A scoping review. *Adv. Exp. Med. Biol.* **2021**, *1327*, 151–160. [CrossRef]
57. Brodowska, A.J.; Nowak, A.; Śmigielski, K. Ozone in the food industry: Principles of ozone treatment, mechanisms of action, and applications: An overview. *Crit. Rev. Food Sci. Nutr.* **2018**, *58*, 2176–2201. [CrossRef]
58. Feng, L.; Zhang, K.; Gao, M.; Shi, C.; Ge, C.; Qu, D.; Zhu, J.; Shi, Y.; Han, J. Inactivation of *Vibrio parahaemolyticus* by aqueous ozone. *J. Microbiol. Biotechnol.* **2018**, *28*, 1233–1246. [CrossRef] [PubMed]
59. Ersoy, Z.G.; Barisci, S.; Turkay, O. Mechanisms of the *Escherichia coli* and *Enterococcus faecalis* inactivation by ozone. *Food Sci. Technol.* **2019**, *100*, 306–313. [CrossRef]
60. Zhang, Y.Q.; Wu, Q.P.; Zhang, J.M.; Yang, X.H. Effects of ozone on membrane permeability and ultrastructure in *Pseudomonas aeruginosa*. *J. Appl. Microbiol.* **2011**, *111*, 1006–1015. [CrossRef] [PubMed]
61. Lall, N.; Henley-Smith, C.J.; Canha, M.N.; Oosthuizen, C.B.; Barrington, D. Viability reagent presto blue in comparison with other available reagents utilized in cytotoxicity and antimicrobial assays. *Int. J. Microbiol.* **2013**, *2013*, 420601. [CrossRef] [PubMed]
62. Riss, T.; Moravec, R.; Niles, A. Development for cell viability and apoptosis for high-throughput screening. In *A Practical Guide to Assay Development and High-Throughput Screening in Drug Discovery*; Chen, T., Ed.; CRC Press: Boca Raton, FL, USA, 2010; pp. 109–110.
63. Riss, T.; Moravec, R.A.; Niles, A.L.; Duellman, S.; Benink, H.A.; Worzella, T.J.; Minor, L.; Markossian, S.; Grossman, A.; Brimacombe, K.; et al. Cell Viability Assays. In *The Assay Guidance Manual*; Sittampalam, G., Ed.; Eli Lilly Co.: Indianapolis, IN, USA; National Center for Advancing Translational Sciences: Bethesda, MD, USA, 2016; pp. 10–12.
64. Präbst, K.; Engelhardt, H.; Ringgeler, S.; Hübner, H. Basic colorimetric proliferation assays: MTT WST and resazurin. *Methods Mol. Biol.* **2017**, *1601*, 1–17. [CrossRef]
65. Sousa, C.S.; Torres, L.M.; Azevedo, M.P.F.; Camargo, T.C.; Graziano, K.U.; Lacerda, R.A.; Turrini, R.N.T. Sterilization with ozone in health care: An integrative literature review. *Rev. Esc. Enfer. USP* **2011**, *45*, 1243–1249. [CrossRef]
66. Rubio-Romero, J.C.; Pardo-Ferreira, M.D.C.; Torrecilla-García, J.A.; Calero-Castro, S. Disposable masks: Disinfection and sterilization for reuse, and non-certified manufacturing, in the face of shortages during the COVID-19 pandemic. *Saf. Sci.* **2020**, *129*, 104830. [CrossRef]
67. EPA. Environmental Protection Agency. Integrated Science Assessment for Ozone and Related Photochemical Oxidant (Final Report, April 2020). 2020. Available online: https://cfpub.epa.gov/ncea/isa/recordisplay.cfm?deid=348522 (accessed on 15 August 2021).
68. Blanco, A.; Ojembarrena, F.B.; Clavo, B.; Negro, C. Ozone potential to fight against SAR-COV-2 pandemic: Facts and research needs. *Environ. Sci. Pollut. Res. Int.* **2021**, *28*, 16517–16531. [CrossRef]
69. Grignani, E.; Mansi, A.; Cabella, R.; Castellano, P.; Tirabasso, A.; Sisto, R.; Spagnoli, M.; Fabrizi, G.; Frigerio, F.; Tranfo, G. Safe and effective use of ozone as air and surface disinfectant in the conjuncture of COVID-19. *Gases* **2021**, *1*, 19–32. [CrossRef]
70. Hudson, J.B.; Sharma, M.; Vimalanathan, S. Development of a practical method for using ozone gas as a virus decontaminating agent. *Ozone Sci. Eng.* **2009**, *31*, 216–223. [CrossRef]
71. McClurkin, J.D.; Maier, D.E.; Ileleji, K.E. Half-life time of ozone as a function of air movement and conditions in a sealed container. *J. Stored Prod. Res.* **2013**, *55*, 41–47. [CrossRef]
72. Dennis, R.; Cashion, A.; Emanuel, S.; Hubbard, D. Ozone gas: Scientific justification and practical guidelines for improvised disinfection using consumer-grade ozone generators and plastic storage boxes. *J. Sci. Med.* **2020**, *2*, 1–15. [CrossRef]
73. Tseng, C.; Li, C. Inactivation of surface viruses by gaseous ozone. *J. Environ. Health* **2008**, *70*, 56–63.
74. Knobling, B.; Franke, G.; Klupp, E.M.; Belmar Campos, C.; Knobloch, J.K. Evaluation of the effectiveness of two automated room decontamination devices under real-life conditions. *Front. Public Health* **2021**, *9*, 618263. [CrossRef] [PubMed]
75. Zoutman, D.; Shannon, M.; Mandel, A. Effectiveness of a novel ozone-based system for the rapid high-level disinfection of health care spaces and surfaces. *Am. J. Infect. Control.* **2011**, *39*, 873–879. [CrossRef]
76. Xu, Y.; Ji, J.; Wu, H.; Pi, F.; Blaženović, I.; Zhang, Y.; Sun, X. Untargeted GC-TOFMS-based cellular metabolism analysis to evaluate ozone degradation effect of deoxynivalenol. *Toxicon* **2019**, *168*, 49–57. [CrossRef]
77. Heß, S.; Gallert, C. Sensitivity of antibiotic-resistant and antibiotic susceptible *Escherichia coli*, *Enterococcus* and *Staphylococcus*, strains against ozone. *J. Water Health* **2015**, *13*, 1020–1028. [CrossRef]
78. Schulz zur Wiesch, P.; Engelstadter, J.; Bonhoeffer, S. Compensation of fitness costs and reversibility of antibiotic resistance mutations. *Antimicrob. Agents Chemother.* **2010**, *54*, 2085–2095. [CrossRef]

79. Von Gunten, U. Ozonation of drinking water: Part II. Disinfection and by-product formation in presence of bromide, iodide, or chlorine. *Water Res.* **2003**, *37*, 1469–1487. [CrossRef]
80. Von Sonntag, C.; Von Gunten, U. *Chemistry of Ozone in Water and Wastewater Treatment from Basic Principles to Applications*; IWA Publishing: London, UK, 2012; p. 306. [CrossRef]
81. Casolari, A. Microbial Death. In *Physiological Models in Microbiology*; Bazin, M.J., Prosser, J.I., Eds.; CRC Press: Boca Raton, FL, USA, 1988; Volume 2, pp. 1–44.
82. Broadwater, W.T.; Hoehn, R.C.; King, P.H. Sensitivity of three selected bacterial species to ozone. *Appl. Microbiol.* **1973**, *26*, 391–393. [CrossRef]
83. Patil, S.; Valdramidis, V.P.; Karatzas, K.A.; Cullen, P.J.; Bourke, P. Assessing the microbial oxidative stress mechanism of ozone treatment through the responses of *Escherichia coli* mutants. *J. Appl. Microbiol.* **2011**, *111*, 136–144. [CrossRef] [PubMed]
84. Xu, P.; Janex, M.L.; Savoye, P.; Cockx, A.; Lazarova, V. Wastewater disinfection by ozone: Main parameters for process design. *Water Res.* **2002**, *36*, 1043–1055. [CrossRef]
85. Patil, S.; Bourke, P.; Frias, J.M.; Tiwari, B.K. Inactivation of *Escherichia coli* in orange juice using ozone. *Inn. Food Sci. Emerg. Technol.* **2009**, *10*, 551–557. [CrossRef]
86. Pak, G.; Salcedo, D.E.; Lee, H.; Oh, J.; Maeng, S.K.; Song, K.G.; Hong, S.W.; Kim, H.C.; Chandran, K.; Kim, S. Comparison of antibiotic resistance removal efficiencies using ozone disinfection under different pH and suspended solids and humic substance concentrations. *Environ. Sci. Technol.* **2016**, *50*, 7590–7600. [CrossRef] [PubMed]
87. Adler, M.G.; Hill, G.R. The kinetics and mechanism of hydroxide iron-catalyzed ozone decomposition in aqueous solutions. *J. Am. Chem. Soc.* **1950**, *72*, 1884–1886. [CrossRef]
88. Hoigne, J.; Bader, H. Ozonation of water: Role of hydroxyl radicals as oxidizing intermediates. *Science* **1975**, *190*, 782–784. [CrossRef]
89. Kang, S.W. Superoxide dismutase 2 gene and cancer risk: Evidence from an updated meta-analysis. *Int. J. Clinic. Exp. Med.* **2015**, *8*, 14647–14655.
90. Imlay, J.A. Cellular defenses against superoxide and hydrogen peroxide. *Annu. Rev. Biochem.* **2008**, *77*, 755–776. [CrossRef]
91. Pomposiello, P.J.; Demple, B. Redox-operated genetic switches: The SoxR and OxyR transcription factors. *Trends. Biotechnol.* **2021**, *19*, 109–114. [CrossRef]
92. Greenberg, J.T.; Monach, P.; Chou, J.H.; Josephy, P.D.; Demple, B. Positive control of a global antioxidant defense regulon activated by superoxide generating agents in *Escherichia coli*. *Proc. Natl. Acad. Sci. USA* **1990**, *87*, 6181–6185. [CrossRef]
93. Delaney, J.M. Requirement of the *Escherichia coli* dnaK gene for thermotolerance and protection against H_2O_2. *J. Gen. Microbiol.* **1990**, *136*, 2113–2118. [CrossRef] [PubMed]
94. Rockabrand, D.; Arthur, T.; Korinek, G.; Livers, K.; Blum, P. An essential role for the *Escherichia coli* DnaK protein in starvation-induced thermotolerance, H2O2 resistance, and reductive division. *J. Bacteriol.* **1995**, *177*, 3695–3703. [CrossRef] [PubMed]
95. Loewen, P.; Hu, B.; Strutinsky, J.; Sparling, R. Regulation in the rpoS regulon of *Escherichia coli*. *Can. J. Microbiol.* **1998**, *44*, 707–717. [CrossRef] [PubMed]
96. Chaffin, D.O.; Taylor, D.; Skerrett, S.J.; Rubens, C.E. Changes in the *Staphylococcus aureus* transcriptome during early adaptation to the lung. *PLoS ONE* **2012**, *7*, e41329. [CrossRef]
97. Hamelin, C.; Chung, Y.S. Optimal conditions for mutagenesis by ozone in *Escherichia coli* K12. *Mutat. Res.* **1974**, *24*, 271–279. [CrossRef]
98. Hamelin, C.; Sarhan, F.; Chung, Y.S. Ozone-induced DNA degradation in different DNA polymerase I mutants of *Escherichia coli* K12. *Biochem. Biophys. Res. Commun.* **1977**, *77*, 220–224. [CrossRef]
99. Hamelin, C.; Sarhan, F.; Chung, Y.S. Induction of deoxyribonucleic acid degradation in *Escherichia coli* by ozone. *Experientia* **1978**, *34*, 1578–1579. [CrossRef]
100. Dodd, M.C. Potential impacts of disinfection processes on eliminating and deactivating antibiotic resistance genes during water and wastewater treatment. *J. Environ. Moni.* **2012**, *14*, 1754–1771. [CrossRef]
101. Scott, D.B.M.; Lesher, E.C. Effect of ozone on survival and permeability of *Escherichia coli*. *J. Bacteriol.* **1963**, *85*, 567–576. [CrossRef]
102. Hunt, N.K.; Mariñas, B.J. Inactivation of *Escherichia coli* with ozone: Chemical and inactivation kinetics. *Water Res.* **1999**, *33*, 263–264. [CrossRef]
103. Han, L.; Patil, S.; Boehm, D.; Milosavljević, V.; Cullen, P.J.; Bourke, P. Mechanisms of inactivation by high-voltage atmospheric cold plasma differ for *Escherichia coli* and *Staphylococcus aureus*. *Appl. Environ. Microbiol.* **2016**, *82*, 450–458. [CrossRef] [PubMed]
104. Yu, W.; Zhang, D.; Graham, N.J.D. Membrane fouling by extracellular polymeric substances after ozone pre-treatment: Variation of nano-particle size. *Water Res.* **2017**, *120*, 146–155. [CrossRef] [PubMed]
105. Halder, S.; Yadav, K.K.; Sarkar, R.; Mukherjee, S.; Saha, P.; Haldar, S.; Karmakar, S.; Sen, T. Alteration of Zeta potential and membrane permeability in bacteria: A study with cationic agents. *Springerplus* **2015**, *4*, 672–686. [CrossRef] [PubMed]
106. Nagayoshi, M.; Kitamura, C.; Fukuizumi, T.; Nishihara, T.; Terashita, M. Antimicrobial effect of ozonated water on bacteria invading dentinal tubules. *J. Endod.* **2004**, *30*, 778–781. [CrossRef] [PubMed]
107. Russell, A.D. Similarities and differences in the responses of microorganisms to biocides. *J. Antimicrob. Chemother.* **2003**, *52*, 750–763. [CrossRef]

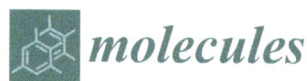

Article

The Effects of Prolonged Storage on ARPE-19 Cells Stored at Three Different Storage Temperatures

Rakibul Islam [1,*], Rima Maria Corraya [1], Lara Pasovic [1,2], Ayyad Zartasht Khan [1], Hans Christian D. Aass [1], Jon Roger Eidet [1,3] and Tor Paaske Utheim [1,3,4,5]

- [1] Department of Medical Biochemistry, Oslo University Hospital, 0450 Oslo, Norway; rimamaria10@gmail.com (R.M.C.); larapasovic@gmail.com (L.P.); a.a.z.khan@studmed.uio.no (A.Z.K.); h.c.aass@medisin.uio.no (H.C.D.A.); j.r.eidet@gmail.com (J.R.E.); utheim2@gmail.com (T.P.U.)
- [2] Department of Surgery, Akershus University Hospital, 1478 Lørenskog, Norway
- [3] Department of Ophthalmology, Oslo University Hospital, 0450 Oslo, Norway
- [4] Department of Ophthalmology, Stavanger University Hospital, 4011 Stavanger, Norway
- [5] Department of Ophthalmology, Sørlandet Hospital Arendal, 4838 Arendal, Norway
- * Correspondence: rakibul.lubikar@gmail.com; Tel.: +47-9483-7512

Academic Editor: Andrea Ragusa
Received: 31 October 2020; Accepted: 4 December 2020; Published: 9 December 2020

Abstract: This study aimed to investigate how prolonged storage of adult retinal pigment epithelial (ARPE-19) cell sheets affects cell metabolism, morphology, viability, and phenotype. ARPE-19 cell sheets were stored at three temperatures (4 °C, 16 °C, and 37 °C) for three weeks. Metabolic status and morphology of the cells were monitored by sampling medium and examining cells by phase-contrast microscopy, respectively, throughout the storage period. Cell viability was analyzed by flow cytometry, and phenotype was determined by epifluorescence microscopy after the storage. Lactate production and glucose consumption increased heavily, while pH dropped considerably, through storage at 37 °C compared to 4 °C and 16 °C. During storage, morphology started to deteriorate first at 4 °C, then at 37 °C, and was maintained the longest at 16 °C. Viability of the cells after three weeks of storage was best preserved at 16 °C, while cells stored at 4 °C and 37 °C had reduced viability. Dedifferentiation indicated by reduced expression of retinal pigment epithelium-specific protein 65 (RPE65), zonula occludens protein 1 (ZO-1), and occludin after three weeks of storage was noticed in all experimental groups compared to control. We conclude that storage temperature affects the metabolic status of ARPE-19 cells and that 16 °C reduces metabolic activity while protecting viability and morphology.

Keywords: retina; storage condition; temperature; regenerative medicine; cell therapy; age-related macular degeneration (AMD); oxidative stress

1. Introduction

The retinal pigment epithelium (RPE) is a monolayer of pigmented cells located between the neurosensory retina and the choroid [1,2]. Loss and dysfunction of RPE cells lead to major pathological changes as seen in age-related macular degeneration (AMD), Stargardt disease, and other macular dystrophies [3]. Transplantation of tissue-engineered RPE cell sheets or suspensions offers the promise of a single-intervention cure [4–7]. A growing body of preclinical studies employing several animal models and various RPE cell sources supports the feasibility of this treatment [8–22]. Several clinical studies have demonstrated promising results [23–26]. Other studies assessing the transplantation of RPE cells derived from different sources are underway [27].

The cells can be delivered to the subretinal space by means of the cell suspension or as an RPE patch [28,29]. However, the preparation of RPE for transplantation in humans is a complex and costly procedure, and upcoming regulatory demands [30] are likely to lead to the establishment of specialized cell processing centers, as described by Oie et al. for human oral mucosal cells [31]. Development of a suitable storage method will be essential to enable the transportation of cell constructs from processing centers to clinics worldwide, thereby ensuring wider access to this novel treatment.

Through several studies [32–36], we and others have explored the feasibility of establishing a xenobiotic-free storage system for RPE cells above freezing temperatures. This would circumvent the need for cryoprotectants, which are known to cause damage to stored cells [37–39]. We showed that storage at 16 °C best preserves adult retinal pigment epithelial (ARPE-19) cells stored for one week compared to eight other temperatures [32]. In the present study, we investigated the effect of storage temperature on the metabolic shift of ARPE-19 cells and evaluated the consequences measured by morphology, viability and phenotypes.

2. Results

2.1. Effect of Three-Week Storage on the Metabolism of Cultured ARPE-19 Cells

To study the effect of storage time and temperature on metabolic parameters (lactate, glucose, pH, pO_2, and pCO_2), the storage medium was sampled every alternate day. Lactate concentration was dramatically increased after storage at 37 °C (0.5–8.6 mmol/L), while it was only slightly increased after storage at 4 °C and 16 °C (0.1–0.5 mmol/L and 0.1–1.4 mmol/L, respectively) (Figure 1A).

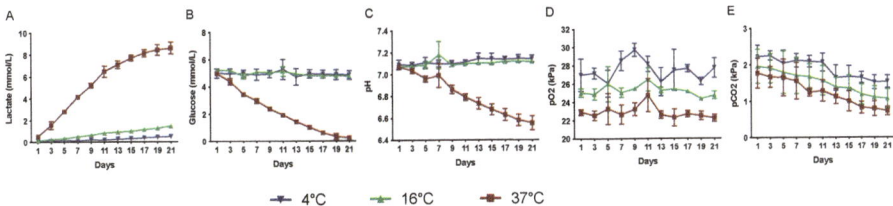

Figure 1. Effect of storage temperature on the metabolic function of RPE cells. The level of lactate (**A**), glucose (**B**), pH (**C**), pO_2 (**D**), and pCO_2 (**E**) in the storage medium was measured every alternate day during the storage period. Data are presented as mean ± standard deviation of the mean. ($n = 8$).

The glucose concentration decreased markedly in cultures stored at 37 °C for three weeks (5.0–0.2 mmol/L), while only a slight reduction was noted in cultures stored at 4 °C and 16 °C (5.0–4.8 mmol/L and 5.2–4.7 mmol/L, respectively) (Figure 1B). The pH was maintained at 7.1 at 4 °C and 16 °C throughout the three weeks of storage but gradually declined at 37 °C storage from 7.1 to 6.6 (Figure 1C). The pO_2 was maintained in all temperature groups throughout the storage period (27.0–27.7 kPa at 4 °C, 25.0–24.7 kPa at 16 °C, and 22.9–22.2 kPa at 37 °C) (Figure 1D). The pCO_2 decreased gradually in all storage groups (2.2–1.5 kPa at 4 °C, 2.0–1.1 kPa at 16 °C, and 1.8–0.7 kPa at 37 °C) (Figure 1E). The partial pressure of both O_2 and CO_2 was inversely proportional to the storage temperature. The metabolic investigations thus show that during the storage duration, the 16 °C conditions kept the measured parameters more stable than the 4 °C and 37 °C groups.

2.2. Effect of Three-Week Storage on the Morphology of Cultured ARPE-19 Cells

To study the morphological effects of storage duration at the three different storage temperatures, phase contrast photomicrographs were captured every alternate day. Prior to storage, cells were generally well apposed and showed typical ARPE morphology (Figure 2A,M,Y).

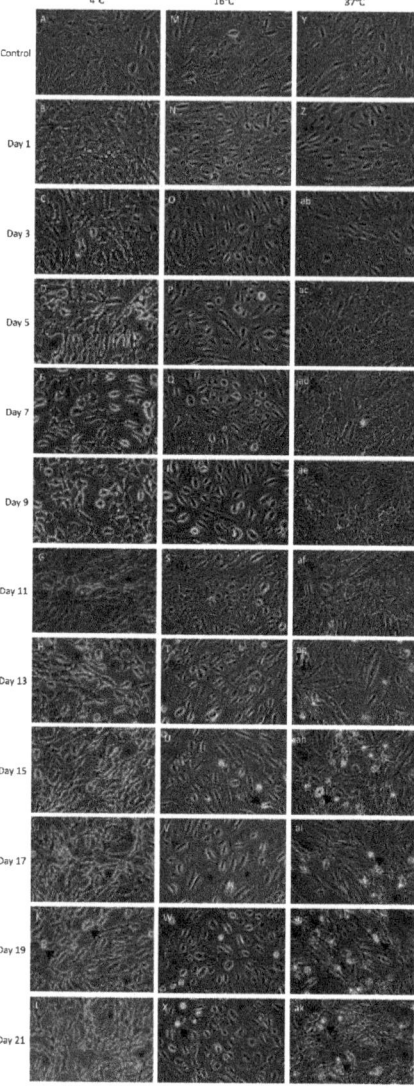

Figure 2. Effect of storage temperature on the morphology of adult retinal pigment epithelial (ARPE-19) cells. Phase-contrast photomicrographs were captured every alternate day during the storage period. Photomicrographs **A**, **M** and **Y** show ARPE-19 cell cultures before storage at three different temperatures. Photomicrograph **B–L**, **N–X**, and **Z–ak** demonstrate the morphology of the ARPE-19 cell cultures following 1 to 21 days of storage at 4 °C, 16 °C and 37 °C, respectively. Black arrows indicate apoptotic cells. Asterisks indicate intercellular spacing (magnification: 400×; $n = 4$).

At the end of the three-week storage period, cells stored at 16 °C showed a morphology most similar to the control. Signs of apoptosis (marked with a black arrow) and intercellular spacing (marked with an asterisk; Figure 2N–X) were infrequently observed at this storage temperature. The majority of cells stored at 4 °C and 37 °C showed signs of cell damage, apoptosis, and necrosis. These signs included extensive loss of cell–cell contact, detachment from the surrounding cells and shrinkage of cytoplasm. In the 4 °C storage group, the deformation of cells was evident from day one (Figure 2B) when the cells started to shrink. In the 37 °C group, cell detachment and fragmentation into apoptotic bodies were observed from day 13 (Figure 2ag–ak). The morphological evidence suggests that both 4 °C and 37 °C storage conditions are suboptimal for maintaining the morphology of the cells, while 16 °C preserved it for the longest duration.

2.3. Effect of Three-Week Storage on the Viability of Cultured ARPE-19 Cells

To assess cell survival after storage at 4 °C, 16 °C and 37 °C for three weeks, cell viability was analyzed by measuring annexin V-binding and PI uptake using flow cytometry (Figure 3A).

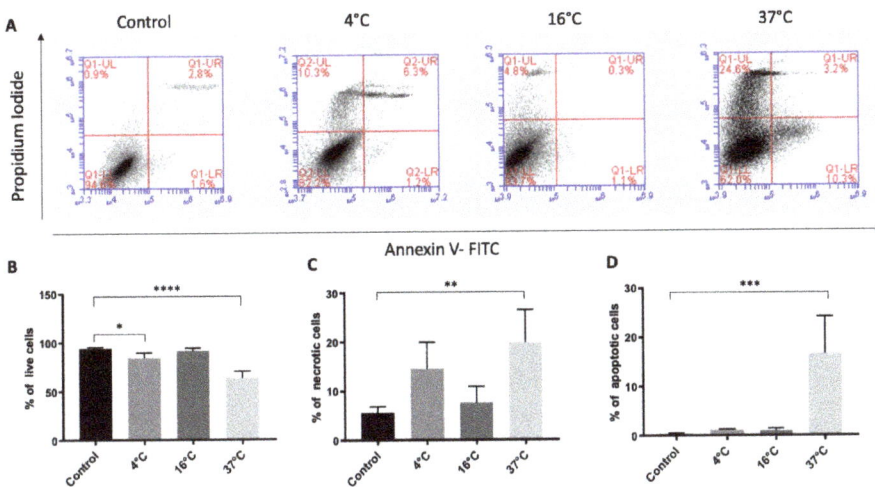

Figure 3. Effect of storage temperature on the viability of ARPE19 cells. Live, necrotic and apoptotic cells were detected by flow cytometry using annexin V and propidium iodide (PI). Cultured ARPE-19 cells were stored at three temperatures for three weeks. Dot plots (**A**) from the flow cytometry analysis were gated based on unstained cells for each experiment (not shown). The cell populations were distributed in four quadrants where the lower left quadrant represents live cells (annexin V and PI-negative), the upper left and right quadrants together represent necrotic cells (only PI-positive as well as both annexin V and PI-positive), while the lower right quadrant represents apoptotic cells (annexin V-positive and PI-negative). Control cells were not stored. The bar chart illustrates the percentages of live (**B**), necrotic (**C**), and apoptotic (**D**) cells. Data are presented as the mean ± standard deviation of the mean of four independent experiments. * $p < 0.05$, ** $p < 0.01$, *** $p < 0.001$, and **** $p < 0.0001$.

Cell viability after three weeks of storage (defined as the percentage of cells that were annexin V- and PI-negative) was significantly reduced at 4 °C (84% ± 5%, $p = 0.047$) and 37 °C (63% ± 6%; $p < 0.001$), but not at 16 °C (91% ± 2%; $p = 0.84$), compared to the control (94% ± 1%) (Figure 3B). Necrotic cells, which were annexin V-negative and PI-positive, were significantly increased at 37 °C (19% ± 6%; $p < 0.001$), but not at 4 °C (14% ± 5%, $p = 0.07$) or 16 °C (7% ± 3%, $p = 0.92$), compared to the control (5% ± 1%) (Figure 3C). Similarly, the percentage of annexin V-positive and PI-negative apoptotic cells was increased only at 37 °C (16% ± 7%; $p < 0.001$), but not at 4 °C (1% ± 0.2%; $p = 0.99$) or 16 °C (1% ± 0.5%; $p = 0.99$), compared to the control (0.2% ± 0.2%) (Figure 3D). The viability analysis thus indicates that among the three storage conditions tested here 16 °C condition is better for preserving cell viability similar to the non-stored cells.

2.4. Effect of Three-Week Storage on the Phenotype of Cultured ARPE-19 Cells

To study the effect of storage temperature on ARPE-19 phenotype following three weeks of storage at 4 °C, 16 °C, and 37 °C, the cells were immunostained with four different markers. The anti-RPE65 antibody was used to target an RPE-selective protein essential for the regeneration of visual pigment [40]. RPE65-expression normalized to control (set to 100%) appeared to be inversely proportional to the storage temperature (4 °C: 50% ± 24%, $p = 0.011$; 16 °C: 29% ± 7%, $p < 0.001$; 37 °C: 19% ± 8%, $p < 0.001$) (Figure 4A,B).

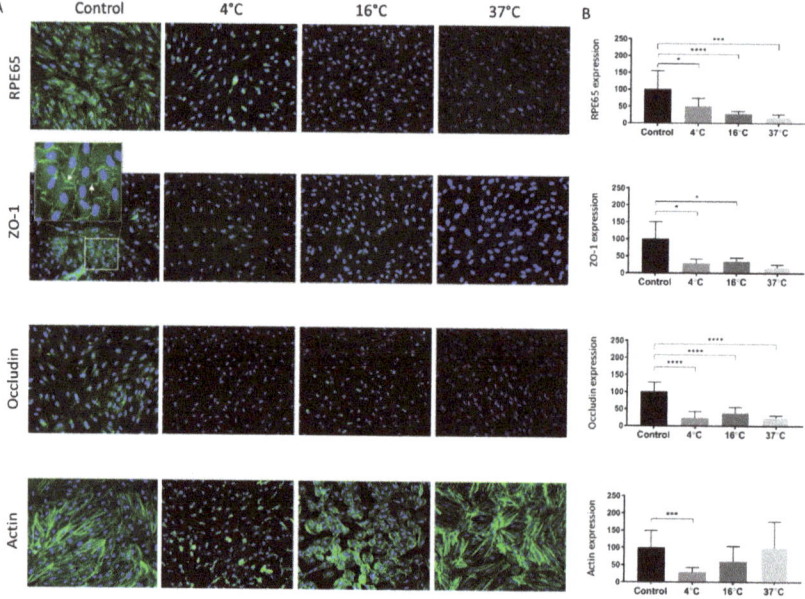

Figure 4. The effect of storage temperature on ARPE-19 cell phenotype. (**A**) The expression of RPE65, ZO-1 (white arrow points within a zoomed inset), occludin and actin in ARPE-19 cell cultures stored for three weeks at 4 °C, 16 °C, or 37 °C was compared with non-stored control cultures. Nuclear DNA was stained with 4′,6-diamidino-2-phenylindole (blue). (**B**) Expression of the markers quantified by measuring the total fluorescence intensity normalized by cell number. The bar charts show the fluorescence intensity of anti-RPE65, anti-ZO-1, anti-occludin, and anti-actin relative to control cultures (100%). Magnification 200×. Data are expressed as mean ± standard deviation of the mean. * $p < 0.05$, *** $p < 0.001$ and **** $p < 0.0001$.

To assess the presence of intercellular tight junctions, staining with anti-ZO-1 and anti-occludin antibodies was performed. The ZO-1 marker localized to cell borders and was present between all apposed cells in the control group, indicating a tight junction organization typical of native RPE (Figure 4A). Compared to the non-stored control (set to 100%; Figure 4A,B) ZO-1-expression was reduced following storage at all storage temperatures (29% ± 13%, $p = 0.035$; 35% ± 10%, $p = 0.0155$ and 17% ± 8%, $p = 0.0510$ for 4, 16 °C and 37 °C, respectively). Occludin, another tight junction marker, was also significantly reduced following storage at all storage temperatures (24% ± 19%, $p < 0.001$; 37% ± 18%, $p < 0.001$; and 24% ± 7, $p < 0.001$; for 4 °C, 16 °C, and 37 °C, respectively) compared to the non-stored control (set to 100%; Figure 4A,B).

Alexa Fluor 568 phalloidin staining was applied for selective labeling of F-actin in order to visualize the cytoskeleton and evaluate the formation of stress fibers. Actin staining revealed a continuous cytoplasmic network of filamentous structures in the control cultures, with the formation of stress fibers seen in some cells (Figure 4A). After storage at 4 °C, there was disorganization and complete loss of actin filamentous structure (Figure 4A). However, in the 16 °C group, actin filaments were less stretched and more circular, whereas the filaments were maintained after storage at 37 °C compared to the control (Figure 4A). Measuring the fluorescence intensity of the filament staining showed that at 4 °C storage it was significantly lower (28% ± 14%; $p < 0.001$) compared to the control (Figure 4B), while, there was no statistically significant difference at 16 °C storage (60% ± 43%; $p = 0.070$) at 37 °C (100% ± 75%; $p > 0.999$) after three weeks (Figure 4A,B).

3. Discussion

In this study, we investigated how prolonged storage of ARPE-19 cell sheets affects cell metabolism, morphology, viability, and phenotype. We found that the temperature affects the metabolic shift over time. Among the three temperature groups, 16 °C kept the metabolic shift low, cell viability high, and morphology preserved. However, the phenotype was not maintained at control levels after storage at any of the temperatures.

Our results demonstrated an increased breakdown of glucose to lactate with a concomitant reduction in pH during storage at 37 °C compared to 4 °C and 16 °C. This is in accordance with earlier findings in stored human-induced pluripotent stem cell-derived retinal pigment epithelium cells [36], epidermal cell sheets [41], cultured human conjunctival cells [42] and human oral keratinocytes [43]. The high lactate/glucose ratio indicates that the glycolytic pathway accounts for a large part of energy production from glucose and could possibly represent a cellular adjustment to avoid an excessive production of damaging reactive oxygen species generated through the oxidative phosphorylation pathway [44]. Lactate concentration at 37 °C storage rose linearly until day 11, after which it started to level off, possibly due to accelerated cell death. In fact, when evaluating the corresponding microscopy images of the same storage group, it appears that apoptotic bodies started to form after day 11. This could be related to the considerable drop in pH at 37 °C storage, which can induce cell apoptosis [45]. Since the storage media is easily accessible without affecting the cells, therefore, the lactate, glucose, and pH values together may be considered as critical quality control parameters for RPE-cells during storage at 37 °C. At 4 °C and 16 °C storage, the changes in the metabolic parameters were not as dramatic as 37 °C. At 4 °C storage, cells exhibited typical signs of apoptosis and necrosis early on during storage without any obvious connection to metabolic parameters. At 4 °C, cells die mainly because of low temperature-related stress [32], whereas, at 37 °C, the primary causes may be associated with accumulation of lactate, pH reduction and associated apoptosis [43,45]. At 16 °C, the morphology of the cells was maintained the longest without dramatic changes in metabolic parameters. Thus, storage at 16 °C reduced the metabolic rate of the cells while not exerting the detrimental effect of low temperature-associated stress [43].

This explanation is corroborated by the post-storage viability, which demonstrated that after 16 °C storage, the live-cell percentage did not significantly differ from non-stored control cells (Figure 3). In a study by Kitahata et al., cell suspension of human-induced pluripotent stem-cell-derived retinal pigment epithelium cells demonstrated a higher percentage of viable cells at 16 °C compared to 4 °C, 25 °C and 37 °C following 24 h of storage [36]. However, our previous study demonstrated the viability of about 50% after one-week storage at 16 °C [32]. This discrepancy can be explained by a change in the viability assessment analysis. In the present study, we used flow cytometry to measure the expression of the apoptotic marker, phosphatidylserine, by binding of annexin V and determine the dead cells by PI staining. Viability was calculated as the percentage of non-stained cells from total acquired cells suspension for the analysis. In the previous study, viability was not assessed in the suspended cells, rather as fluorescence intensity of calcein-acetoxymethyl ester staining on adherent cells determined by a microplate fluorometer.

The RPE is a highly specialized tissue performing several functions that are crucial for sight, including phagocytosis of shed photoreceptor outer segments, regeneration of visual cycle pigments, and transport of nutrients and fluid between the choroid and neuroretina [3,46]. These traits are affected by macular disease and could be remedied by transplanted tissue. It is, therefore, important that transplanted cells display differentiated RPE properties. The ARPE-19 cell line is a widely employed model for the study of RPE biology. While it displays significant functional differentiation [47,48], it does not mirror all characteristics of native RPE, and its phenotype is highly dependent on culture conditions [49–52]. However, the use of serum-free media and plastic substrates, which are employed herein, have been shown to reduce dedifferentiation in culture [49,53]. Earlier, we showed that ARPE-19 cells stored at 16 °C for one week are capable of maintaining the expression of the RPE differentiation marker RPE65 [32]. The current results demonstrated a reduced RPE65 expression at 16 °C following three weeks' storage compared to one-week storage, which may indicate dedifferentiation of ARPE-19 cells with increasing storage duration. Similarly, we earlier showed maintained expression of the tight junction markers ZO-1 and occludin after one-week storage of ARPE-19 cells [32,33]. The expression of these markers is not maintained after three weeks' storage. The effect of storage on cell phenotype has been described previously for several cell types. Studies have demonstrated that cultured limbal cells can be stored for one week in an organ culture medium at 23 °C with intact phenotype [54]. Similarly, cultured human oral keratinocytes can be stored under the conditions described herein for one week without signs of differentiation [43]. Microarray analysis demonstrated upregulation of tight junction proteins after one-week storage at 37 °C compared to 12 °C, indicating an increased synthesis of tight junctions in HOK cells stored at 37 °C [55]. In cultured epidermal cell sheets stored at different temperatures for two weeks, there was a tendency of increased expression of differentiation markers at all temperatures except for 12 °C [56]. Based on these observations, it seems that the phenotypic plasticity during storage varies between different cell types.

In the present study, there were also changes in the distribution of the actin cytoskeleton, which is important for cell adhesion, morphogenesis, and phagocytosis. Contractile actomyosin bundles called stress fibers assemble following mechanical stress and are common in cultured epithelial cells [57,58]. Actin staining revealed a continuous cytoplasmic network of filamentous structures in the control cultures, with the formation of stress fibers seen in some cells. These features were maintained after storage at 37 °C. After storage at 4 °C and 16 °C, however, there was a disruption of the actinic cytoskeleton. Disrupted staining patterns of the actin cytoskeleton, tight junctions, and adherens junctions in the RPE in relation to elevated reactive oxygen species were previously reported elsewhere. [59] ARPE-19 cells stored at 16 °C for one week displayed a similar distribution with a predominantly circumferential actin arrangement and fewer elongated cells than control cultures [32].

Replacement of the diseased RPE is on the verge of becoming a reality in regenerative therapies to cure age-related macular degenerative diseases. The successful outcome with the first two patients from a clinical study by transplanting cultured cell sheet has demonstrated the potential effectiveness of the therapy [26]. The development of complementary storage techniques for RPE transplants is likely to have a large medical impact as it allows flexibility in scheduling surgery and can widen patients' access to future applications of regenerative therapy.

We conclude from our study that the storage temperature affects the metabolic status of ARPE-19 cells and that 16 °C is superior for keeping the metabolic activity low while protecting the viability and morphology. Our study infers the importance of monitoring metabolic parameters as quality control of the stored ARPE-19 cells.

4. Materials and Methods

4.1. Cell Culture Media and Reagents

ARPE-19 cells were obtained from the American Type Culture Collection (ATCC) (Manassas, VA, USA). Dulbecco's Modified Eagle's Medium: nutrient mixture F12 (hereafter named DMEM:F12), fetal bovine serum (FBS), bovine serum albumin (BSA), trypsin-EDTA, 4-(2-hydroxyethyl)-1-piperazineethanesulfonic acid (HEPES), sodium bicarbonate, gentamycin, phosphate-buffered saline (PBS), penicillin, streptomycin, 4′,6-diamidino-2-phenylindole (DAPI), propidium iodide (PI), Tween-20 and PAP pen were purchased from Sigma-Aldrich (St. Louis, MO, USA). Fluorescein isothiocyanate (FITC)-labeled annexin V (to bind PS), annexin V-binding buffer containing 10 mM HEPES (pH 7.4), 140 mM NaCl, and 2.5 mM $CaCl_2$, were purchased from Becton Dickinson Biosciences (BD), Belgium. Minimum essential medium (MEM) was purchased from Invitrogen (Carlsbad, CA, USA). Pipettes, 25 cm^2 flasks, 15 mL and 50 mL centrifugation tubes, 1 L glass bottles, and pipette tips were supplied by VWR International (West Chester, PA, USA). Vacuum filtration rapid filter mix was supplied by BioNordika (Oslo, Norway). Mouse anti-RPE65, rabbit anti-occludin, FITC-conjugated goat anti-mouse IgG and FITC-conjugated goat anti-rabbit IgG antibodies were obtained from Abcam (Cambridge, UK). Mouse anti-ZO-1 and Alexa Fluor 568 phalloidin were purchased from Life Technologies (Carlsbad, CA, USA).

4.2. Culture of ARPE-19 Cells

Human ARPE-19 cells were routinely cultured in 95% air and 5% CO_2 at 37 °C in DMEM:F12 containing 10% FBS, 50 units/mL penicillin and 50 µg/mL streptomycin. The cells at passage 6 were seeded (120,000 cells/flask) in 25 cm^2 culture flasks with filter closer. The culture medium was changed every other day, and confluent cultures were obtained on the sixth day. Control cultures, which were not subjected to subsequent storage, were immediately prepared for the various analyses.

4.3. Storage of ARPE-19 Cells

After the six-days culture period, the T25 flasks were removed from the incubator, and the culture medium was replaced by a storage medium consisting of 9.53 g MEM, 25 mM HEPES, 600 mg/L sodium bicarbonate and 50 µg/mL gentamycin in 1 L distilled water. The filter cap of the flasks was changed to a solid cap to avoid evaporation during storage. Thereafter, the cultures were randomized for storage at three temperatures (4 °C, 16 °C and 37 °C) for three weeks in storage containers without CO_2 supply. The storage containers have been described previously [32]. The stability of the temperature inside the storage containers has been reported [60] and was controlled regularly throughout all experiments.

4.4. Metabolic Analysis

Samples of the storage medium (2 mL) were taken every alternate day from day 1 to day 21 and were analyzed using a Radiometer ABL 700 blood gas analyzer (Radiometer, Bronshoj, Denmark) at room temperature. The following parameters were studied: pH, glucose, lactate, partial pressure of oxygen (pO_2) and partial pressure of carbon dioxide (pCO_2). The experiment was repeated eight times ($n = 8$).

4.5. Morphology Analysis

Morphology of the stored ARPE-19 cell cultures was assessed by light microscopy every alternate day during the storage period. The experiment was repeated four times ($n = 4$). Photomicrographs were captured at 400× magnification using a Leica DM IL LED microscope and a Canon EOS 5D Mark II camera.

4.6. Viability Analysis

Viability after three weeks of storage was analyzed by a flow cytometer (BD Accuri C6 flow cytometer, Becton Dickinson, CA, USA) using FITC-conjugated annexin V and PI. Annexin V binds selectively to phosphatidylserine (in the presence of calcium ions), which is anchored at the cytosolic face of the plasma membrane in viable cells. During the early phases of apoptosis, phosphatidylserine is re-localized to the outer surface of the plasma membrane, where it can be detected with fluorescently labeled annexin V [61]. Apoptotic cells were defined as annexin V-positive and PI-negative. PI passes through permeable cell membranes of necrotic cells and stains double-stranded DNA. Viable cells were defined as both annexin V- and PI-negative.

The analysis was performed according to the protocol provided by the supplier and repeated four times ($n = 4$). Briefly, RPE cells were trypsinized and centrifuged at room temperature. The supernatant was aspirated from the cell pellet, which was resuspended in 200 µL of annexin V-binding buffer containing annexin V-FITC (1 µL/mL) and incubated for 25 min at room temperature. PI dye (10 µg/mL) was added for further 5-min incubation at room temperature before the suspension was analyzed using a flow cytometer.

4.7. Phenotype Analysis

Cells were cultured in T25 flasks and stored at 4 °C, 16 °C and 37 °C for three weeks, as described above. Samples were subsequently prepared for immunocytochemical characterization with 30 min of 4% formaldehyde fixation at room temperature followed by one hour of permeabilization and blocking in PBS containing 1% BSA and 0.01% Tween-20. Control cells were processed for immunocytochemistry immediately after the six-day culture period. Anti-RPE65 (1:50), anti-ZO-1 (1:50) and anti-occludin (1:50) antibodies were diluted in blocking solution (PBS with 1% BSA). In the negative controls, primary antibodies were substituted with PBS. Samples were incubated for one hour at room temperature. FITC-conjugated goat anti-mouse secondary antibodies (diluted 1:200 in blocking solution) and FITC-conjugated goat anti-rabbit secondary antibodies (1:250) were added for one hour at room temperature. Specimens were washed three times in PBS, and 1 µg/mL DAPI was added during the last wash to stain the nuclear DNA. To visualize the actin cytoskeleton, samples were fixed, blocked, and permeabilized as described above and stained with 100 units/mL, which is equivalent to approximately 20 µM Alexa Fluor 568 phalloidin. After incubating for 1 h at room temperature, specimens were washed in PBS and stained with DAPI.

The samples were studied using a Nikon Eclipse Ti fluorescence microscope and photographed at ×200 magnification with a DS-Qi1 black-and-white camera. Identical exposure length and gain were maintained for all compared samples, and the image brightness was within the dynamic range of the camera. The experiments were repeated four times ($n = 4$).

The photomicrographs were then objectively assessed using ImageJ software (National Institutes of Health, Bethesda, MD, USA) as described previously [62], with some modifications. In brief, for DAPI count, 16-bit photomicrographs of DAPI-stained nuclei were converted to 8-bit images before being auto-thresholded to binary photos using the "Make Binary" function in ImageJ. Touching cell nuclei were separated by the "Watershed" command. Cell debris and other smaller cellular particles were excluded from analysis on the basis of size by the "Analyze Particle" function. For phenotypic quantification, unevenly transmitted light was subtracted from all 16-bit photomicrographs using the "Subtract Background (rolling = 50)" command in ImageJ before the total fluorescence intensity was measured. Finally, the total fluorescence intensity in each photomicrograph was divided by the number of DAPI-stained nuclei in each corresponding DAPI-photomicrograph. By using this method, we were able to normalize for differences in cell density in each photomicrograph.

4.8. Statistical Analysis

A one-way analysis of variance with Tukey's post hoc comparisons (SPSS ver. 19.0 or GraphPad prism 8.2.1) was used for statistical evaluation of the results. P values below 0.05 were considered significant.

Author Contributions: Conceptualization, T.P.U., J.R.E., R.M.C., R.I.; methodology, R.M.C., R.I., H.C.D.A.; software, A.Z.K.; formal analysis, R.I., A.Z.K.; investigation, R.M.C., R.I.; resources, T.P.U.; writing—original draft preparation, R.I., R.M.C., L.P.; writing—review and editing, R.I., R.M.C., L.P., A.Z.K., H.C.D.A., J.R.E., T.P.U.; visualization, R.I., H.C.D.A.; supervision, J.R.E., T.P.U.; project administration, R.M.C. and R.I.; funding acquisition, T.P.U. All authors have read and agreed to the published version of the manuscript.

Funding: This research received no external funding.

Conflicts of Interest: The authors declare no conflict of interest. The funders had no role in the design of the study; in the collection, analyses, or interpretation of data; in the writing of the manuscript, or in the decision to publish the results.

References

1. Marmorstein, A.D. The Polarity of the Retinal Pigment Epithelium. *Traffic* **2001**, *2*, 867–872. [CrossRef]
2. De Jong, P.T.V.M. Age-related macular degeneration. *N. Engl. J. Med.* **2006**, *355*, 1474–1485. [CrossRef]
3. Hicks, D.; Hamel, C.P. The Retinal Pigment Epithelium in Health and Disease. *Curr. Mol. Med.* **2010**, *10*, 802–823. [CrossRef]
4. Vaajasaari, H.; Ilmarinen, T.; Juuti-Uusitalo, K.; Rajala, K.; Onnela, N.; Narkilahti, S.; Suuronen, R.; Hyttinen, J.; Uusitalo, H.; Skottman, H. Toward the defined and xeno-free differentiation of functional human pluripotent stem cell–derived retinal pigment epithelial cells. *Mol. Vis.* **2011**, *17*, 558–575.
5. Alexander, P.; Thomson, H.A.J.; Luff, A.J.; Lotery, A.J. Retinal pigment epithelium transplantation: Concepts, challenges, and future prospects. *Eye* **2015**, *29*, 992–1002. [CrossRef]
6. Nazari, H.; Zhang, L.; Zhu, D.; Chader, G.J.; Falabella, P.; Stefanini, F.R.; Rowland, T.J.; Clegg, D.O.; Kashani, A.H.; Hinton, D.R.; et al. Stem cell based therapies for age-related macular degeneration: The promises and the challenges. *Prog. Retin. Eye Res.* **2015**, *48*, 39. [CrossRef]
7. Mandai, M.; Watanabe, A.; Kurimoto, Y.; Hirami, Y.; Morinaga, C.; Daimon, T.; Fujihara, M.; Akimaru, H.; Sakai, N.; Shibata, Y.; et al. Autologous Induced Stem-Cell–Derived Retinal Cells for Macular Degeneration. *N. Engl. J. Med.* **2017**, *376*, 1038–1046. [CrossRef]
8. Crafoord, S.; Algvere, P.V.; Seregard, S.; Kopp, E.D. Long-term outcome of RPE allografts to the subretinal space of rabbits. *Acta Ophthalmol. Scand.* **1999**, *77*, 247–254. [CrossRef] [PubMed]
9. Lund, R.D.; Adamson, P.; Sauvé, Y.; Keegan, D.J.; Girman, S.V.; Wang, S.; Winton, H.; Kanuga, N.; Kwan, A.S.L.; Beauchène, L.; et al. Subretinal transplantation of genetically modified human cell lines attenuates loss of visual function in dystrophic rats. *Proc. Natl. Acad. Sci. USA* **2001**, *98*, 9942–9947. [CrossRef]
10. Wang, H.; Leonard, D.S.; Castellarin, A.; Tsukahara, I.; Ninomiya, Y.; Yagi, F.; Cheewatrakoolpong, N.; Sugino, I.K.; Zarbin, M. Short-term study of allogeneic retinal pigment epithelium transplants onto debrided Bruch's membrane. *Investig. Ophthalmol. Vis. Sci.* **2001**, *42*, 2990–2999.
11. Coffey, P.J.; Girman, S.; Wang, S.M.; Hetherington, L.; Keegan, D.J.; Adamson, P.; Greenwood, J.; Lund, R.D. Long-term preservation of cortically dependent visual function in RCS rats by transplantation. *Nat. Neurosci.* **2001**, *5*, 53–56. [CrossRef] [PubMed]
12. Girman, S.V.; Wang, S.; Lund, R.D. Cortical visual functions can be preserved by subretinal RPE cell grafting in RCS rats. *Vis. Res.* **2003**, *43*, 1817–1827. [CrossRef]
13. Haruta, M.; Sasai, Y.; Kawasaki, H.; Amemiya, K.; Ooto, S.; Kitada, M.; Suemori, H.; Nakatsuji, N.; Ide, C.; Honda, Y.; et al. In vitro and in vivo characterization of pigment epithelial cells differentiated from primate embryonic stem cells. *Investig. Opthalmol. Vis. Sci.* **2004**, *45*, 1020–1025. [CrossRef] [PubMed]
14. McGill, T.; Lund, R.; Douglas, R.; Wang, S.; Lu, B.; Prusky, G. Preservation of vision following cell-based therapies in a model of retinal degenerative disease. *Vis. Res.* **2004**, *44*, 2559–2566. [CrossRef]
15. Del Priore, L.V.; Tezel, T.H.; Kaplan, H.J. Survival of allogeneic porcine retinal pigment epithelial sheets after subretinal transplantation. *Investig. Opthalmol. Vis. Sci.* **2004**, *45*, 985–992. [CrossRef]
16. Wang, S.; Lu, B.; Wood, P.; Lund, R.D. Grafting of ARPE-19 and Schwann Cells to the Subretinal Space in RCS Rats. *Investig. Opthalmol. Vis. Sci.* **2005**, *46*, 2552–2560. [CrossRef]
17. Lund, R.D.; Wang, S.; Klimanskaya, I.; Holmes, T.; Ramos-Kelsey, R.; Lu, B.; Girman, S.; Bischoff, N.; Sauvé, Y.; Lanza, R. Human Embryonic Stem Cell–Derived Cells Rescue Visual Function in Dystrophic RCS Rats. *Cloning Stem Cells* **2006**, *8*, 189–199. [CrossRef]
18. Yaji, N.; Yamato, M.; Yang, J.; Okano, T.; Hori, S. Transplantation of tissue-engineered retinal pigment epithelial cell sheets in a rabbit model. *Biomaterials* **2009**, *30*, 797–803. [CrossRef]
19. Carr, A.-J.F.; Vugler, A.A.; Hikita, S.T.; Lawrence, J.M.; Gias, C.; Chen, L.L.; Buchholz, D.E.; Ahmado, A.; Semo, M.; Smart, M.J.K.; et al. Protective Effects of Human iPS-Derived Retinal Pigment Epithelium Cell Transplantation in the Retinal Dystrophic Rat. *PLoS ONE* **2009**, *4*, e8152. [CrossRef]
20. Hu, Y.; Liu, L.; Lu, B.; Zhu, D.; Ribeiro, R.; Diniz, B.; Thomas, P.B.; Ahuja, A.K.; Hinton, D.R.; Tai, Y.-C.; et al. A Novel Approach for Subretinal Implantation of Ultrathin Substrates Containing Stem Cell-Derived Retinal Pigment Epithelium Monolayer. *Ophthalmic Res.* **2012**, *48*, 186–191. [CrossRef]

21. Li, Y.; Tsai, Y.-T.; Hsu, C.-W.; Erol, D.; Yang, J.; Wu, W.-H.; Davis, R.J.; Egli, D.; Tsang, S.H. Long-term Safety and Efficacy of Human-Induced Pluripotent Stem Cell (iPS) Grafts in a Preclinical Model of Retinitis Pigmentosa. *Mol. Med.* **2012**, *18*, 1312–1319. [CrossRef] [PubMed]
22. Sun, J.; Mandai, M.; Kamao, H.; Hashiguchi, T.; Shikamura, M.; Kawamata, S.; Sugita, S.; Takahashi, M. Protective Effects of Human iPS-Derived Retinal Pigmented Epithelial Cells in Comparison with Human Mesenchymal Stromal Cells and Human Neural Stem Cells on the Degenerating Retina inrd1mice. *Stem Cells* **2015**, *33*, 1543–1553. [CrossRef]
23. Schwartz, S.D.; Hubschman, J.-P.; Heilwell, G.; Franco-Cardenas, V.; Pan, C.K.; Ostrick, R.M.; Mickunas, E.; Gay, R.; Klimanskaya, I.; Lanza, R. Embryonic stem cell trials for macular degeneration: A preliminary report. *Lancet* **2012**, *379*, 713–720. [CrossRef]
24. Schwartz, S.D.; Regillo, C.D.; Lam, B.L.; Eliott, D.; Rosenfeld, P.J.; Gregori, N.Z.; Hubschman, J.-P.; Davis, J.L.; Heilwell, G.; Spirn, M.; et al. Human embryonic stem cell-derived retinal pigment epithelium in patients with age-related macular degeneration and Stargardt's macular dystrophy: Follow-up of two open-label phase 1/2 studies. *Lancet* **2015**, *385*, 509–516. [CrossRef]
25. Schwartz, S.D.; Tan, G.; Hosseini, H.; Nagiel, A. Subretinal Transplantation of Embryonic Stem Cell–Derived Retinal Pigment Epithelium for the Treatment of Macular Degeneration: An Assessment at 4 Years. *Investig. Opthalmol. Vis. Sci.* **2016**, *57*, ORSFc1–ORSFc9. [CrossRef]
26. Da Cruz, L.; Fynes, K.; Georgiadis, O.; Kerby, J.; Luo, Y.H.; Ahmado, A.; Vernon, A.; Daniels, J.T.; Nommiste, B.; Hasan, S.M.; et al. Phase 1 clinical study of an embryonic stem cell–derived retinal pigment epithelium patch in age-related macular degeneration. *Nat. Biotechnol.* **2018**, *36*, 328–337. [CrossRef]
27. Bracha, P.; A Moore, N.; A Ciulla, T. Induced pluripotent stem cell-based therapy for age-related macular degeneration. *Expert Opin. Biol. Ther.* **2017**, *17*, 1113–1126. [CrossRef]
28. Ramsden, C.M.; Powner, M.B.; Carr, A.-J.F.; Smart, M.J.K.; Da Cruz, L.; Coffey, P.J. Stem cells in retinal regeneration: Past, present and future. *Deversity* **2013**, *140*, 2576–2585. [CrossRef]
29. Ramsden, C.M.; Da Cruz, L.; Coffey, P. Stemming the Tide of Age-Related Macular Degeneration: New Therapies for Old Retinas. *Investig. Opthalmol. Vis. Sci.* **2016**, *57*. [CrossRef]
30. Daniels, J.T.; Secker, G.A.; Shortt, A.J.; Tuft, S.J.; Seetharaman, S. Stem cell therapy delivery: Treading the regulatory tightrope. *Regen. Med.* **2006**, *1*, 715–719. [CrossRef]
31. Oie, Y.; Nozaki, T.; Takayanagi, H.; Hara, S.; Hayashi, R.; Takeda, S.; Mori, K.; Moriya, N.; Soma, T.; Tsujikawa, M.; et al. Development of a Cell Sheet Transportation Technique for Regenerative Medicine. *Tissue Eng. Part C Methods* **2014**, *20*, 373–382. [CrossRef] [PubMed]
32. Pasovic, L.; Utheim, T.P.; Maria, R.; Lyberg, T.; Messelt, E.B.; Aabel, P.; Chen, D.F.; Chen, X.; Eidet, J.R. Optimization of Storage Temperature for Cultured ARPE-19 Cells. *J. Ophthalmol.* **2013**, *2013*, 11. [CrossRef] [PubMed]
33. Pasovic, L.; Eidet, J.R.; Brusletto, B.S.; Lyberg, T.; Utheim, T.P. Effect of Storage Temperature on Key Functions of Cultured Retinal Pigment Epithelial Cells. *J. Ophthalmol.* **2015**, *2015*, 10. [CrossRef] [PubMed]
34. Pasovic, L.; Eidet, J.R.; Olstad, O.K.; Chen, D.F.; Lyberg, T.; Utheim, T.P. Impact of Storage Temperature on the Expression of Cell Survival Genes in Cultured ARPE-19 Cells. *Curr. Eye Res.* **2016**, *42*, 134–144. [CrossRef]
35. Khan, A.Z.; Utheim, T.P.; Reppe, S.; Sandvik, L.; Lyberg, T.; Roald, B.B.-H.; Ibrahim, I.B.; Eidet, J.R. Cultured Human Retinal Pigment Epithelial (hRPE) Sheets: A Search for Suitable Storage Conditions. *Microsc. Microanal.* **2018**, *24*, 147–155. [CrossRef]
36. Kitahata, S.; Tanaka, Y.; Hori, K.; Kime, C.; Sugita, S.; Ueda, H.; Takahashi, M. Critical Functionality Effects from Storage Temperature on Human Induced Pluripotent Stem Cell-Derived Retinal Pigment Epithelium Cell Suspensions. *Sci. Rep.* **2019**, *9*, 2891. [CrossRef]
37. Wang, A.W.; Zhang, H.; Ikemoto, I.; Anderson, D.J.; Loughlin, K.R. Reactive oxygen species generation by seminal cells during cryopreservation. *Urology* **1997**, *49*, 921–925. [CrossRef]
38. Honda, S.; Weigel, A.; Hjelmeland, L.M.; Handa, J.T. Induction of Telomere Shortening and Replicative Senescence by Cryopreservation. *Biochem. Biophys. Res. Commun.* **2001**, *282*, 493–498. [CrossRef]
39. Pegg, D.E. The History and Principles of Cryopreservation. *Semin. Reprod. Med.* **2002**, *20*, 005–014. [CrossRef]
40. Ahmado, A.; Carr, A.-J.; Vugler, A.A.; Semo, M.; Gias, C.; Lawrence, J.M.; Chen, L.L.; Chen, F.K.; Turowski, P.; Da Cruz, L.; et al. Induction of Differentiation by Pyruvate and DMEM in the Human Retinal Pigment Epithelium Cell Line ARPE-19. *Investig. Opthalmol. Vis. Sci.* **2011**, *52*, 7148–7159. [CrossRef]

41. Jackson, C.J.; Aabel, P.; Eidet, J.R.; Messelt, E.B.; Lyberg, T.; Von Unge, M.; Utheim, T.P. Effect of Storage Temperature on Cultured Epidermal Cell Sheets Stored in Xenobiotic-Free Medium. *PLoS ONE* **2014**, *9*, e105808. [CrossRef]
42. Eidet, J.R.; Utheim, Ø.A.; Islam, R.; Lyberg, T.; Messelt, E.B.; Dartt, D.A.; Utheim, T.P. The Impact of Storage Temperature on the Morphology, Viability, Cell Number and Metabolism of Cultured Human Conjunctival Epithelium. *Curr. Eye Res.* **2015**, *40*, 30–39. [CrossRef] [PubMed]
43. Islam, R.; Jackson, C.J.; Eidet, J.R.; Messelt, E.B.; Corraya, R.M.; Lyberg, T.; Griffith, M.; Dartt, D.A.; Utheim, T.P. Effect of Storage Temperature on Structure and Function of Cultured Human Oral Keratinocytes. *PLoS ONE* **2015**, *10*, e0128306. [CrossRef] [PubMed]
44. Slikker, W.; Desai, V.G.; Duhart, H.; Feuers, R.; Imam, S.Z. Hypothermia enhances bcl-2 expression and protects against oxidative stress-induced cell death in chinese hamster ovary cells. *Free. Radic. Biol. Med.* **2001**, *31*, 405–411. [CrossRef]
45. Park, H.J.; Lyons, J.C.; Ohtsubo, T.; Song, C.W. Acidic environment causes apoptosis by increasing caspase activity. *Br. J. Cancer* **1999**, *80*, 1892–1897. [CrossRef] [PubMed]
46. Marmor, M.F. Control of subretinal fluid: Experimental and clinical studies. *Eye* **1990**, *4*, 340–344. [CrossRef]
47. Dunn, K.; Aotaki-Keen, A.; Putkey, F.; Hjelmeland, L. ARPE-19, A Human Retinal Pigment Epithelial Cell Line with Differentiated Properties. *Exp. Eye Res.* **1996**, *62*, 155–170. [CrossRef]
48. Dunn, K.C.; Marmorstein, A.D.; Bonilha, V.L.; Rodriguez-Boulan, E.; Giordano, F.; Hjelmeland, L.M. Use of the ARPE-19 cell line as a model of RPE polarity: Basolateral secretion of FGF5. *Investig. Ophthalmol. Vis. Sci.* **1998**, *39*, 6.
49. Tian, J.; Ishibashi, K.; Honda, S.; A Boylan, S.; Hjelmeland, L.M.; Handa, J.T. The expression of native and cultured human retinal pigment epithelial cells grown in different culture conditions. *Br. J. Ophthalmol.* **2005**, *89*, 1510–1517. [CrossRef]
50. Luo, Y.; Zhuo, Y.; Fukuhara, M.; Rizzolo, L.J. Effects of Culture Conditions on Heterogeneity and the Apical Junctional Complex of the ARPE-19 Cell Line. *Investig. Opthalmol. Vis. Sci.* **2006**, *47*, 3644–3655. [CrossRef]
51. Geisen, P.; McColm, J.R.; King, B.M.; Hartnett, M.E. Characterization of Barrier Properties and Inducible VEGF Expression of Several Types of Retinal Pigment Epithelium in Medium-Term Culture. *Curr. Eye Res.* **2006**, *31*, 739–748. [CrossRef] [PubMed]
52. Samuel, W.; Jaworski, C.; Postnikova, O.A.; Kutty, R.K.; Duncan, T.; Tan, L.X.; Poliakov, E.; Lakkaraju, A.; Redmond, T.M. Appropriately differentiated ARPE-19 cells regain phenotype and gene expression profiles similar to those of native RPE cells. *Mol. Vis.* **2017**, *23*, 60–89. [PubMed]
53. Tian, J.; Ishibashi, K.; Handa, J.T. The expression of native and cultured RPE grown on different matrices. *Physiol. Genom.* **2004**, *17*, 170–182. [CrossRef] [PubMed]
54. Utheim, T.P.; Raeder, S.; Utheim, Ø.A.; Cai, Y.; Roald, B.; Drolsum, L.; Lyberg, T.; Nicolaissen, B. A novel method for preserving cultured limbal epithelial cells. *Br. J. Ophthalmol.* **2006**, *91*, 797–800. [CrossRef] [PubMed]
55. Utheim, T.P.; Islam, R.; Fostad, I.G.; Eidet, J.R.; Sehic, A.; Olstad, O.K.; Dartt, D.A.; Messelt, E.B.; Griffith, M.; Pasovic, L. Storage Temperature Alters the Expression of Differentiation-Related Genes in Cultured Oral Keratinocytes. *PLoS ONE* **2016**, *11*, e0152526. [CrossRef]
56. Jackson, C.; Eidet, J.R.; Reppe, S.; Aass, H.C.D.; Tønseth, K.A.; Roald, B.; Lyberg, T.; Utheim, T.P. Effect of Storage Temperature on the Phenotype of Cultured Epidermal Cells Stored in Xenobiotic-Free Medium. *Curr. Eye Res.* **2015**, *41*, 757–768. [CrossRef]
57. Pellegrin, S.; Mellor, H. Actin stress fibres. *J. Cell Sci.* **2007**, *120*, 3491–3499. [CrossRef]
58. Tojkander, S.; Gateva, G.; Lappalainen, P. Actin stress fibers—assembly, dynamics and biological roles. *J. Cell Sci.* **2012**, *125*, 1855–1864. [CrossRef]
59. Narimatsu, T.; Ozawa, Y.; Miyake, S.; Kubota, S.; Hirasawa, M.; Nagai, N.; Shimmura, S.; Tsubota, K. Disruption of Cell-Cell Junctions and Induction of Pathological Cytokines in the Retinal Pigment Epithelium of Light-Exposed Mice. *Investig. Opthalmol. Vis. Sci.* **2013**, *54*, 4555–4562. [CrossRef]
60. Eidet, J.R.; Pasovic, L.; Maria, R.; Jackson, C.J.; Utheim, T.P. Objective assessment of changes in nuclear morphology and cell distribution following induction of apoptosis. *Diagn. Pathol.* **2014**, *9*, 92. [CrossRef]

61. Vermes, I.; Haanen, C.; Steffens-Nakken, H.; Reutellingsperger, C. A novel assay for apoptosis Flow cytometric detection of phosphatidylserine expression on early apoptotic cells using fluorescein labelled Annexin V. *J. Immunol. Methods* **1995**, *184*, 39–51. [CrossRef]
62. Khan, A.Z.; Utheim, T.P.; Jackson, C.J.; Reppe, S.; Lyberg, T.; Eidet, J.R. Nucleus Morphometry in Cultured Epithelial Cells Correlates with Phenotype. *Microsc. Microanal.* **2016**, *22*, 612–620. [CrossRef] [PubMed]

Sample Availability: Samples of the compounds are not available from the authors.

Publisher's Note: MDPI stays neutral with regard to jurisdictional claims in published maps and institutional affiliations.

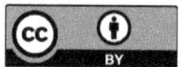

© 2020 by the authors. Licensee MDPI, Basel, Switzerland. This article is an open access article distributed under the terms and conditions of the Creative Commons Attribution (CC BY) license (http://creativecommons.org/licenses/by/4.0/).

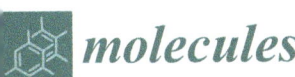

Review

Cystic Fibrosis and Oxidative Stress: The Role of CFTR

Evelina Moliteo [1], Monica Sciacca [1], Antonino Palmeri [1], Maria Papale [1], Sara Manti [1,2], Giuseppe Fabio Parisi [1,*] and Salvatore Leonardi [1]

1. Pediatric Respiratory Unit, Department of Clinical and Experimental Medicine, San Marco Hospital, University of Catania, Viale Carlo Azeglio Ciampi sn, 95121 Catania, Italy
2. Pediatric Unit, Department of Human and Pediatric Pathology "Gaetano Barresi", AOUP G. Martino, University of Messina, Via Consolare Valeria, 1, 98124 Messina, Italy
* Correspondence: gf.parisi@policlinico.unict.it; Tel.: +39-09-5479-4181

Abstract: There is substantial evidence in the literature that patients with cystic fibrosis (CF) have higher oxidative stress than patients with other diseases or healthy subjects. This results in an increase in reactive oxygen species (ROS) and in a deficit of antioxidant molecules and plays a fundamental role in the progression of chronic lung damage. Although it is known that recurrent infection–inflammation cycles in CF patients generate a highly oxidative environment, numerous clinical and preclinical studies suggest that the airways of a patient with CF present an inherently abnormal proinflammatory milieu due to elevated oxidative stress and abnormal lipid metabolism even before they become infected. This could be directly related to cystic fibrosis transmembrane conductance regulator (CFTR) deficiency, which appears to produce a redox imbalance in epithelial cells and extracellular fluids. This review aims to summarize the main mechanism by which CFTR deficiency is intrinsically responsible for the proinflammatory environment that characterizes the lung of a patient with CF.

Keywords: cystic fibrosis; oxidative stress; cystic fibrosis transmembrane conductance regulator; antioxidant

1. Introduction

Cystic fibrosis (CF) is still today the most common lethal genetic disease with autosomal recessive inheritance in the Caucasian population, with a prevalence of 1 case per 2500 live births [1]. The disease is caused by a mutation in the cystic fibrosis transmembrane conductance regulator (CFTR) gene that causes the CFTR protein to become dysfunctional. When the protein is not working correctly, there is reduced transport of chloride ions with consequent dysregulation of epithelial lining fluid (mucus) transport in the lung, pancreas and other organs [2].

There are more than 2000 different mutations in the gene encoding the CFTR protein [3]. Among these, seven main groups have been identified based on the type of DNA alteration that characterizes the mutation. Class I mutations induce a block of protein synthesis. Class II mutations, of which the more common F508del mutation is part, synthesize a misfolded CFTR protein, leading to the failure of maturation and trafficking to the cell surface. Mutations of class III, also termed as "gating defect", affect the activation of ion transport function, while mutations of class IV reduce the number of chloride ions transported through pore channels. Class V mutations allow the synthesis of the protein in reduced quantities. Class VI mutations produce unstable CFTR with a short half-life. Class VII mutations, recently introduced, interfere with mRNA splicing, leading to the absence of full-length mature RNA, so the CFTR protein is totally absent, as occurs in class I mutations [4–7].

The presence of so many mutations reflects the extremely variable phenotypes: some subjects have a severe clinical presentation, and their life expectancy is dependent on lung or liver transplantation. On the other extreme, there are patients who manifest the pathology later in life, or early but with mild symptoms or even without any [8].

Among the different organs affected, in the lungs, the accumulation of thick mucus decreases the ciliary mucus clearance function, favoring colonization by numerous germs, first bacteria, leading to infection, inflammation and other complications. The inflammation is a self-amplifying process: a vicious circle is established and constitutes a chronic challenge to the integrity of airway epithelial cells [9]. Oxidative stress is a key element contributing to persistent cellular damage and preventing proper airway remodeling.

Oxidative stress is a complex process in which excess reactive oxygen species (ROS) affect, either directly or indirectly, all structural and functional components of cells at a molecular level [10–12]. This arises because the production of these chemical species is increased and/or because the physiological defense capacity towards them, thanks to the antioxidant system, is reduced. Changes in the balance between oxidant and antioxidant substances are considered a normal part of cell physiology; many cellular signaling pathways, in fact, are regulated by changes in redox balance [13]. In CF patients, malabsorption of dietary antioxidants, induced by exocrine pancreatic insufficiency and by a decrease in bile acids, and the inability of cells with the CFTR mutation to efflux glutathione (GSH) play an essential role in the systemic redox imbalance already exacerbated by the excessive release of oxidants by neutrophils [14]. This sustained redox imbalance leads to the establishment of an oxidizing environment that causes the oxidation of proteins, DNA, lipids and other metabolites with the consequent alteration of various signaling pathways [13].

In consideration of the pathogenetic mechanism described above, it is logical that the optimization of the antioxidant and anti-inflammatory status represents an important goal in patients with CF. There is substantial evidence that antioxidant supplementation positively influences the outcome of CF patients, especially in terms of a reduction in pulmonary exacerbation, but the efficacy is limited and transient [15,16]. New therapeutic strategies are therefore necessary and are under study.

CFTR-targeted therapeutics, mainly responsible for the increase in life expectancy that has occurred in recent years, in association with antioxidant and anti-inflammatory therapies, appear to be the only weapon to reduce the underlying inflammatory state that leads to progressive lung damage.

Ivacaftor was the first drug able to act on the causes of the disease by improving the function of the defective protein. It is suitable for gating mutations (class III) in the CFTR gene. Lumacaftor/ivacaftor was the first drug used for the defect in the processing and transport of the CFTR protein in patients with CF with a double copy of the F508del mutation. Last but not least, we can mention the triple combination elaxacaftor/tezacaftor/ivacaftor, which works as a modulator of the CFTR protein that is defective and therefore responsible for the symptoms of the disease [17–19].

This review aims to summarize the main mechanism by which CFTR deficiency is intrinsically responsible for the proinflammatory environment that characterizes the lung of a patient with CF.

A combination of antioxidant, anti-inflammatory and CFTR-targeted therapeutics could be required for full correction of the CF phenotype to decrease the basic inflammatory status, improving the disease outcome.

2. Literature Search Methodology

Literature searches for specific research were conducted using the PubMed database with keywords such as "cystic fibrosis", "oxidative stress", "cystic fibrosis transmembrane conductance regulator" and "antioxidant". We included review articles, meta-analyses, case–control studies, case reports and letters to the editor, including only papers over the last 10 years and published in English. Only studies specifically correlating oxidative stress and cystic fibrosis were considered. The review was completed by searching for bibliographic references and definitions of the topic described above.

3. Evidence from Literature

One of the main determinants of progressive lung damage in CF is represented by chronic oxidative stress, which leads to the establishment of an intrinsically proinflammatory environment. The mechanisms behind this are still partially unknown, but several studies have shown the direct implication of CFTR protein dysfunction, mainly in the lungs, but also in extrapulmonary tissues such as the pancreas and intestine [20].

Several molecular mechanisms have been proposed to explain the link between CFTR deficiency and oxidative stress (Figure 1).

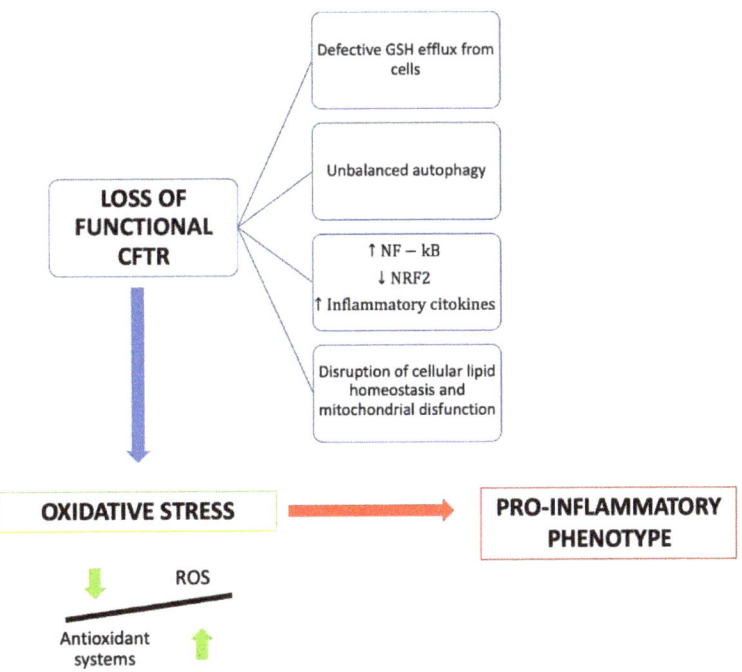

Figure 1. Summary of the consequences of the loss of functional CFTR in cystic fibrosis patients.

There is some evidence that the efflux of GSH out of cells is a chloride-dependent mechanism involving the CFTR channel. Indeed, CFTR shares a structural similarity with ABCC proteins, which normally export glutathione and/or glutathione S-conjugates [13]. Glutathione (GSH) is a tripeptide with antioxidant properties consisting of cysteine, glycine and glutamic acid. It represents the first-line defense of the lung against oxidative stress-induced damage, and its availability inside the cell is fundamental to sustaining a good redox state. The ratio between reduced and oxidized glutathione is an indicator of the cellular redox state and describes the antioxidative capacity of cells [21].

Unsurprisingly, in patients with CF, low CFTR activity is correlated with GSH deficiency, resulting in an altered extracellular ratio between oxidized and reduced glutathione [22–24]; oxidized glutathione species are significantly elevated, and there is an inadequate response to neutrophil-mediated oxidative stress during infections. Rather, the reactive oxidant species produced by neutrophils, including myeloperoxidase (MPO)-derived hypochlorous acid, contribute to the oxidation of glutathione, leading to a vicious cycle. Dickerhof N et al. demonstrated that the pharmacological inhibition of MPO by orally administered AZM198 decreases oxidative stress and improves infection outcomes in mice with CF-like inflammation without interfering with the clearance of bacteria [25]. Still, few studies have been conducted or are ongoing on the beneficial effects of direct

GSH supplementation in CF. For example, Calabrese et al. studied the possible beneficial effects of long-term treatment with inhaled glutathione [26]. Hewson et al. established that exogenous administration of γ-glutamylcysteine (GGC), the immediate precursor of glutathione, can increase intracellular levels of total glutathione and protect CF cells from lipopolysaccharide (LPS)-induced cell damage [27].

It has also been demonstrated that the administration of N-acetylcysteine (NAC), the acetylated form of the amino acid L-cysteine and a precursor to glutathione, is able to reduce the redox imbalance, increasing the GSH level. Furthermore, an influence of NAC on nuclear factor kappa-light-chain-enhancer of activated B cells (NFkB) activation was observed [14].

Mutated CFTR is associated with the alteration of some signal transduction pathways at a cellular level, such as that of NFkB, required for the transcription of various proinflammatory molecules. NFkB overexpression is an intrinsic underlying feature of the patient with cystic fibrosis and is exacerbated by hyperproduction of ROS and by bacterial stimulation on the cell surface that induces further activation. Moreover, the CFTR mutation is also associated with reduced production of peroxisome proliferator-activated receptor (PPAR), a transcription factor that normally counteracts the action of NFKB [14,20]. This results in increased production of oxidizing molecules and proinflammatory cytokines such as IL-1, TNF, IL-6 and IL-17A.

In normal cell physiology, under conditions of increased oxidant production, a series of pathways are activated that play an active role in the suppression of inflammatory signaling. Among these, the most important is the Nuclear factor erythroid 2-related factor 2 (Nrf2) pathway, an antagonist of proinflammatory transcription factors such as NFkB. Following the hyperactivation of the inflammatory response, the Kelch-like-ECH-associated protein 1 (KEAP1) protein, which normally binds Nrf2 in the cytoplasm of cells, oxidizes and dissociates from Nrf2, allowing its subsequent transcriptional activation, which leads to the production of over 200 antioxidant and detoxifying proteins; these include heme oxygenase-1 (HO-1), NAD(P)H quinone oxidoreductase 1 (NQO1), glutamate–cysteine ligase (GCL) and glutathione S transferase (GST). Nrf2-mediated HO-1 expression is also regulated by transcription factor BTB (TF BTB) and CNC Homology 1 (Bach1), which suppress HO-1 expression [26,28]. The heme oxygenase-1/carbon monoxide (HO-1/CO) pathway is essential to ensure a controlled immune response and effective bactericidal activity by monocytes and macrophages. The blunt activation of this pathway in CF patients therefore contributes to hyperinflammation and defective host defense against bacteria. Recent studies have shown that the administration of controlled doses of CO can induce HO1 by reducing lung hyperinflammation and oxidative stress [29]. Furthermore, CO stimulates autophagy [29], the cellular mechanism that is fundamental to efficient bacterial clearance by immune cells. Recent works prove that CFTR deficiency in macrophages and neutrophils results in an inability to kill bacteria and, thus, in limited autophagy activity [30].

There is much evidence that the Nrf2 pathway is dysfunctional in cells with mutated CFTR [13,28,29].

Laselva et al. demonstrated that the administration of dimethyl fumarate (DMF), an activator of the Nrf2 pathway, drastically reduced both the basal and stimulated expression of proinflammatory cytokines while also exerting an antioxidant effect [30].

Borcherding et al. demonstrated that the CFTR modulators VX-809 (Lumacaftor) and VX-661 (Tezacaftor) significantly increase Nrf2 activity in CF patients [31]; this could represent one of the mechanisms through which CFTR modulators mitigate the inflammatory response and oxidative stress.

Pellullo et al., in their study, used mRNA extracted from nasal epithelial cells to analyze the expression levels of the genes involved in oxidative stress. They found that the expression of Nrf2 mRNA and its targets, such as HO-1 and miR-125b, is upregulated in the nasal epithelia cells of CF patients compared to healthy subjects. This suggests that the protective mechanisms against oxidative stress may be functional but not sufficient to counteract the hyperproduction of ROS and the oxidative stress that characterizes the pathology. Moreover, the authors found that elevated HO-1 and miR-125b levels are associated with an improved FEV1 value, so they could be considered potential predictive biomarkers of CF clinical outcomes. The wide expression range of these markers could partly explain the phenotypic variability of CF, beyond the mutations of the CFTR gene itself [28].

Another mechanism that links CFTR deficiency and oxidative stress and that contributes to CF airways' chronic damage is the alteration of lipid metabolism [29]. Thanks to several studies, it has been found that CF airway pathology is related to alterations in fatty acids, ceramides and cholesterol, but their role in the etiopathogenesis of CF pulmonary pathology is unclear.

An increased ratio of long-chain to very long chain ceramide species (LCC/VLCC), abnormalities in sphingosine phosphate (S1P) metabolism and, consequently, abnormal lipid levels in the blood and lungs are hallmarks of CF. Lipid synthesis is increased, whereas their catabolism is reduced, contributing to inflammation, oxidative stress and impaired autophagy. In this view, dyslipidemia should be considered a contributor to CF airways' chronic damage, and thus, lipid metabolism should become an important therapeutic target [32–34].

Signorelli et al. have shown that modulating the synthesis of sphingolipids and hindering the accumulation of ceramide with Myrocin (Myr), a sphingolipid synthesis inhibitor, significantly reduces the accumulation of lipids, promotes the oxidation of fatty acids and reduces inflammation and oxidative stress, and it restores the defensive response against pathogen infection, which is defective in CF [35].

Veltman et al. examined the consequences of CFTR deficiency on lipid metabolism, highlighting how the alterations concerning the metabolism of fatty acids and ceramide induce a state of chronic oxidative stress, but also, in turn, chronic oxidative stress can cause a great imbalance in the metabolism of lipids. The new CFTR-modulating drugs considerably reduce the alterations of lipid balance, confirming the role of CFTR as a regulator of cellular lipid balance [36].

4. Discussion

The role of oxidative stress in the progression of lung injury in CF patients has been widely recognized and very well described in the literature (Table 1). It has been shown that in patients with CF, there is an important deficit of antioxidant molecules and an increase in oxidative stress [24,37]. The sustained imbalance between oxidant and antioxidant species induces chronic inflammation, which is the key element contributing to persistent cellular damage and preventing proper airway remodeling. Both hereditary and acquired factors, such as CFTR deficiency and persistent infections, contribute to abnormal and self-sustaining lung inflammation in CF.

Table 1. Summary of the main studies pointing towards the involvement of oxidative stress in CF disease.

Authors	Type of Study	Aim of the Study	Materials and Methods	Main Findings
Checa et al. 2021 [10]	Research article	To identify oxidative stress modulators in CF airway epithelial cells	Unbiased genome-wide RNAi screen using a randomized siRNA library	The usefulness of combining unbiased genome-wide knockdown to uncover new genes/pathways involved in oxidative stress to identify and characterize new drugs.

Table 1. Cont.

Authors	Type of Study	Aim of the Study	Materials and Methods	Main Findings
Guerini et al. 2022 [14]	Review	To show the potential role of N-acetylcysteine in preventing and eliminating biofilms as an anti-inflammatory and antioxidant drug.	NA	It is possible to establish that this molecule offers great hope for the treatment of this disease.
Ciofu et al. 2014 [15]	Cochrane systematic review	To synthesize existing data on the effect of antioxidants such as vitamin C, vitamin E, ß-carotene, selenium and glutathione in CF disease.	Randomized controlled studies and quasi-randomized controlled studies of people with cystic fibrosis comparing antioxidants to placebo or standard care.	Intensive antibiotic treatment and other drugs used in CF patients make it very difficult to evaluate the usefulness of antioxidant therapy. Based on the available evidence, glutathione (administered either orally or by inhalation) appears to improve lung function.
Sagel et al. 2018 [16]	Research article	To evaluate the effects of an oral antioxidant-enriched multivitamin supplement in CF disease and clinical outcomes.	Multicenter randomized, double-blind, controlled trial; 73 pancreatic-insufficient subjects with CF 10 years of age and older with an FEV1 between 40% and 100% predicted were randomized to 16 weeks of an antioxidant-enriched multivitamin or control multivitamin without antioxidant enrichment.	Antioxidant supplementation was safe and well tolerated. It increased systemic antioxidant concentrations with a modest reduction in systemic inflammation after 4 weeks. Antioxidant treatment was also associated with a lower risk of first pulmonary exacerbation.
Bergeron et al. 2021 [17]	Review	To summarize the current knowledge of CF genetics and therapies restoring CFTR function, particularly CFTR modulators and gene therapy.	NA	There is hope that the treatment burden can be decreased using highly effective CFTR modulator therapy.
Wu et al. 2003 [21]	Research article	To analyze the role of glutathione in antioxidant defense, nutrient metabolism and regulation of cellular events.	NA	New knowledge on the efficient utilization of dietary protein or precursors for GSH synthesis and its nutritional status is critical for the development of effective therapeutic strategies to treat CF.
Zhao et al. 2019 [22]	Systematic review and meta-analysis	To explore the influence of glutathione versus placebo on pulmonary function in cystic fibrosis.	NA	Glutathione improved pulmonary function in CF, as shown by the increase in FEV1.

Table 1. Cont.

Authors	Type of Study	Aim of the Study	Materials and Methods	Main Findings
Dickerhof et al. 2017 [23]	Original article	To establish whether oxidative stress or glutathione status could be associated with bronchiectasis and whether glutathione deficiency could be linked to CF or a consequence of oxidative stress.	A total of 263 children and infants, out of which 205 had CF and 58 did not. Collectively, they provided 635 BAL samples.	Glutathione deficiency exists in the lower respiratory tract during early stages of cystic fibrosis lung disease, and treatments targeting glutathione have potential benefits for CF patients.
Causer et al. 2020 [24]	Systematic review and meta-analysis.	To evaluate the concentrations of proinflammatory molecules and antioxidant substances in the serum or plasma of CF and non-CF control patients.	Mean contents of blood biomarkers from people with clinically stable CF and non-CF controls were used to calculate the standardized mean difference (SMD) and 95% confidence intervals (95% CI).	Protein carbonyls, F2-isoprostane 8- iso-prostaglandin F2α and malondialdehyde were significantly higher, and vitamins A, β-carotene and albumin were significantly lower in the plasma or serum of people with CF versus controls.
Dickerhof et al. 2020 [25]	Research article	To investigate whether the 2-thioxanthine inhibitor AZM198, when given orally, can inhibit myeloperoxidases in airways of βENaC mice and block oxidative stress without compromising the host's defense mechanisms.	Transgenic β-epithelial sodium channel (βENaC)- overexpressing mice (n = 10) were infected with $Burkholderia\ multivorans$ and treated twice daily with the MPO inhibitor AZM198.	Blocking hypochlorous acid production in epithelia during pulmonary infections through inhibition of MPO improves morbidity in mice with CF-like lung inflammation without interfering with clearance of bacteria. Inhibition of MPO is an approach to limit oxidative stress in cystic fibrosis lung disease in humans.
Calabrese et al. 2014 [26]	Research article	To evaluate the effect of inhaled GSH in patients with CF.	A total of 54 adult and 51 pediatric patients were randomized to receive inhaled GSH or placebo twice daily for 12 months.	In the pediatric group, a 12-month treatment with inhaled GSH did not lead to any significant increase in FEV1 from baseline. Inhaled GSH has positive effects in CF patients with moderate lung disease.
Hewson et al. 2020 [27]	Research article	To demonstrate that novel antioxidant therapy with the immediate precursor to glutathione, γ-glutamylcysteine (GGC), ameliorates LPS-induced cellular stress in vitro.	Human airway basal epithelial cells were obtained by brushing the nasal inferior turbinate and from bronchoalveolar lavage fluid during bronchoscopy. Proteomic analysis identified perturbations in several pathways related to cellular respiration, transcription, stress responses and cell–cell junction signaling.	Administration of exogenous γ-glutamylcysteine to CF airway epithelium in vitro can increase total intracellular glutathione levels and protect cells from LPS-induced cellular damage.

Table 1. Cont.

Authors	Type of Study	Aim of the Study	Materials and Methods	Main Findings
Pelullo et al. 2020 [28]	Research article	To evaluate if oxidative stress and the aberrant expression levels of genes and microRNAs (miRNAs/miRs) implicated in detoxification may be associated with a better clinical outcome.	Used total RNA extracted from nasal epithelial cells and analyzed the expression levels of oxidative stress genes and one miRNA using quantitative PCR in a representative number of patients with CF compared with healthy individuals.	The activation of an inducible oxidative stress response to protect airway cells against reactive oxygen species injuries in CF patients. The correlations of HO-1 and miR-125b expression with an improved FEV1 value suggested that these factors may synergistically protect airway cells from oxidative stress damage, inflammation and apoptosis.
Di Pietro Caterina et al. 2020 [29]	Review	Blunted heme oxygenase-1 activation in CF-affected cells contributes to hyperinflammation and reduction in the host defense against infections. They discussed potential cellular mechanisms that may lead to decreased heme oxygenase-1 induction in CF cells.	NA	Induction of heme oxygenase-1 may be beneficial for the treatment of CF lung disease. They discussed recent studies highlighting how endogenous heme oxygenase-1 can be induced by administration of controlled doses of CO to reduce lung hyperinflammation, oxidative stress, bacterial infection and dysfunctional ion transport, which are all hallmarks of CF lung disease.
Laselva et al. 2021 [30]	Research article	To understand the role of dimethyl fumarate as an anti-inflammatory and antioxidant drug in CF, they focused on the effect of dimethyl fumarate on CF-related cytokine expression, ROS measurements and CFTR channel function.	Human immortalized bronchial epithelial cells:	Dimethyl fumarate reduced the inflammatory response to LPS stimulation in both CF and non-CF bronchial epithelial cells and restored the LPS-mediated decrease in Kaftrio-TM-mediated CFTR function in CF cells bearing the most common mutation.
Borcherding et al. 2019 [31]	Research article	To determine the effects of CFTR modulation on Nrf2 in primary non-CF and CF human bronchial epithelial cells.	They used primary non-CF or CF human bronchial epithelial cells.	The primary finding of this study is that the F508del CFTR correctors VX809 and VX661 reverse the dysregulation of Nrf2 activity in primary human CF epithelial cells, and that this rescue is CFTR function-dependent.
Nandy Mazumdar et al. 2021 [32]	Research article	Examined the role of BACH1 globally in the oxidative stress response in the airway epithelium and also its role in modulating CFTR expression.	RNA from confluent cultures was extracted with TRIzol (Invitrogen), and cDNA was prepared with the TaqMan reverse transcription kit.	BACH1 regulates CFTR gene expression by modulating locus architecture through its occupancy of enhancers and structural elements, and depletion of BACH1 alters the higher-order chromatin structure. BACH1 may have a dual effect on CFTR expression by direct occupancy of CREs at physiological oxygen (~8%) while indirectly modulating expression under conditions of oxidative stress.

Table 1. Cont.

Authors	Type of Study	Aim of the Study	Materials and Methods	Main Findings
Scholte et al. 2019 [34]	Research article	To determine whether lipid pathway dysregulation is also observed in BALF from children with CF and to identify biomarkers of early lung disease and potential therapeutic targets.	A comprehensive panel of lipids that included sphingolipids, oxylipins, isoprostanes and lysolipids, all bioactive lipid species known to be involved in inflammation and tissue remodeling, were measured in BALF from children with CF and age-matched non-CF patients with unexplained inflammatory disease	Several lipid biomarkers of early CF lung disease were identified, which point toward potential disease therapeutic approaches used to complement CFTR modulators.
Signorelli et al. 2021 [35]	Research article	To demonstrate that Myriocin modulates the transcriptional profile of CF cells in order to restore autophagy, activate an antioxidative response, stimulate lipid metabolism and reduce lipid peroxidation.	They labeled the cells by means of a fluorescent probe with a high affinity for neutral lipids. We compared CF to healthy cells.	Lipid synthesis is increased in CF, whereas their catabolism is reduced, contributing to inflammation, oxidative stress and impaired autophagy. Myriocin, an inhibitor of sphingolipid synthesis, significantly reduces inflammation. Targeting sphingolipids' de novo synthesis may counteract lipid accumulation by modulating the CF altered transcriptional profile, thus restoring autophagy and lipid metabolism homeostasis.
Veltman et al. 2021 [36]	Research article	To examine the impact of CFTR deficiency on lipid metabolism and proinflammatory signaling in airway epithelium using a mass spectrometric protein array.	They used CF mouse lung and well-differentiated bronchial epithelial cell cultures of CFTR knockout pigs and CF patients.	Protein array analysis revealed differential expression and shedding of cytokines and growth factors from CF epithelial cells compared to non-CF cells, consistent with sterile inflammation and tissue remodeling under basal conditions.
Olveira et al. 2017 [37]	Research article	To assess oxidation biomarkers and levels of inflammation to determine whether there is an association between these parameters and the intake of macrolides.	Cross-sectional study with clinically stable CF patients and healthy controls. Serum and plasma inflammatory and oxidative stress biomarkers were measured: interleukin-6, reactive C protein, tumor necrosis alpha, glutathione peroxidase, total antioxidant capacity, catalase and superoxide dismutase, together with markers of lipid peroxidation.	Inflammation and oxidation biomarkers were increased in patients with CF compared with controls. The use of azithromycin was associated with reduced TNF-α levels and did not influence oxidation parameters.

The central role of CFTR deficiency has been increasingly recognized in recent years. Mutations in the CFTR gene appear to make CF epithelial cells more susceptible to inflammation compared with healthy cells; for this reason, once an infection is introduced, it triggers the onset of mucosal damage and chronic airway infection. CFTR dysfunction, in fact, not only alters ion exchange and fluid secretion in the lungs but also causes the dysregulation of several signaling pathways, generating an innate oxidative state that, over time, could promote the loss of lung epithelial cell integrity. Impaired extracellular glutathione transport, alterations in lipid metabolism, dysregulation of the main pro- and anti-inflammatory signaling pathways and unbalanced autophagy are the main molecular mechanisms correlated with CFTR dysfunction in CF. Starting from this consolidated knowledge, numerous research groups have identified targets and strategies aimed at reducing the exaggerated immune response that causes chronic inflammation in CF, without altering the natural defenses against infection. Currently used drugs, such as steroidal and non-steroidal anti-inflammatories, mucolytics and antibiotics, reduce inflammation, improving the natural history of the disease; however, there are a lot of concerns about their chronic use because of their immunosuppressive effects that compromise the host's defenses [29].

New therapeutic approaches are therefore needed and are currently being evaluated, with the aim of reducing the proinflammatory response in CF, preserving the host defense against microorganisms. The most promising results come from the use of CFTR modulators, which, in the last several years, have radically changed the natural history of CF. In our review, we found that the excellent results from the use of these drugs are related not only to the restoration of physiological ion exchanges, which improve mucociliary clearance, but also, given the close correlation between CFTR deficiency and oxidative stress, to the reduction in the basic inflammatory status that characterizes CF patients. Further studies are needed to confirm, through the evaluation of specific markers, whether CF patients treated with modulators have a significant reduction in oxidative stress. However, these therapies are targeted for specific mutations characterizing CF, and it is not known how long they will have this crucial role in containing the inflammatory response. Future therapeutic perspectives should include the use of additional antioxidant and anti-inflammatory drugs, in combination with CFTR modulators, which specifically target the altered signaling pathway, in order to obtain a more selective response without altering the local tissue defenses.

5. Conclusions

Mutations in the CFTR gene produce an inherently proinflammatory cellular environment, in addition to repeated infections that set the stage for chronic airway infection and progressive loss of lung function. Although the molecular mechanisms underlying it are not fully understood, this aspect represents a central feature of the disease and, consequently, an important therapeutic target.

Author Contributions: Conceptualization, E.M., M.S. and A.P.; methodology, S.M. and M.P., validation, G.F.P. and S.L.; formal analysis, E.M., M.S. and A.P.; investigation, S.M. and M.P.; resources, G.F.P.; data curation, E.M., M.S. and A.P.; writing—original draft preparation, E.M., M.S. and A.P.; writing—review and editing, S.M., M.P. and G.F.P.; visualization, S.L.; supervision, G.F.P. and S.L. All authors have read and agreed to the published version of the manuscript.

Funding: This research received no external funding.

Institutional Review Board Statement: Not applicable.

Informed Consent Statement: Not applicable.

Data Availability Statement: Not applicable.

Conflicts of Interest: The authors declare no conflict of interest.

References

1. Burgel, P.-R.; Bellis, G.; Olesen, H.V.; Viviani, L.; Zolin, A.; Blasi, F.; Elborn, J.S.; ERS/ECFS Task Force on Provision of Care for Adults with Cystic Fibrosis in Europe. Future trends in cystic fibrosis demography in 34 European countries. *Eur. Respir. J.* **2015**, *46*, 133–141. [CrossRef]
2. Manti, S.; Parisi, G.F.; Papale, M.; Marseglia, G.L.; Licari, A.; Leonardi, S. Type 2 inflammation in cystic fibrosis: New insights. *Pediatr. Allergy Immunol.* **2022**, *33*, 15–17. [CrossRef] [PubMed]
3. The Clinical and Functional Translation of CFTR (CFTR2). Available online: https://www.cftr2.org/ (accessed on 12 June 2022).
4. De Boeck, K. Cystic fibrosis in the year 2020: A disease with a new face. *Acta Paediatr.* **2020**, *109*, 893–899. [CrossRef] [PubMed]
5. Shteinberg, M.; Haq, I.J.; Polineni, D.; Davies, J.C. Cystic fibrosis. *Lancet* **2021**, *397*, 2195–2211. [CrossRef]
6. Farinha, C.M.; Callebaut, I. Molecular mechanisms of cystic fibrosis–how mutations lead to misfunction and guide therapy. *Biosci. Rep.* **2022**, *42*, BSR20212006. [CrossRef] [PubMed]
7. Parisi, G.F.; Cutello, S.; Di Dio, G.; Rotolo, N.; La Rosa, M.; Leonardi, S. Phenotypic expression of the p.Leu1077Pro CFTR mutation in Sicilian cystic fibrosis patients. *BMC Res. Notes* **2013**, *6*, 461. [CrossRef] [PubMed]
8. Parisi, G.F.; Di Dio, G.; Franzonello, C.; Gennaro, A.; Rotolo, N.; Lionetti, E.; Leonardi, S. Liver disease in cystic fibrosis: An update. *Hepat. Mon.* **2013**, *13*, e11215. [CrossRef]
9. Leonardi, S.; Parisi, G.F.; Capizzi, A.; Manti, S.; Cuppari, C.; Scuderi, M.G.; Rotolo, N.; Lanzafame, A.; Musumeci, M.; Salpietro, C. YKL-40 as marker of severe lung disease in cystic fibrosis patients. *J. Cyst. Fibros.* **2016**, *15*, 583–586. [CrossRef]
10. Checa, J.; Martínez-González, I.; Maqueda, M.; Mosquera, J.L.; Aran, J.M. Genome-Wide RNAi Screening Identifies Novel Pathways/Genes Involved in Oxidative Stress and Repurposable Drugs to Preserve Cystic Fibrosis Airway Epithelial Cell Integrity. *Antioxidants* **2021**, *10*, 1936. [CrossRef]
11. Spicuzza, L.; Parisi, G.F.; Tardino, L.; Ciancio, N.; Nenna, R.; Midulla, F.; Leonardi, S. Exhaled markers of antioxidant activity and oxidative stress in stable cystic fibrosis patients with moderate lung disease. *J. Breath Res.* **2018**, *12*, 026010. [CrossRef]
12. Manti, S.; Marseglia, L.; D'Angelo, G.; Cuppari, C.; Cusumano, E.; Arrigo, T.; Gitto, E.; Salpietro, C. "Cumulative Stress": The Effects of Maternal and Neonatal Oxidative Stress and Oxidative Stress-Inducible Genes on Programming of Atopy. *Oxid. Med. Cell. Longev.* **2016**, *2016*, 8651820. [CrossRef] [PubMed]
13. Ziady, A.G.; Hansen, J. Redox balance in cystic fibrosis. *Int. J. Biochem. Cell Biol.* **2014**, *52*, 113–123. [CrossRef] [PubMed]
14. Guerini, M.; Condrò, G.; Friuli, V.; Maggi, L.; Perugini, P. N-acetylcysteine (NAC) and Its Role in Clinical Practice Management of Cystic Fibrosis (CF): A Review. *Pharmaceuticals* **2022**, *15*, 217. [CrossRef]
15. Ciofu, O.; Smith, S.; Lykkesfeldt, J. Antioxidant supplementation for lung disease in cystic fibrosis. *Cochrane Database Syst. Rev.* **2019**, *10*, CD007020. [CrossRef] [PubMed]
16. Sagel, S.D.; Khan, U.; Jain, R.; Graff, G.; Daines, C.L.; Dunitz, J.M.; Borowitz, D.; Orenstein, D.M.; Abdulhamid, I.; Noe, J.; et al. Effects of an Antioxidant-enriched Multivitamin in Cystic Fibrosis. A Randomized, Controlled, Multicenter Clinical Trial. *Am. J. Respir. Crit. Care Med.* **2018**, *198*, 639–647. [CrossRef] [PubMed]
17. Bergeron, C.; Cantin, A.M. New Therapies to Correct the Cystic Fibrosis Basic Defect. *Int. J. Mol. Sci.* **2021**, *22*, 6193. [CrossRef]
18. Guimbellot, J.S.; Taylor-Cousar, J.L. Combination CFTR modulator therapy in children and adults with cystic fibrosis. *Lancet Respir. Med.* **2021**, *9*, 677–679. [CrossRef]
19. King, J.A.; Nichols, A.-L.; Bentley, S.; Carr, S.B.; Davies, J.C. An Update on CFTR Modulators as New Therapies for Cystic Fibrosis. *Pediatr. Drugs* **2022**, *24*, 321–333. [CrossRef]
20. Mitri, C.; Xu, Z.; Bardin, P.; Corvol, H.; Touqui, L.; Tabary, O. Novel Anti-Inflammatory Approaches for Cystic Fibrosis Lung Disease: Identification of Molecular Targets and Design of Innovative Therapies. *Front. Pharmacol.* **2020**, *11*, 1096. [CrossRef]
21. Wu, G.; Fang, Y.-Z.; Yang, S.; Lupton, J.R.; Turner, N.D. Glutathione metabolism and its implications for health. *J. Nutr.* **2004**, *134*, 489–492. [CrossRef]
22. Zhao, J.; Huang, W.; Zhang, S.; Xu, J.; Xue, W.; He, B.; Zhang, Y. Efficacy of Glutathione for Patients With Cystic Fibrosis: A Meta-analysis of Randomized-Controlled Studies. *Am. J. Rhinol. Allergy* **2020**, *34*, 115–121. [CrossRef] [PubMed]
23. Dickerhof, N.; Pearson, J.F.; Hoskin, T.S.; Berry, L.J.; Turner, R.; Sly, P.D.; Kettle, A.J.; Arest, C.F. Oxidative stress in early cystic fibrosis lung disease is exacerbated by airway glutathione deficiency. *Free Radic. Biol. Med.* **2017**, *113*, 236–243. [CrossRef] [PubMed]
24. Causer, A.; Shute, J.K.; Cummings, M.H.; Shepherd, A.; Gruet, M.; Costello, J.; Bailey, S.; Lindley, M.; Pearson, C.; Connett, G.; et al. Circulating biomarkers of antioxidant status and oxidative stress in people with cystic fibrosis: A systematic review and meta-analysis. *Redox Biol.* **2020**, *32*, 101436. [CrossRef] [PubMed]
25. Dickerhof, N.; Huang, J.; Min, E.; Michaëlsson, E.; Lindstedt, E.-L.; Pearson, J.F.; Kettle, T.; Day, B.J. Myeloperoxidase inhibition decreases morbidity and oxidative stress in mice with cystic fibrosis-like lung inflammation. *Free Radic. Biol. Med.* **2020**, *152*, 91–99. [CrossRef] [PubMed]
26. Calabrese, C.; Tosco, A.; Abete, P.; Carnovale, V.; Basile, C.; Magliocca, A.; Quattrucci, S.; De Sanctis, S.; Alatri, F.; Mazzarella, G.; et al. Randomized, single blind, controlled trial of inhaled glutathione vs placebo in patients with cystic fibrosis. *J. Cyst. Fibros.* **2015**, *14*, 203–210. [CrossRef]

27. Hewson, C.K.; Capraro, A.; Wong, S.L.; Pandzic, E.; Zhong, L.; Fernando, B.S.M.; Awatade, N.T.; Hart-Smith, G.; Whan, R.M.; Thomas, S.R.; et al. Novel Antioxidant Therapy with the Immediate Precursor to Glutathione, γ-Glutamylcysteine (GGC), Ameliorates LPS-Induced Cellular Stress in In Vitro 3D-Differentiated Airway Model from Primary Cystic Fibrosis Human Bronchial Cells. *Antioxidants* **2020**, *9*, 1204. [CrossRef]
28. Pelullo, M.; Savi, D.; Quattrucci, S.; Cimino, G.; Pizzuti, A.; Screpanti, I.; Talora, C.; Cialfi, S. miR-125b/NRF2/HO-1 axis is involved in protection against oxidative stress of cystic fibrosis: A pilot study. *Exp. Ther. Med.* **2021**, *21*, 585. [CrossRef]
29. Di Pietro, C.; Öz, H.H.; Murray, T.S.; Bruscia, E.M. Targeting the Heme Oxygenase 1/Carbon Monoxide Pathway to Resolve Lung Hyper-Inflammation and Restore a Regulated Immune Response in Cystic Fibrosis. *Front. Pharmacol.* **2020**, *11*, 1059. [CrossRef]
30. Laselva, O.; Allegretta, C.; Di Gioia, S.; Avolio, C.; Conese, M. Anti-Inflammatory and Anti-Oxidant Effect of Dimethyl Fumarate in Cystic Fibrosis Bronchial Epithelial Cells. *Cells* **2021**, *10*, 2132. [CrossRef]
31. Borcherding, D.C.; Siefert, M.E.; Lin, S.; Brewington, J.; Sadek, H.; Clancy, J.P.; Plafker, S.M.; Ziady, A.G. Clinically-approved CFTR modulators rescue Nrf2 dysfunction in cystic fibrosis airway epithelia. *J. Clin. Investig.* **2019**, *129*, 3448–3463. [CrossRef]
32. NandyMazumdar, M.; Paranjapye, A.; Browne, J.; Yin, S.; Leir, S.-H.; Harris, A. BACH1, the master regulator of oxidative stress, has a dual effect on CFTR expression. *Biochem. J.* **2021**, *478*, 3741–3756. [CrossRef] [PubMed]
33. Favia, M.; de Bari, L.; Bobba, A.; Atlante, A. An Intriguing Involvement of Mitochondria in Cystic Fibrosis. *J. Clin. Med.* **2019**, *8*, 1890. [CrossRef]
34. Scholte, B.J.; Horati, H.; Veltman, M.; Vreeken, R.J.; Garratt, L.W.; Tiddens, H.A.W.M.; Janssens, H.M.; Stick, S.M.; Australian Respiratory Early Surveillance Team for Cystic Fibrosis (AREST CF). Oxidative stress and abnormal bioactive lipids in early cystic fibrosis lung disease. *J. Cyst. Fibros.* **2019**, *18*, 781–789. [CrossRef] [PubMed]
35. Signorelli, P.; Pivari, F.; Barcella, M.; Merelli, I.; Zulueta, A.; Cas, M.D.; Rosso, L.; Ghidoni, R.; Caretti, A.; Paroni, R.; et al. Myriocin modulates the altered lipid metabolism and storage in cystic fibrosis. *Cell. Signal.* **2021**, *81*, 109928. [CrossRef]
36. Veltman, M.; De Sanctis, J.B.; Stolarczyk, M.; Klymiuk, N.; Bähr, A.; Brouwer, R.W.; Oole, E.; Shah, J.; Ozdian, T.; Liao, J.; et al. CFTR Correctors and Antioxidants Partially Normalize Lipid Imbalance but not Abnormal Basal Inflammatory Cytokine Profile in CF Bronchial Epithelial Cells. *Front. Physiol.* **2021**, *12*, 619442. [CrossRef] [PubMed]
37. Olveira, C.; Padilla, A.; Dorado, A.; Contreras, V.; Garcia-Fuentes, E.; Rubio-Martin, E.; Porras, N.; Doña, E.; Carmona, A.; Olveira, G. Inflammation and Oxidation Biomarkers in Patients with Cystic Fibrosis: The Influence of Azithromycin. *Eurasian J. Med.* **2017**, *49*, 118–123. [CrossRef]

MDPI
St. Alban-Anlage 66
4052 Basel
Switzerland
www.mdpi.com

Molecules Editorial Office
E-mail: molecules@mdpi.com
www.mdpi.com/journal/molecules

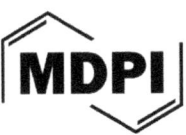

Disclaimer/Publisher's Note: The statements, opinions and data contained in all publications are solely those of the individual author(s) and contributor(s) and not of MDPI and/or the editor(s). MDPI and/or the editor(s) disclaim responsibility for any injury to people or property resulting from any ideas, methods, instructions or products referred to in the content.

www.ingramcontent.com/pod-product-compliance
Lightning Source LLC
LaVergne TN
LVHW070731100526
838202LV00013B/1211